OLD REMEDIES FOR MODERN LIVING

OLD REMEDIES FOR MODERN LIVING
An Encyclopaedia of Forgotten Herbal Cures

SAMANTHA ALMOND

First published 2025 by
Aeon Books Ltd

The right of Samantha Almond to be identified as the author of this work has been asserted in accordance with §§ 77 and 78 of the Copyright Design and Patents Act 1988.

All rights reserved. No part of this publication may be reproduced, stored in a retrieval system, or transmitted, in any form or by any means, electronic, mechanical, photocopying, recording, or otherwise, without the prior written permission of the publisher.

British Library Cataloguing in Publication Data

A C.I.P. for this book is available from the British Library

ISBN-978-1-80152-174-1

Printed in Great Britain

www.aeonbooks.co.uk

DISCLAIMER

The information contained in this book is intended for educational and informational purposes only. While every effort has been made to ensure the accuracy and reliability of the content, the author is not responsible for any errors, omissions, or outcomes related to the use of the information in this book.

Foraging for wild plants and using herbal medicines can involve risks, including the possibility of misidentifying plants, allergic reactions, or adverse health effects. Not all plants are safe for human consumption or medicinal use, and some may be toxic. It is strongly recommended that readers seek advice from a qualified herbalist, botanist, or healthcare professional before attempting to forage or use any plant for medicinal purposes.

This book does not provide medical advice, and it is not a substitute for professional healthcare. Always consult a licensed healthcare provider before using herbal remedies, especially if you are pregnant, nursing, taking medications, or have existing health conditions.

PREFACE

The journey to writing this book began several years ago when I began visiting the Forest of Dean. It was late April and the smell of the Wild garlic that grows abundantly in the forest was overwhelming. As an avid researcher and lover of the natural world and its gifts, my natural response was to read everything I could find about the plant.

I soon discovered that in addition to its delicious flavour, Wild garlic has multiple amazing health and ecological benefits. It has a long history in the region, as it thrives in ancient woodland and is likely to have been gathered by the forest's past communities, going as far back as the Celts and Britons, both for its flavourful addition to food and for its health benefits, such as supporting digestion and treating infections.

With my curiosity peaked I then wanted to know more about other plants in the area. I began to find a great amount of folklore connected to the plants as well as many details of their historical medicinal uses. This led me in turn, to the works of Nicholas Culpeper (1616–1654), sometimes called the 'father' of medical herbalism. Through his work, I felt as though I was uncovering a wealth of largely forgotten knowledge. Culpeper was a man far ahead of his time and believed that medical knowledge should be available to everyone. In 1652, he wrote *The English Physician* (later known as *Culpeper's Herbal*), making herbal knowledge available to the masses for a few pennies; he also supplied plant medicines at very low cost to poor Londoners, often teaching them how to find and use the plants themselves, much to the outrage of the expensive and exclusive physicians and apothecaries of the day.

Having combed the historical writings, I then wanted to compare these to modern scientific publications and began to scour public databases, sift through journal articles, and collate the knowledge accumulated by experts from around the world. Public resources like PubMed have been invaluable, offering a treasure trove of peer-reviewed studies that helped inform and shape the content of this book.

In spite of the great advances of modern scientific medicine, many people still prefer plant-based natural cures over synthetic pharmaceuticals. The World Health Organisation estimates that, at the end of the 20th century, about 80% of the world's population received their primary healthcare from traditional medicines, which mainly used plant extracts or their active ingredients (Tahir et al., 2023). I am certainly one of those who prefers natural remedies, and this book aims to provide a resource that shows the usefulness of plants that are often now dismissed as weeds and reveals their ongoing usefulness to a broad audience, from students to seasoned professionals.

While *Culpeper's Herbal* has been my main source for the historical uses of the plants, you will find mention of other important historical works, such as Pliny's *Naturalis Historia*, Dioscorides' *De Materia Medica*, Hildegard of Bingen's *Physica* and John Gerard's *Herball*. However, there is not a lot of 'older' information in relation to some of the plants and so it was Culpeper that I constantly returned to and cross-referenced. Despite his writings being over 350 years old, when I compared many of his findings to modern scientific publications, he was and is amazingly accurate. It is simply that our modern-day scientists now have the knowledge and technology to discover why the plants have the effects that they do. Please remember, however, that research into many of these plants is in its infancy and may still be restricted to *in vitro* (laboratory) and *in vivo* (animal) tests rather than clinical studies on humans.

Where herbal remedies still differ from allopathic medicine is that they are often not a quick fix. Their effects are cumulative and, in many cases, focus on assisting the body's ability to adapt and heal itself. The enduring popularity of herbal medicines may be explained by their tendency to work with minimal toxic side effects, but as mentioned previously, the information provided here is not intended to be a substitute for any medical treatment.

It is also important to point out that these recipes are intended for personal use. If you are in the UK and intend to sell any of your preparations, you will need to bear in mind the regulations under The Human Medicines Regulations 2012.

All of the plants in this book are those that I have found in my local area and researched. Some may differ to other geographical areas but most are found in the wild in the UK. So, if you are intending to wild harvest your herbs, please make certain of your identification prior to harvesting any plant as ingestion, application or other use of some plants may cause serious illness or even death. The photographs in this book were taken by me as part of my research and are not intended as a guide to identification.

Please, please harvest sustainably and only for your own personal use. Harvest only from a large growing patch. Do not harvest single standing plants that are not part of a plant community. Never take more than 10% from a site. It should look like you did not take anything at all, and your impact should be negligible. If there is not enough to harvest that day, just enjoy the plants that are growing, show your respect and gratitude and leave.

All of the stated dosages are taken from Bartram's *Encyclopedia of Herbal Medicine* (1998) unless otherwise stated.

A standard tisane is 1tsp in 250ml water, and a standard tincture is 1:5, which is one part marc (herb) to 5 parts menstruum (liquid).

No project of this magnitude can be accomplished alone, and I am deeply grateful to those who supported, encouraged and contributed to this journey. First and foremost, my love and gratitude go to my partner, Adrian, for his unwavering belief in me and his patience with the countless "treasures" I've brought home from the Forest. I am also immensely thankful to my incredibly supportive family, who always show genuine interest in whichever plant I've chosen to enlighten them about. A special thanks to my sister, Luisa, for encouraging me to transform my copious volumes of notes into this book.

Finally, to you, the reader: thank you for picking up this book. Whether you are just starting your journey or already well-versed in the subject, I hope the pages that follow not only inform but also inspire you to think critically and explore the world around you with curiosity and enthusiasm.

This book is dedicated to all those who believe in the power of nature, knowledge and the value of sharing it. I hope that this work provides you with an enriching perspective on local plants and their environments and a deeper appreciation and understanding of the natural world around you.

Samantha Almond
www.theherbalforager.co.uk
October 2024

CONTENTS

PREFACE

Agrimony – *Agrimonia eupatoria* 1
    Agrimony recipes 5
Anemone – *Anemonoides nemorosa* ... 7
    Anemone recipes 10
Angelica (Wild) – *Angelica sylvestris*. 11
    Angelica recipes 16
Avens – *Geum urbanum* 17
    Avens recipes 21
Bedstraws – *Galium verum/mollugo* .. 23
    Bedstraw recipes 26
Betony – *Betonica officinalis* 27
    Betony recipes 31
Bindweed – *Calystegia sepium/arvensis* 33
    Bindweed recipes 36
Bistort – *Bistorta officinalis* 37
    Bistort recipes 40
Black horehound – *Ballota nigra* 41
    Black horehound recipes 46
Bugle – *Ajuga reptans* 47
    Bugle recipes 50
Burdock – *Arctium lappa/minus* 51
    Burdock recipes 56
Burnet – *Sanguisorba minor/officinalis*.. 57
    Burnet recipes 60
Buttercup – *Ranunculus spp.* 61
    Buttercup recipes 65
Celandine (Greater) – *Chelidonium majus* 67
    Greater celandine recipes 71

Celandine (Lesser) – *Ranunculus ficaria* 73
    Lesser celandine recipes 75
Centaury – *Centaurium erythraea* 77
    Centaury recipes 80
Chickweed – *Stellaria media* 81
    Chickweed recipes 85
Cinquefoils – *Potentilla spp.* 87
    Cinquefoil recipes 92
Cleavers – *Galium aparine* 93
    Cleavers recipes 97
Clover – *Trifolium spp.* 99
    Clover recipes 102
Coltsfoot – *Tussilago farfara* 103
    Coltsfoot recipes 107
Columbine – *Aquilegia vulgaris* 109
    Columbine recipes 111
Comfrey – *Symphytum officinale* 113
    Comfrey recipes 116
Cow parsley (Chervil – *Anthriscus sylvestris*) 119
    Cow parsley recipes 122
Cowslip – *Primula veris* 123
    Cowslip recipes 127
Cranesbill – *Geranium spp.* 129
    Cranesbill recipes 132
Daisy – *Bellis perennis* 133
    Daisy recipes 138
Dandelion – *Taraxacum officinale* 139
    Dandelion recipes 143

Deadnettles – *Lamium spp.* 145
   Deadnettle recipes 148
Dog's mercury – *Mercurialis perennis* 149
   Dog's mercury recipes 152
Eyebright – *Euphrasia officinalis* 153
   Eyebright recipes 157
Feverfew – *Tanacetum parthenium* ... 159
   Feverfew recipes 162
Figwort – *Scrophularia nodosa/
auriculata* 163
   Figwort recipes 167
Fleabane – *Pulicaria dysenterica* 169
   Fleabane recipes 172
Fumitory, Common – *Fumaria
officinalis* 173
   Fumitory recipes 177
Garlic mustard – *Alliaria petiolata* ... 179
   Garlic mustard recipes 181
Goldenrod – *Solidago virgaurea* 183
   Goldenrod recipes 187
Ground elder – *Aegopodium podagraria* 189
   Ground elder recipes 191
Ground ivy – *Glechoma hederacea* 193
   Ground ivy recipes 196
Groundsel – *Senecio vulgaris* 197
   Groundsel recipes 200
Hawkweed, Mouse-ear – *Pilosella
officinarum* 201
   Hawkweed recipes 205
Heartsease – *Viola tricolor* 207
   Heartsease recipes 210
Hedge parsley – *Torilis japonica* 211
   Hedge parsley recipes 214
Hemlock – *Conium maculatum* 215
   Hemlock recipes 218

Hemp agrimony – *Eupatorium
cannabinum* 219
   Hemp agrimony recipes 222
Herb Robert – *Geranium
robertianum* 223
   Herb Robert recipes 226
Hogweed – *Heracleum sphondylium* .. 227
   Hogweed recipes 230
Honeysuckle – *Lonicera spp.* 231
   Honeysuckle recipes 235
Hops – *Humulus lupulus* 237
   Hops recipes 241
Horsetail – *Equisetum arvense* 243
   Horsetail recipes 246
Knapweed – *Centaurea nigra/scabiosa* 247
   Knapweed recipes 251
Lady's mantle – *Alchemilla vulgaris* .. 253
   Lady's mantle recipes 256
Lady's smock – *Cardamine pratensis* . 257
   Lady's smock recipes 260
Loosestrife (Yellow) – *Lysimachia
vulgaris* 261
   Yellow loosestrife recipes 265
Mallow – *Malva sylvestris* 267
   Mallow recipes 270
Meadowsweet – *Filipendula ulmaria*. 271
   Meadowsweet recipes 275
Mint (Wild) – *Mentha spp.* 277
   Mint recipes 280
Mistletoe – *Viscum album* 281
   Mistletoe recipes 285
Mugwort – *Artemisia vulgaris* 287
   Mugwort recipes 291
Mullein – *Verbascum thapsus* 293
   Mullein recipes 296
Nettle (Stinging) – *Urtica dioica* 297
   Nettle recipes 303

Pineappleweed – *Matricaria discoidea*................................305
    Pineappleweed recipes 308
Plantain – *Plantago lanceolata/major* . 309
    Plantain recipes......................313
Prickly lettuce – *Lactuca serriola*.......315
    Prickly lettuce recipes 318
Scarlet pimpernel – *Anagallis arvensis* . 319
    Scarlet pimpernel recipes 322
Self-heal – *Prunella vulgaris*...........323
    Self-heal recipes 327
Shepherd's purse – *Capsella bursa-pastoris*...................................329
    Shepherd's purse recipes 332
Solomon's seal – *Polygonatum spp.*.....333
    Solomon's seal recipes 337
Sorrels – *Rumex spp* 339
    Sorrel recipes 344
Speedwell – *Veronica spp.*...............345
    Speedwell recipes...................348
Spurges – *Euphorbia spp.*................349
    Spurge recipes 352
Stitchwort, Greater – *Stellaria holostea* . 353
    Stitchwort recipes 356
St John's wort – *Hypericum spp.* 357
    St John's wort recipes 363
Sweet woodruff – *Galium odoratum* .. 365
    Sweet woodruff recipes 367
Tansy – *Tanacetum vulgare* 369
    Tansy recipes 372
Toadflax – *Linaria vulgaris*...........373
    Toadflax recipes 376
Usnea – *Usnea barbata* 377
    Usnea recipes 381
Vervain – *Verbena officinalis*...........383
    Vervain recipes 386
Violet – *Viola odorata* 387
    Violet recipes 392
Willowherbs – *Epilobium spp.* 393
    Willowherb recipes.................398
Woundwort – *Stachys spp.* 399
    Woundwort recipes................403
Yarrow – *Achillea millefolium* 405
    Yarrow recipes 409
Yellow dock – *Rumex crispus*..........411
    Yellow dock recipes................414

BIBLIOGRAPHY......................415
INDEX 441

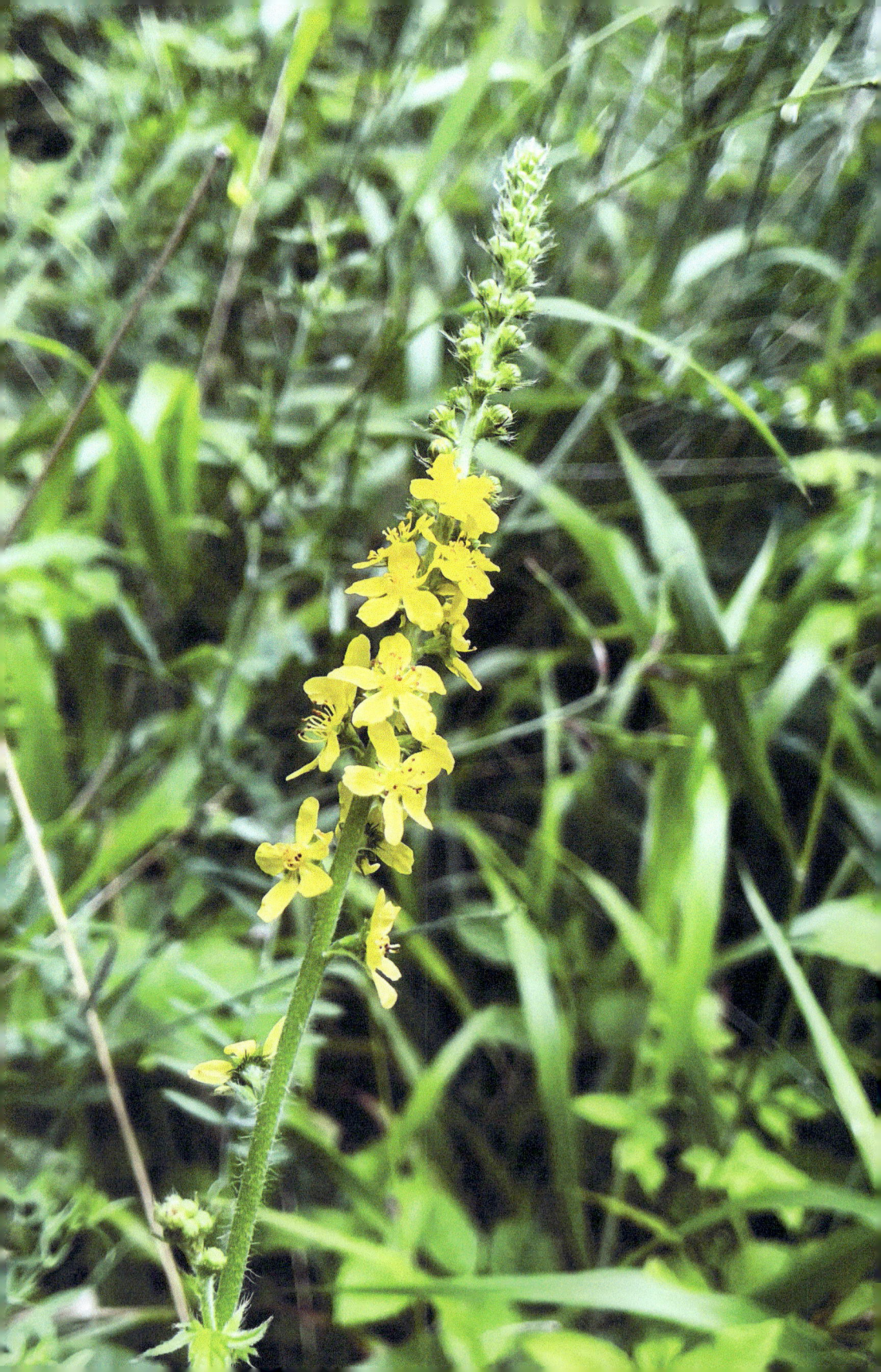

AGRIMONY
Agrimonia eupatoria

Agrimonia eupatoria, commonly known as Agrimony, is native to the UK and belongs to the Rose family. It grows in grasslands, woodland edges, meadows and disturbed areas such as roadsides. In traditional herbal medicine, Agrimony has been used as a remedy for gastrointestinal issues.

HISTORICAL USES

The Anglo-Saxons called the plant Garclive and used it to heal wounds, snake bites, warts, etc. The herb was also mentioned in the *Old English Herbarium* from the 10th century (Cameron, 2006; Voights, 1979; Watkins *et al.*, 2012).

In the time of Chaucer, the name appears as Egrimoyne, and it was used with Mugwort and vinegar for 'a bad back' and 'alle woundes'. It was at one time included in the London *Materia Medica* as a wound-healing herb. According to John Gerard (1545–1612), Pliny, the 1st-century Roman author, naturalist and natural philosopher, called it a 'herb of princely authoritie' and Dioscorides, the Greek physician of the same era stated that it was not only 'a remedy for them that have bad livers', but also 'for such as are bitten with serpents'.

ETYMOLOGY OF COMMON NAME
Agrimony is derived from the Greek *argemos*, meaning a white speck on the eye which this plant was supposed to cure.

PLANT LORE
Once known as 'fairy's wand', it is thought to induce sleep if placed under a pillow and protect against nightmares and psychic attacks.

USE
All parts.

EDIBILITY
The leaves, flowers and stems are edible, but mostly enjoyed as a tea.

HARVEST
In summer before the seeds appear.

MEDICINAL PROPERTIES
Diuretic, anti-inflammatory, astringent, digestive, antibacterial, antidiabetic and hepatic.

ACTIVE CONSTITUENTS
Tannins, flavonoids, coumarins, phenolic acids, polysaccharides, essential oils, bitters.

LEFT: AGRIMONY

Culpeper's Herbal agreed:

> It openeth and cleanseth the liver, helpeth the jaundice, and is very beneficial to the bowels, healing all inward wounds, bruises, hurts, and other diſtempers. The decoction of the herb made with wine ... helps them that have foul, troubled, or bloody water, and makes them part with clear urine speedily; it also helpeth the cholic, cleanseth the breaſt, and rids away the cough. A draught of the decoction, taken warm before the fit, firſt relieves, and in time rids away the tertian or quartan agues [malaria]. The leaves and seeds taken in wine ſtays the bloody flux; outwardly applied, being ſtamped with old swine's grease, it helpeth old sores, cancers, and inveterate ulcers, and draweth forth thorns and splinters of wood, nails, or any other such thing gotten into the flesh: it helpeth to ſtrengthen members that be out of joint: and being bruised and applied, or the juice dropped in it, helpeth foul and impoſthumed [abscessed] ears.

Fray's Golden Recipes for the Use of All Ages, dated 1897, stated that the best comforter for a depressed or desponding mind is equal parts of Agrimony and Rosemary, made and used in the manner of tea.

According to Mrs Grieve's *A Modern Herbal* (1931):

> Dr Hill, who from 1751 to 1771 published several works on Herbal medicine, recommends 'an infusion of 6 oz. of the crown of the root in a quart of boiling water, sweetened with honey and half a pint drank three times a day', as an effectual remedy for jaundice. It gives tone to the syſtem and promotes assimilation of food.

MODERN RESEARCH

Also known as 'church steeples' owing to its slender spikes of yellow flowers, there has been a moderate amount of research on this small herb, stemming from its wide historical use in folk medicine. Research has found the following properties attributed to Agrimony:

Diuretic

Culpeper refers to the ability of Agrimony to cause 'them to make water clear and speedily', and in 1989, it was shown that administration of Agrimony infusions and decoctions increased urine and prevented losses of electrolytes, and K^+ ions in rats (Giachetti *et al.*, 1989), no doubt owing to its tannin content.

Astringent

Also as a result of a high tannin content, Agrimony is very astringent, which is why the Ancient Greeks and Anglo-Saxons found it good for drying up and healing wounds (Jahodář, 2010). Infusions made from Agrimony leaves were also traditionally taken for their anti-diarrhoeal effects or as a gargle for oral and throat inflammation (ESCOP, 2005). Agrimony's astringent actions may also be useful in the gut, particularly in cases of ulcers and colitis.

Anti-inflammatory and vulnerary

In addition to its tannins, Agrimony also contains phenolic acids, including caffeic acid, chlorogenic acid and ellagic acid. These acids have been shown to have anti-inflammatory effects by inhibiting inflammatory enzymes and reducing the production of inflammatory mediators. In 1982, Agrimony was used to treat 35 patients suffering from chronic gastroduodenitis. After 25 days of therapy, 75% of patients claimed to be free from pain, 95% from dyspeptic symptoms and 76% from palpitation pains. Gastroscopy indicated that haemorrhagic changes had healed. As an anti-inflammatory, it may also be useful as Culpeper points out for 'Cholic'.

Antidiabetic

Agrimony has also been found to aid diabetes, with a 1998 study showing that it demonstrated the presence of antihyperglycaemic, insulin-releasing and insulin-like activity. This finding has been confirmed by further studies in 2016 by Kuczmannová *et al*.

Anti-hepatic

Confirming the historical use mentioned by Dioscorides, Gerard, Culpeper and Hill of Agrimony for the liver, an 8-week study between January and July 2013 on 80 subjects with elevated alanine transaminase levels (one of the signs of liver disease) showed a significant reduction in levels at 8 weeks post treatment compared with the placebo group. There were no reported severe adverse events during this study, and total protein, albumin, blood urea nitrogen, creatine and cholesterol levels were normal in both groups. Agrimony extract was therefore deemed safe and well tolerated for liver complaints without severe adverse events.

Antibacterial

Agrimony was known to Culpeper to help 'them that have foul, troubled or bloody water', and it has been used traditionally for urinary tract infections. A study of 40 women with vaginal trichomoniasis showed that a decoction of Agrimony extract inhibited the growth of gram-positive bacteria (Wang et al., 1953). When a cotton ball treated with the herb was inserted into the vagina for 3 to 4 hours, 37 of the women were cured with one treatment. In another study using a decoction of Agrimony inhibited the growth of *Mycobacterium tuberculosis* (Peter-Horvath, 1965) and even destroyed resistant strains.

A 2015 study found there was marked antibacterial activity against *Staphylococcus aureus* and *α-haemolytic Streptococci*, as well as potential antiviral activity against hepatitis B. During the study, wound-healing time decreased by just under 30% faster than fucidin ointment. This again confirms that the historical writers as far back as the Anglo-Saxons were well-advised in using Agrimony as a vulnerary.

Anticancerogenic

Miyamoto et al. (1988) investigated the effect of agrimoniin, a tannin contained in *Agrimony* and results indicated that it is a potent anti-tumour compound which can enhance the immune response on tumour cells and some cells of the immune system. In 1992, it was found that agrimoniin is able to induce interleukin (IL)-1 production *in vitro* (human peripheral blood mononuclear cells) and in vivo (mouse adherent peritoneal exudate cells), and accordingly the anti-tumour effects can be justified.

TOPICAL USES

Owing to its astringent, antibacterial and anti-inflammatory effects, an infusion or decoction can be used as a wash for acne, wounds, sores, rashes, eczema and psoriasis or as a gargle for sore throats and nasal mucus. As Culpeper rightly pointed out, Agrimony's astringent properties will also draw out thorns and splinters while a weak infusion can be used as an eyewash for conjunctivitis.

DOSAGE

Tisane – 1tsp/5g, 3 times per day.
Tincture – 1:45 45%, 1–4ml, 3 times per day – 20 drops = 1ml/1tsp = 5ml.

PRECAUTIONS

The intake of large quantities of Agrimony can cause digestive complaint and constipation. It should also be avoided by those with autoimmune disease and anyone on blood thinners and diabetic drugs. It is not suitable for children or those who are pregnant or lactating.

Agrimony recipes

Medicinal recipes

Agrimony tisane
Pour 250ml boiling water over 1tsp/5g of the dried herb and allow to steep for 10–15 minutes. Use for gastrointestinal disorders. For sore throats use the tisane as a gargle, and for conjunctivitis use a weak tisane (2tsp/10g to 500ml water) as an eyewash.

Agrimony compress
Soak a cloth in a tisane of the dried herb and apply 2–3 times a day for acne, wounds, splinters and sores.

Agrimony decoction
Quoting from *Harold Ward's Herbal Manual* (1936):

Agrimony is an old remedy for debility, as it gives tone to the whole system. It is administered as a decoction of one ounce (28g) to 1 1/2 pints (850ml) water, simmered down to 1 pint, in half teacupful or larger doses, and may be sweetened with honey or black treacle if desired. Use also for diarrhoea, cystitis, bronchitis and UTI's, etc.

Agrimony infused tincture 1:5 45%
If you are using 40% alcohol, ie vodka, make a simple tincture by covering 1 part herb to 5 parts fluid.

If you are using Everclear or other 100% proofs, then use the following method for a specific tincture:

- 100g dried Agrimony
- 225ml alcohol
- 275ml water

Split the dried herb into to equal 50g parts. Cover one 50g part with 225ml of the alcohol. Then steep/infuse another 50g part in 275ml of water for 15 minutes. Strain thoroughly and top up if the water is less than 275ml. Add the infusion to the alcohol mix and leave for 14 days before straining. Use for cystitis, UTIs, bronchitis and heavy menstrual bleeding, up to 4 ml 3 times per day (in juice if necessary).

Agrimony oxymel
An oxymel makes hard-to-take herbs much easier to stomach. Agrimony is a bitter and so this recipe works well. Fill your jar a quarter full of herbs and then use the ratio of 1 part honey to 3 parts apple cider vinegar. Stir, seal and leave to steep/infuse for two weeks. Strain out the liquid into another jar and then take 2 spoonfuls diluted with water at each dose. Use for gastrointestinal disorders, UTIs and heavy menstrual bleeding.

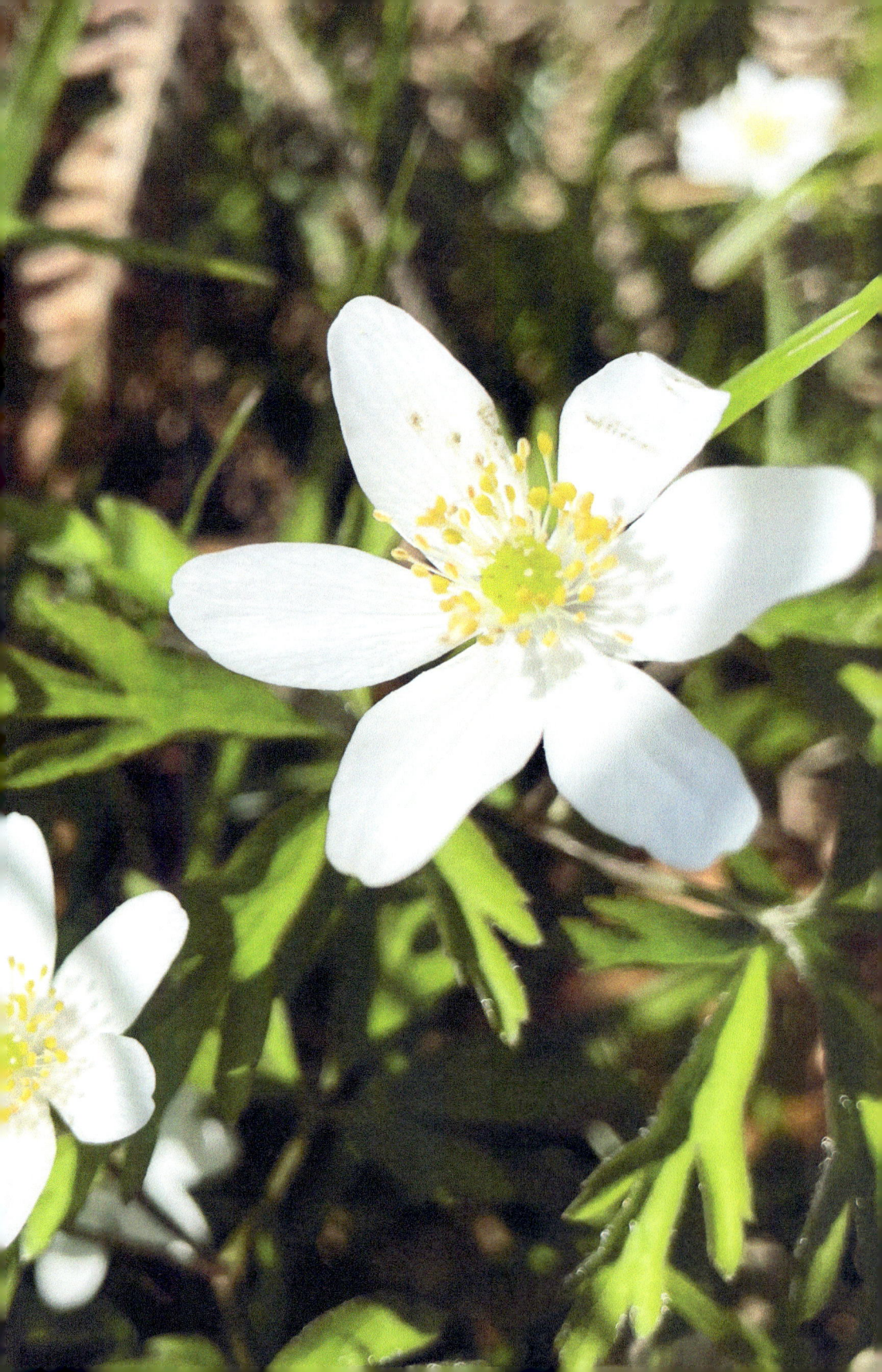

ANEMONE
Anemonoides nemorosa

Anemonoides nemorosa, commonly called Wood anemone or Windflower, is native to the UK and belongs to the Buttercup family, *Ranunculaceae*. Wood anemones typically grow in deciduous woodlands, shady areas, and meadows. They are known for their delicate, star-shaped flowers that bloom in early spring.

HISTORICAL USES

The Romans plucked Anemones as a charm against fever, and Greek legends say that Anemos, the Wind, sends his namesakes the Anemones, in the earliest spring days as the heralds of his coming. Pliny affirmed in *Naturalis Historia* that the flowers only open when the wind blows, hence their name of Windflower, and in the 1st century CE, Dioscorides recommended in *De Materia Medica* that the plant be used in external treatments for eye inflammation and ulcers.

Gerard and Culpeper, our chosen 16th and 17th-century writers, agreed with Dioscorides. Culpeper said '… *the body being bathed with the decoction of them* [the leaves], *cures the leprosy: the leaves being stamped, and the juice snuffed up the nose, purgeth the head mightily; so doth the root, being chewed in the mouth, for it procureth much spitting, and bringeth*

ETYMOLOGY OF COMMON NAME
Anemone comes from ancient Greek *anemos* meaning 'wind' because, in Culpeper's words, *the flowers never open but when the wind bloweth. Pliny is my author; if it be not so, blame him.*

PLANT LORE
Fairies are said to take shelter in the closing petal of Anemone during rain, while in ancient Greek mythology, the Anemone was believed to have sprung from the tears of Aphrodite as she mourned the death of Adonis.

USE
All aerial parts.

EDIBILITY
Not edible!

HARVEST
In spring.

MEDICINAL PROPERTIES
Antispasmodic, stimulant, analgesic, antimicrobial, anticancerogenic, anti-inflammatory.

ACTIVE CONSTITUENTS
Alkaloids, flavonoids, triterpenoid saponins, phenolic acids, tannins, glycosides, essential oils.

away many watery and phlegmatic humors, and is therefore excellent for the lethargy… Being made into an ointment, and the eyelids anointed with it, it helps inflammations of the eyes … The same ointment is excellent good to cleanse malignant and corroding ulcers.'

In his book *Herbal Simples* (second edition 1897), William Fernie to some extent echoed Culpeper, noting that '*A tincture is made with spirit of wine from the entire plant, collected when in flower. This tincture is remarkably beneficial in disorders of the mucous membranes, alike of the respiratory and of the digestive passages.*

MODERN RESEARCH

We now know that the main active substance of Anemone is protoanemonin, a volatile oil that is poisonous. However, during the drying process, protoanemonin is converted into anemonin, which has medicinal properties that support the historical findings as follows:

Antispasmodic

Anemonin has been used as a remedy for asthma, whooping cough and uterine bleeding such as endometriosis. Demonstrating this, extract of Anemone has shown antispasmodic activity in rabbit small intestine. Furthermore, in small doses, anemonin acts as a central nervous system depressant, lowering heart rate and respiration. This depressant activity combined with the antispasmodic activity may account for the effect on digestive and respiratory distress, reported by Fernie [see *Journal of Restorative Medicine*, 2(1) (10 January 2013): 109–13].

Stimulant and analgesic

Culpeper and Gerard agree that Anemone is good for lethargy, and it is interesting to note that the Nez Perce and Teton Sioux Native Americans used the plant *Clematis hirsutissima* as a horse restorative to increase the stamina and speed of the horse. The one thing Clematis and Anemone have in common is anemonin. The Clematis root was crushed and used as a smelling salt to revive exhausted horses. The Flathead Indians of western Montana also used *Clematis hirsutissima* as a remedy for headaches, just as Culpeper and Gerard describe for purging the head.

Antimicrobial

The use of Anemone to clean and heal sores and ulcers as described by Culpeper is based on the protoanemonin content, which has been shown to be effective against both gram-positive and gram-negative bacteria such as *Escherichia coli* and *Staphylococcus aureus* as well as fungal species such as *Mycobacterium tuberculosis*, *Bacillus subtilis*, *Klebsiella pneumoniae* and *Candida albicans*.

Anticancerogenic

In 2019, an investigation of the mode of cell death by Anemone extract on cervical cancer cells was carried out. The results showed that Anemone produced a delay in the early mitosis phase of the cell cycle, and apoptosis (programmed cell death) was confirmed after 24 and 48 hours. The results imply that Anemone may have potential anti-proliferative properties.

Anti-inflammatory

A 2009 study found that anemonin can inhibit the release of cytokines, proteins secreted by the immune system that promote inflammation, and alleviate excessive inflammatory responses while having a therapeutic effect on endotoxaemia (blood toxins) (Fostok et al., 2009). This was confirmed by two studies in 2022, the first of which, designed to assess antioxidant and cytotoxic activity on the inflammation process, showed general anti-inflammatory activity as well as confirming again that anemonin acts against the formation of cancers; the second showed that anemonin relieved the symptoms of ulcerative colitis in mice. These results suggest that Wood anemone extracts could help cells, tissues, and organs restore to normal function.

TOPICAL USES

The herb is used externally for rheumatism, gout, skin diseases and as an antiseptic; its juice is used against warts. I have not found any information to substantiate the use of Anemone on the eyes.

DOSAGE

Tincture – 1:1 – 3–4 drops with a tbsp water.

PRECAUTIONS

Fresh Wood anemone can severely irritate the stomach and intestines. Skin contact can cause slow-healing blisters and burns. *Anemone nemorosa* is not recommended with kidney inflammation and is not suitable for children or those who are pregnant or lactating.

Anemone recipes

Medicinal recipes

NB: Wood anemone must be dried before use to remove toxins.

Anemone tisane

Add 200ml of boiling water to 1 teaspoon of dried herb and leave for 30 minutes, drain, rub 10ml into the skin of painful places once per day. After application wash hands carefully with soap.

Anemone cold infusion

Make a tisane as above and then leave for 20 hours, before filtering. Use 2 tablespoons 3 times per day in compresses for rheumatism and gout by soaking a cloth in the infusion as a wash for dermatitis or poor wound-healing.

Anemone poultice

- 1tsp dried leaves
- 2tsp coconut oil
- cheesecloth or cotton bandage

Powder the leaves and mix with a little water, then add the coconut oil to make a paste. Spread the paste evenly over the desired area and wrap with the cloth or bandage. Use for pain relief in joints, to heal wounds and burns and to calm inflammation.

Anemone infused extract – 1:1

- 100g of dried root
- 1l alcohol

Cover the dried Anemone with the alcohol. Leave for 7–10 days before straining. Can be used for internal and external pains and wounds.

ANGELICA (WILD)
Angelica sylvestris

Angelica sylvestris, commonly known as Wild or Wood angelica, is a plant native to the UK. It belongs to the *Apiaceae* family, which also includes Parsley, Celery and Carrots, and is typically found in damp, marshy areas, along riverbanks and in woodland clearings. Wild angelica has a long history of medicinal and culinary uses and was cultivated around the 10th century into the familiar Garden angelica (*Angelica archangelica*).

HISTORICAL USES

Angelica was used at least 500 years ago, during the Ottoman period, as part of a remedy called Mesir. Mesir paste was used to relieve many kinds of pain from headache to stomach pain and includes Ginger, Black chuglam, Cumin and Angelica. Each of the ingredients of Mesir paste separately have been used in Turkish folk medicine for centuries.

By the 1500s the preference was for the cultivated Garden angelica, about which John Gerard said in his *Herball*:

The root is a singular remedy against poison, and against the plague, and all infections taken by evil and corrupt air. It openeth the liver and spleen: draweth down the terms, driveth out or expelleth the secondine [placenta]. *The decoction of the root made in wine, is good against the cold shivering of*

ETYMOLOGY OF COMMON NAME
Named because it blooms on the day of Michael the Archangel (8 May, old style).

PLANT LORE
In European folklore, it was sometimes hung around the home or carried as an amulet to guard against negative energies and malevolent forces. It is named after the archangel Michael, who, according to legend, appeared in a vision to a monk and revealed the plant's ability to cure the plague.

USE
All parts.

EDIBILITY
The stems can be eaten fresh but are traditionally candied.

HARVEST
In the summer for stems and leaves and autumn for the root and seeds.

MEDICINAL PROPERTIES
Analgesic, antispasmodic, anti-inflammatory, digestive, carminative emmenagogue, expectorant, antimicrobial, anticancerogenic and anxiolytic.

ACTIVE CONSTITUENTS
Coumarins, phenolic acids, essential oils, flavonoids, polysaccharides.

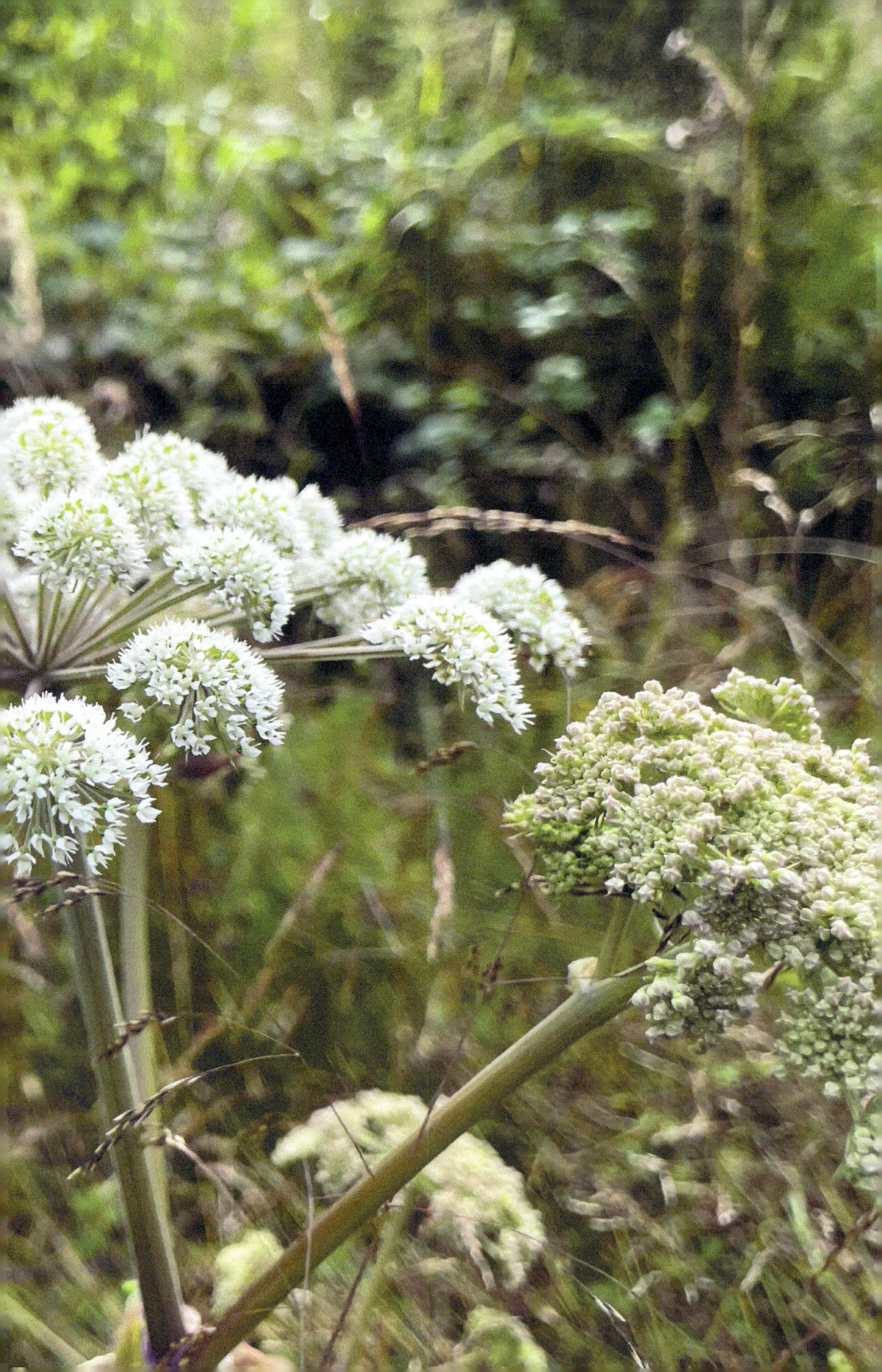

ANGELICA (WILD)

agues. It attenuateth and maketh thin, gross and tough phlegm: the root being used green, and while it is full of juice, helpeth them that be asthmatic, dissolving and expectorating the stuffings therein, by cutting off and cleansing the parts affected, reducing the body to health again; but when it is dry it worketh not so effectually. It is a most singular medicine against surfeiting and loathsomeness to meat: it helpeth concoction in the stomach and is right beneficial to the heart: it cureth the bitings of mad dogs, and all other venomous beasts. The wild kinds are not of such force in working, albeit they have the same virtues attributed unto them.

Culpeper's Herbal also recommended a decoction of the root:

> *... drank two or three spoonfuls at a time, to ease pains and torments of cold and wind, so that the body be not bound ... taken with some of the root in powder, at the beginning, helps the pleurisy [pain around the lungs], as also all other diseases of the lungs and breast, as coughs, phthisic, and shortness of breath; and a syrup of the stalks do the like. It helps pains of the cholic, the stranguary and stoppage of the urine, procures women's courses, and expels the afterbirth, opens the stoppings of the liver and spleen, and eases all windiness and inward swellings. The juice, or water, being dropped into the eyes or ears, helps dimness of sight and deafness; the juice put into the hollow teeth, eases their pains.*

MODERN RESEARCH

Angelica, as can be seen, has a long history of medicinal use. Modern research into Angelica is also largely in relation to the cultivated variety, but the wild variety can be used in the same way as follows:

Analgesic, antispasmodic and anti-inflammatory

Angelica has been used in Chinese medicine as an ingredient to treat arthritis and rheumatism and as an anti-inflammatory herb (Sarker and Nahar, 2004; Jung et al., 2007). In 2009 Song et al. identified a polysaccharide substance in the root that possesses significant analgesic activity, and shortly thereafter, ligustilide was identified as the component responsible for both analgesic and anti-inflammatory effects (Su et al., 2011). Its inclusion in remedies such as Mesir paste is therefore verified, and it continues to be used as a pain remedy in Turkey and China.

Digestive and carminative

The historical writers are accurate in their use of Angelica for the stomach. Owing to the angelicin it contains, it acts as an aromatic bitter, which helps stimulate digestion and metabolism but is also anti-flatulent, so it also eases indigestion, bloating and gas.

Expectorant

As the above also note, it also has an expectorant effect. This again is on account of the angelicin, which has a stimulating effect on the lungs and can help soothe asthma, coughs, bronchitis, and colds or flu; this is particularly true of the root and seed.

Emmenagogue

The same stimulating effect of the angelicin will also affect the uterus and promote menstruation. *Angelica sinensis*, another member of the same family, is officially listed in the *Chinese Pharmacopoeia* (as Dong Quai) and is one of the most commonly used Chinese traditional drugs in the treatment of menstrual disorders, menorrhagia and rheumatalgia (Liu et al., 2000). Given post-partum the same effect will release the placenta, as indicated by both Gerard's and Culpeper's references to the expelling of the placenta.

Diuretic

The seed will also encourage diuresis and has demonstrated anti-inflammatory, bacteriostatic and fungistatic properties, so it may well therefore be useful in cystitis, confirming Culpeper's assertion that it helps 'stoppage of the urine'.

Antimicrobial

In addition to the above effects, Angelica may also kill harmful bacteria, viruses and fungi. In a 2016 study the *in vitro* antimicrobial activity of the roots of Wild angelica, as a component of the traditional Mesir paste, were found to have activity against several gram-positive and gram-negative microorganisms, especially *Enterococcus faecium*, *Listeria monocytogenes*, *Bacillus subtilis*, *Staphylococcus epidermidis* and *Staphylococcus aureus*.

Furthermore, a 2017 study reported that compounds in Angelica (in this instance the cultivated garden version), including imperatorin, also exhibit antiviral activity against the *Herpes simplex* (cold sore) virus and coxsackievirus, which causes digestive illness.

Anticancerogenic

Anticancer effects have also been reported, in February 2019, on breast cancer, with the conclusion that, 'Altogether, we have reported for the first time the potential of the Angelica as a cell death inducer in breast cancer cells. The property found to be the constituent was again angelicin.

Anxiolytic

Finally, there's some compelling evidence from animal studies that Angelica may help reduce anxiety. Rat studies noted that coumarins isolated from Angelica and its constituents imperatorin and isoimperatorin have the potential to reduce anxiety. However, the mixture of the two constituents has more significant activity than the individual components.

TOPICAL USES

Owing to its antifungal properties the powdered dried root can be used for athlete's foot and a decoction can be used to treat ulcers, bites, gout and sciatica. It also works to calm the epidermis and heal problems such as eczema and breakouts, making a great bath additive for this purpose.

DOSAGE

Decoction – 1tbsp/15g of root to a 500ml of boiled water. Drink half a cup, 3 times per day.
Tincture – 1:5 50% – ½tsp–2ml – 20 drops = 1ml/1tsp = 5ml.

PRECAUTIONS

Not for use during pregnancy or heavy menstruation, nor by those with diabetes or on warfarin. May cause skin photosensitivity with prolonged use and also increases stomach acid. Not suitable for children or those who are pregnant or lactating.

Angelica recipes

Medicinal recipes

Angelica tisane

Pour 250ml boiling water over 2tsp/10g of the leaf and allow to steep for 10–15 minutes. Serve with sugar and lemon if necessary. Use for soothing bloat, tension, colds, coughs, rheumatism and urinary disorders.

Angelica decoction

Place 15g Angelica root and leaf in a pan. Add 500ml of water. Bring the water to a gentle boil, reduce heat and simmer for 20–40 minutes. Remove from heat and allow to cool a bit. Carefully strain off the herbs and drink as desired. Use for easing menstrual pain, bloating, gas, asthma, bronchitis, colds and flu. Can also be used as an antibacterial wash for the face, to prevent acne and be added to baths for eczema.

Angelica decocted tincture: 1:5 50%

If you are using 40% alcohol, ie vodka, make a simple tincture by covering 1 part herb to 5 parts fluid.

If you are using Everclear or other 100% proof, use the following method:

- 100g dried Angelica root
- 250ml alcohol
- 250ml water

Divide your Angelica root into two equal 50g parts. Cover 50g dried powdered root with 250ml of the alcohol. Then place the other 50g of dried root in 250ml of water. Bring the water to a gentle boil, reduce heat and simmer for 20–40 minutes. Remove from heat and allow to cool a bit. Strain thoroughly and top up if the water is less than 250ml. Add the decoction to the alcohol mix and leave for 14 days before straining. Use for heartburn, flatulence, loss of appetite, arthritis, circulation problems, nervousness and anxiety, fever and insomnia.

Angelica bath oil

- 100g of dried and powdered root
- 2 tbsp of alcohol, such as Everclear
- 1l of rapeseed oil

Place the root in a jar with the alcohol and allow to steep for 10 minutes before adding the oil. Leave for 4 weeks and then strain. Use as a bath or massage oil for eczema and other skin irritations.

AVENS
Geum urbanum

Geum urbanum, commonly known as Wood avens or Herb Bennet, is native to the UK. It belongs to the *Rosaceae* family, which also includes roses and strawberries. Wood avens is commonly found in hedgerows, woodlands and other shady or damp habitats. It has a long history of use in traditional herbal medicine. In medieval times, it was believed to have various medicinal properties and was used to treat ailments such as digestive disorders, fevers and wounds.

HISTORICAL USES

The other name for Wood avens, 'Herb Bennet', is derived from St Benedict of Nursia, reflecting the plant's long-standing association with healing and protection. Benedictine monks are said to have cultivated Wood avens in their gardens for its medicinal and protective properties, making it an important part of monastic medicine, used in various remedies and elixirs.

A cordial against the plague was made by boiling Avens roots in wine. Nicholas Culpeper also recommended it for the diseases of the chest, for pains and stitches in the sides and to expel crude and raw humours from the belly. He said it '… *dissolves inward congealed blood occasioned by falls and*

ETYMOLOGY OF COMMON NAME
Avens is from Middle English *avance*, *anancia*, *enancia* and signifies an antidote, because it was thought to ward off the Devil and evil spirits.

PLANT LORE
In medieval European folklore, Wood avens was believed to have protective properties that could ward off evil spirits and negative influences. It was often hung in homes and churches to keep these malevolent forces at bay.

USE
All parts.

EDIBILITY
The young leaves can be added to salads and the root, if harvested in early spring, imparts a clove flavour when added to soups, stews and beverages.

HARVEST
In spring and summer. Large roots are best.

MEDICINAL PROPERTIES
Antiseptic, astringent, digestive, antibacterial, cardiogenic, neuroprotective and febrifuge.

ACTIVE CONSTITUENTS
Tannins, phenolic acids, essential oils, flavonoids, polysaccharides.

bruises and the spitting of blood, if the roots either green or dried be boiled in wine and drunk ... It helpeth digeſtion, warmeth a cold ſtomach and openeth obſtructions of liver and spleen.'

Robert Thornton's *Family Herbal* (1814) recommended Avens in intermittent fevers, dysentery and chronic diarrhoeas, flatulent colic, affections of the primae viae (stomach), asthmatic symptoms, and cases of debility.

In his *Herbal Manual* (1936) Harold Ward wrote that the properties of Avens make for success in the treatment of diarrhoea and dysentery '... *The tonic effect upon the glands of the ſtomach and alimentary tract point to its helpfulness in dyspepsia. In general debility continued use has had good results. The aſtringent qualities may also be utilised in cases of relaxed throat. Although wineglass-ful doses three or four times daily of the 1 ounce to 1 pint infusion are usually prescribed, Avens may be taken freely, and is, indeed, used by country people in certain diſtricts as a beverage in place of tea or coffee.'*

MODERN RESEARCH

Wood avens is another plant with a long history of use. Its other name is Herb Bennet or the Blessed herb because the plant was widely used in medieval herbal medicine. Research has confirmed the following medicinal properties of Avens:

Astringent and digestive

Avens contains tannins, which are responsible for the astringent properties noted by the historical authors in the plant's use for dissolving congealed blood and treating dysentery and diarrhoea. The bitter properties also stimulate the appetite and trigger gastric secretion and bowel movements, namely 'to expel crude and raw humours from the belly', while the essential oil in the rhizome has antispasmodic action and inhibits gas formation and irritation of the stomach. This explains how it 'warmeth a cold stomach and openeth obstructions of liver and spleen'. It is also, as a result, a good remedy for IBS and Crohn's.

Antibacterial

In addition to confirming the effects described by the historical texts, further activity was studied in 2016 on bacterial growth. Results revealed that methanolic extracts of Avens leaves showed maximum activity against all the test bacteria including *Pseudomonas aeruginosa*, followed by *Escherichia coli* (the cause of most infections in the digestive and urinary tracts of humans

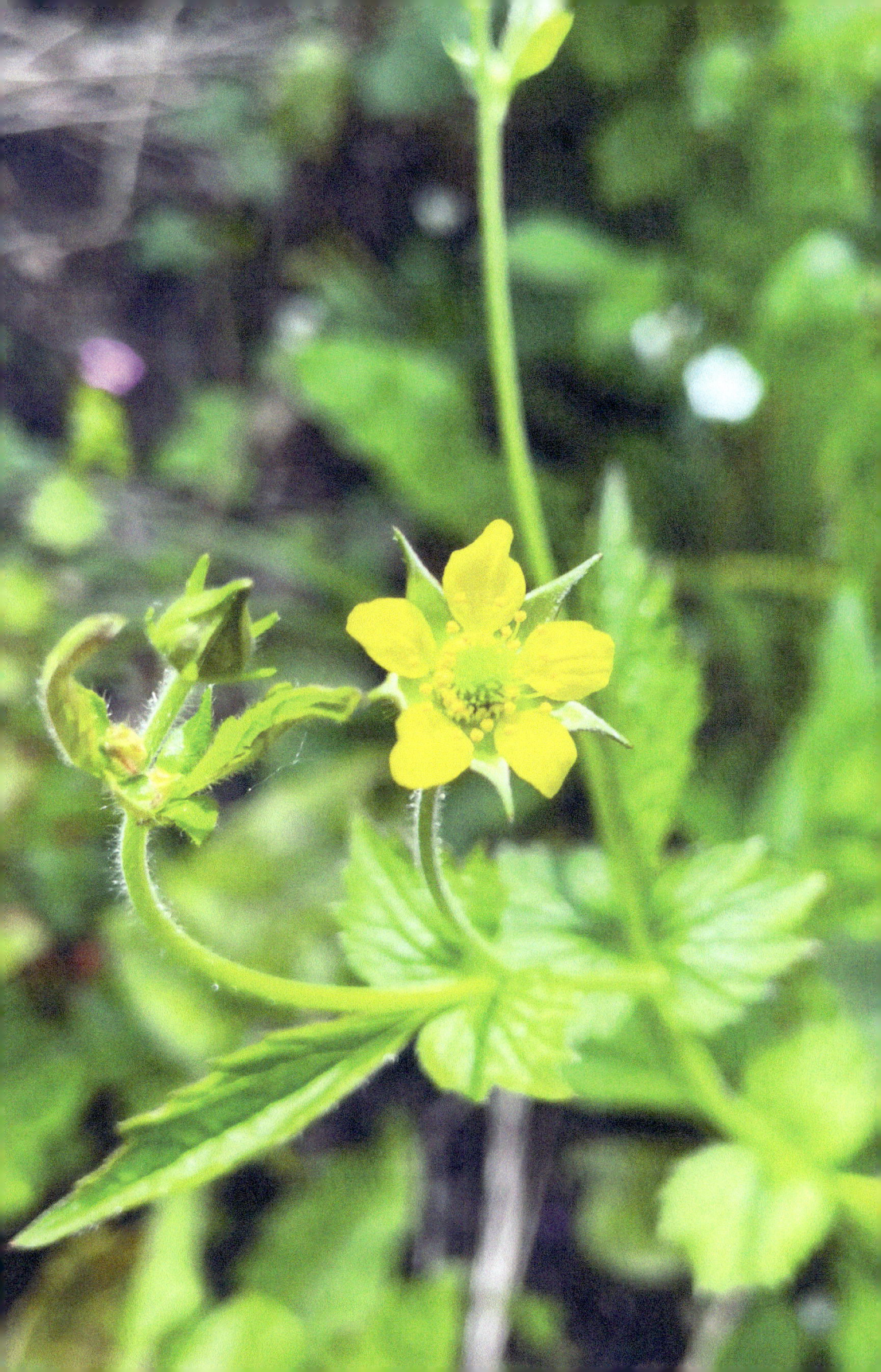

and animals), *Bacillus subtilis* and *Staphylococcus aureus*.

Cardiogenic

In 2018, a study was undertaken to investigate the cardiogenic effects of extracts of Wood avens on cultured stem cells. The methanolic extracts of the root and aerial parts showed no toxic effects on cells but effectively increased the levels of some essential cardiogenic markers, probably owing to ellagic and gallic acid derivatives. These findings indicate that Avens potentially may have a therapeutic role to play in cardiac medicine.

Neuroprotective

A promising study was carried out in May 2019 on two Parkinson's disease hallmarks, Lewy bodies and Lewy neurites, which consist of proteins that clump together and consequently no longer transmit correctly. The results showed that Wood avens inhibits the rapid contractions that cause clumping and even partly disintegrates preformed protein clumps.

TOPICAL USES

We know that the tannins in Avens make it a great astringent and so it is useful as a gargle to heal mouth ulcers and for infections of the pharynx and larynx.

A 2022 study into the antimicrobial potential of rhizome extracts confirmed potential for the topical treatment of acne and use in preparations such as creams or facial steam baths against inflamed skin.

DOSAGE

Tisane – 1–2tsp/5–10g. Drink half a cup, 3 times per day.

It is best to consume this plant between meals because when taken for a long period of time it could possibly cause intestinal irritation.

PRECAUTIONS

Because of its high tannin content Avens should not be used in excessive doses or for a long period of time. Not suitable for children or those who are pregnant or lactating.

Avens recipes

Medicinal recipes

Wood avens tisane
Pour 250ml boiling water over 1tsp/5g of the dried leaf and allow to steep for 10-15 minutes. Use for diarrhoea, nausea and other stomach complaints as well as a gargle for mouth ulcers and throat infections.

Wood avens compress
Soak a cloth in a tisane of the dried herb and apply 2-3 times a day to heal acne.

Wood avens powder
The root is best harvested in the spring, since this is when it is most fragrant. Much of the fragrance can be lost on drying, so dry with great care and then store in an airtight container. For use as a styptic for heavy bleeding, an initial dose of 2-3tsp of powder is administered, after which the treatment is continued with 1tsp/5g of powder 4 times a day for 5 straight days.

Wood avens decoction
Take 15g of the powdered root or herb to 500ml of water. Boil for 20 minutes, strain and allow to cool. Use as a gargle to treat gingivitis, bad breath and sore throats, 3 times per day for 1-2 weeks. For cases of diarrhoea, IBS and Crohn's the dosage is increased to 4 times per day.

Avens and Agrimony syrup
- 250ml Avens tisane
- 250ml Agrimony tisane
- 500g sugar
- 25ml tincture, optional (preservative)

Warm your tisanes over a low heat and bring to a simmer. Then cover partially and reduce the liquid down to half its original volume, ie. 250ml. Add the sugar and stir constantly, but do not let the mix boil. Remove the syrup from the heat and add the tinctures at a ratio of 5%. Syrups keep for up to 2 years unopened. After opening, store in the refrigerator and use within 1 month. Use for ulcerative colitis, diarrhoea, diverticulitis, Crohn's disease. A general dosage is a dessertspoon taken 1 to 3 times a day with increased frequency during an acute phase of symptoms.

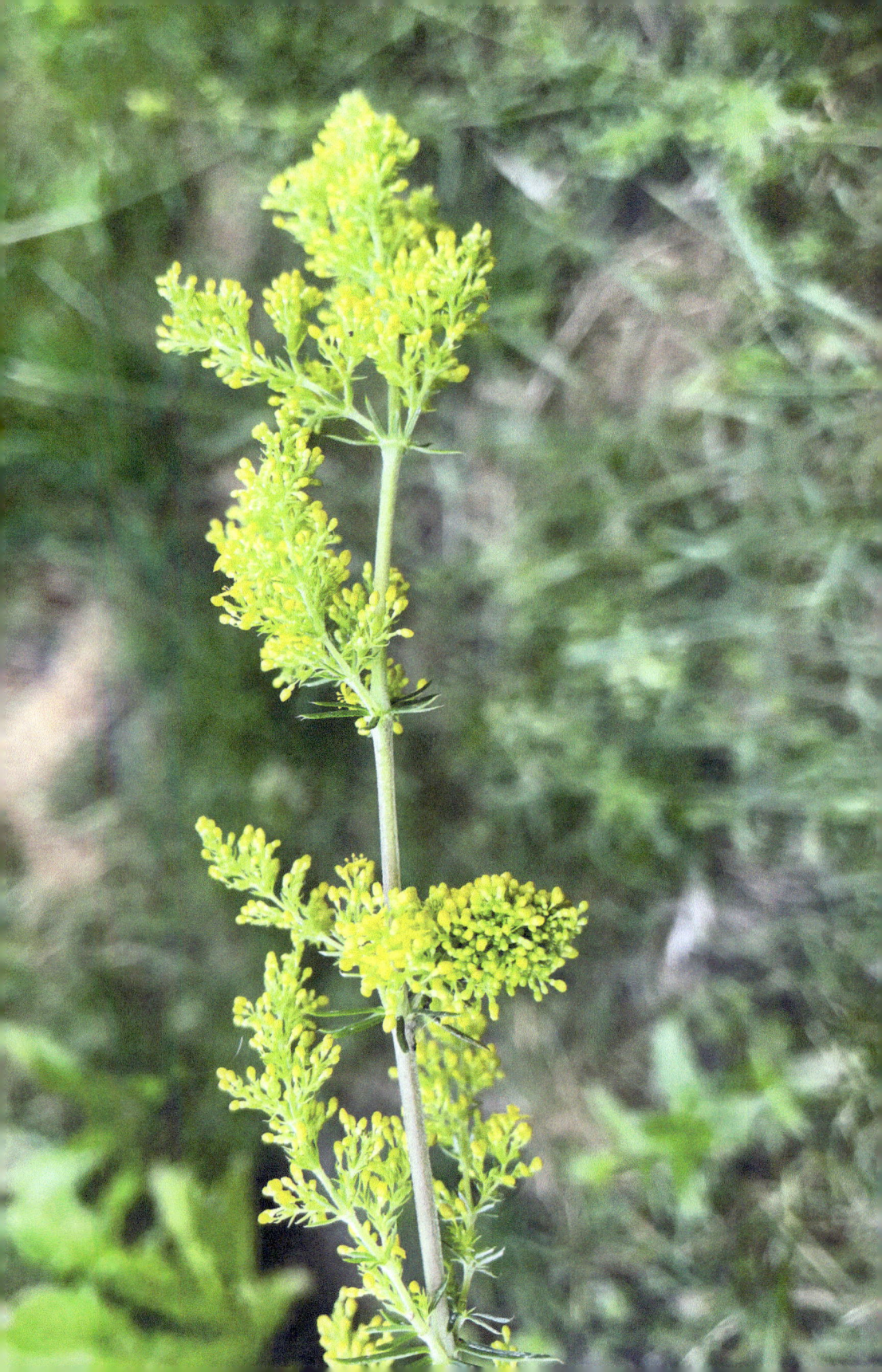

BEDSTRAWS
Galium verum/mollugo

In the UK, several species of *Galium*, commonly known as bedstraw, can be found, including Cleavers (*Galium aparine*) and Woodruff (*Galium odoratum*), which have their own chapters in this book. Hedge bedstraw (*Galium mollugo*) and Lady's bedstraw (*Galium verum*), meanwhile, were originally used to stuff mattresses and pillows and can be found in grasslands and meadows. Both are part of the Madder family, *Rubiaceae*.

HISTORICAL USES

Both Lady's bedstraw and Hedge bedstraw were part of the European herbal tradition, and their uses extended beyond the medicinal. Lady's bedstraw was used in traditional cheese making. The plant's flowers were added to milk to coagulate it, providing a source of rennet for curdling; also, being part of the Madder family, both were used as a natural dye for textiles. The flowers of Lady's bedstraw produced a yellow or greenish hue while the roots of Hedge bedstraw yielded red and brown dyes.

While always stating that the plants have a long history of use as diuretics, the medicinal data are a little short on detail, although Nicholas Culpeper said, '*The decoction, being drank, is good*

ETYMOLOGY OF COMMON NAME
Derived from the tradition of stuffing straw mattresses with the plant.

PLANT LORE
A tea made from Lady's bedstraw was said to calm the terrifying battle frenzy of the Celtic hero Cúchulainn. In European folklore, placing bedstraw around the home or in bedding was thought to ward off evil spirits and prevent nightmares.

USE
All aerial parts.

EDIBILITY
The leaves can be eaten raw or cooked, and the seed is also edible. The chopped-up plant can be used as a rennet substitute in cheese.

HARVEST
In spring and summer.

MEDICINAL PROPERTIES
Astringent, antioxidant, anticancerogenic, anti-ischaemic, anti-inflammatory, antimicrobial and diuretic.

ACTIVE CONSTITUENTS
Coumarins, tannins, flavonoids, anthraquinones, polysaccharides, alkaloids, essential oils.

LEFT: LADY'S BEDSTRAW

to fret and break the stone, provoke urine, stay inward bleedings, and to heal inward wounds. The herb or flower bruised, and put up into the nostrils, stayeth their bleeding likewise; the flowers and the herb being made into an oil, by being set in the sun, and changed after it hath stood ten or twelve days; or into an ointment being boiled in Axungia [lard] *or oil with some wax melted therein after it is strained, do help burning with fire or scalding with water. The same, or the decoction of the herb and flower, is good to bathe the feet of travellers and lacquais* [footmen], *whose long running causesth weariness and stiffness in their sinews and joints. If the decoction be used warm, and the joints afterwards anointed with the ointment, it helpeth the dry scab, and the itch in children.'*

MODERN RESEARCH

Galium species have been traditionally used for the treatment of many diseases and conditions. As stated above, they are renowned for use in milk coagulation, which is the reason the plant is also known as 'Yogurt herb'. In parts of Scotland the plant is still used in cheese manufacturing.

Gallium mullogo, the Hedge bedstraw, is less studied than the Lady's bedstraw, *Galium verum*, but taking into consideration similar chemical composition, we may assume that this species exerts similar activity to Lady's bedstraw as follows:

Diuretic

As Culpeper said, the plant has diuretic effects and can be used to clear toxins and stones from the kidneys (ie. break the stone and provoke urine). Because it is related to Cleavers, it is interchangeable with that plant and so it is useful for people suffering from a lymphatic system disorder.

Anticancerogenic

According to a detailed survey by Jonathan Hartwell in the 1970s (*Plants Used Against Cancer: A Survey*), Lady's bedstraw has been traditionally used in Europe and North America for the treatment of cancerous ulcers or breast cancer. Amirghofran et al. showed in 2006 that the plant has a cytotoxic effect on leukaemia cells, while and Zhao et al. isolated from it diosmetin, a flavone that showed protective effects on the thymus gland in mice. The cytotoxicity of Lady's bedstraw was evaluated against laryngeal cancer cells in 2013 and 2014 and found to be potentially useful as a preventive or a therapeutic approach in head and neck cancers. The treatment of tongue cancer with Lady's bedstraw is also supported by reports of patients with tongue and larynx carcinoma being successfully treated with the tea of this plant.

A 2022 study returned to the anti-cancer studies of the plant and reported that a methanol extract of Lady's bedstraw produced a significant decrease of cell viability in colon cancer and fibroblast cell lines. The percentage of dead cells in the experimental group increased significantly when compared to the control group, which may extend its use in the body.

Antioxidant

Bedstraw was found to exhibit very potent antioxidant activities, largely owing to its caffeic and chlorogenic acid content as well as vitamins C, E and β-carotene (Prior, 2003). The conclusion of the studies was that this plant is a good source of phenols that can avert the damage of cells resulting from free-radical oxidation reactions.

Anti-ischaemic

Because it is rich in antioxidants, Lady's bedstraw was studied in 2018 for its potential in reducing post-ischaemic myocardial dysfunction, which occurs when blood flow to the heart is reduced, preventing the heart muscle from receiving enough oxygen. An echocardiographic examination of heart function demonstrated that after 4 weeks of treatment the plant extract reduced left ventricular enlargement, and considerably improved cardiac function.

Antimicrobial

In a study of the antimicrobial activity of extracts of bedstraws, it has been found that the ethanol extract exhibits the highest activity. *Bacillus subtilis*, the cause of pneumonia and septicaemia, was the most susceptible bacteria, and results indicate the potential of the plant in the development of antibacterial agents.

Anti-inflammatory

The anti-inflammatory activity of bedstraws is based on the caffeic and chlorogenic acid contained in the plants, which have the ability to prevent a number of cell reactions in the inflammatory process. In a study of paw oedema in mice, the anti-inflammatory effect reached significant results in one hour and suppressed inflammation by 37%, which exceeded the results in the control group by 1.5 times. This may well be the reason that Culpeper recommends it for treatment of tired or sore feet and joints.

TOPICAL USES

Culpeper alluded to the fact that bedstraw topical ointment may be useful in the treatment of skin disorders, and being both antimicrobial and anti-inflammatory as well as a potent antioxidant, these will help to calm the skin and help it to heal. Caffeic acid is also believed to enhance collagen production, which will help heal wounds and improve the appearance of the skin.

DOSAGE

Tisane – 1–2tsp/5–10g. Drink freely

PRECAUTIONS

None found, but it is not suitable for children or those who are pregnant or lactating.

Bedstraw recipes

Medicinal recipes

Lady's bedstraw tisane
Pour 250ml boiling water over 1-2tsp/5-10g of the dried leaf and allow to steep for 15 minutes. Use as a diuretic and tonic.

Lady's bedstraw compress
Soak a cloth in a tisane of the dried herb and apply 2-3 times a day to improve the appearance of skin.

Lady's bedstraw poultice
- 1tsp fresh root (if using dried you will need to moisten with water first)
- 2tsp coconut oil
- cheesecloth or cotton bandage

Finely grate the root into a pulp and add the coconut oil to make a paste. Spread the paste evenly over the desired area and wrap with the cloth or bandage. Use to heal wounds and burns and to calm inflammation.

Lady's bedstraw bath
- 50g Lady's bedstraw herb
- 1l water
- Steep the herb in the water for 15 minutes, then strain and add to the bathwater to ease psoriasis.

Lady's bedstraw infused honey
- Fresh Lady's bedstraw flowers
- Honey

Harvest fresh Lady's bedstraw flowers, ensuring they are clean and free of pesticides. Fill a clean, dry jar with the Lady's bedstraw flowers. Pour honey over the flowers, making sure they are completely submerged. Seal the jar and let it sit in a warm, dark place for several weeks to allow the flavours to infuse. Then strain out the flowers and use as a sweetener in teas or desserts.

BETONY
Betonica officinalis

Betonica officinalis, commonly known as Betony or Wood betony, is a woodland plant belonging to the mint family, *Lamiaceae*. Betony has a long history of use in traditional herbal medicine. It was considered a panacea in medieval times and was believed to have a wide range of medicinal properties.

HISTORICAL USES

Wood betony was held in high repute not only in the Middle Ages, but also by the Greeks who extolled its qualities. It also appears in the *Leechbook of Bald*, an Anglo-Saxon medical text, as a treatment for a broken head *'For broken head, take betony, bruise it and lay it on the head above, then it unites the wound and healeth it'*.

An old Italian proverb, 'Sell your coat and buy Betony', and an equally old Spanish one, 'He has as many virtues as Betony', show what value was placed on its remedial properties. Antonius Musa, chief physician to the Emperor Augustus, filled a whole volume with its many virtues, saying it cured forty-seven different disorders; hence the proverb 'You have more virtues than Betony'.

Hildegard of Bingen (1098–1179) wrote in her *Physica* … *'A woman who suffers inordinately with great menstruation at the wrong time should place*

ETYMOLOGY OF COMMON NAME
The name *Betonica* is from the Celtic ben, head, and tonic, in allusion to the usefulness of the herb against infirmities of the head.

PLANT LORE
Betony was burned at summer solstice for purification and protection. It was believed that it grew in places frequented by fairies and that gathering it on Midsummer's Eve could grant protection and blessings from the fae.

USE
All aerial parts

EDIBILITY
The leaves are generally used as a tisane substitute for black tea

HARVEST
When in flower

MEDICINAL PROPERTIES
Hepatobiliary, analgesic, antioxidant, amenorrhoeal, alterative, anti-inflammatory.

ACTIVE CONSTITUENTS
Iridoid glycosides, flavonoids, triterpenoids, phenolic acids, essential oils.

Betony in wine, so that the flavour passes into it and drink it often'.

John Gerard (1545–1612) advised us in his *Herball* that '... *a conserve made of the flowers and sugar, is good for many things, especially for the headache. A dram weight of the root of Betony dried, and taken with mead or honeyed water, procureth vomit, and bringeth forth gross and tough humours, as divers of our age do report. The powder of the dried leaves drunk in wine is good for them that spit or piss blood, and cureth all inward wounds, especially the green leaves boiled in wine and given. The powder taken with meat looseth the belly very gently, and helpeth them that have the falling sickness* [epilepsy] *with madness and headache. It is singular against all pains of the head: it killeth worms in the belly; helpeth the ague: it cleanseth the mother* [womb]*, and hath great virtue to heal the body, being hurt within by bruising or such like.'*

Culpeper's *Herbal* held that *'Betony helpeth those that cannot digest their meat, those that have weak stomachs, or sour belchings. It helpeth the jaundice, falling sickness, the palsy, convulsions, shrinking of the sinews, the gout, those that are inclined to dropsy* [odoema] *and those that have continuous pains in their head.'*

In *Medicina Britannica* of 1666, we read, '*I have known the most obstinate headaches cured by daily breakfasting for a month or six weeks on a decoction of Betony, made with new milk, and strained.'*

Finally, Robert Turner, a physician writing in the latter half of the 17th century, recounted nearly thirty complaints for which Betony was considered efficacious, and added *'I shall conclude with the words I have found in an old manuscript under the virtues of it:* '*More than all this have been proved of Betony.'*

MODERN RESEARCH

I'm not sure there is a herb that has been held in higher repute than Betony, and yet in modern herbal medicine, you do not see it used that often. Betony fell out of favour because it can take a long time of continuous use to see results. It helps the body to heal itself cumulatively, and this cumulative effect is referred to by David Hoffmann in 2003 (*Medical Herbalism*) when he said, *Its underlying action appears to be through toning and strengthening the nervous system while simultaneously soothing nervous tension.* Properties confirmed by modern research are:

Hepatobiliary

Supporting Culpeper's findings that the herb could be used to treat jaundice, according to the online Bastyr University *Materia Medica*, 49 patients with obstructive jaundice who underwent surgery because they were unresponsive to conventional therapy, were given a Betony preparation before and after the operation. Under the influence of the preparation, a more rapid normalisation of the indices of homeostasis, ie blood pressure, core body temperature, heart rate, respiratory

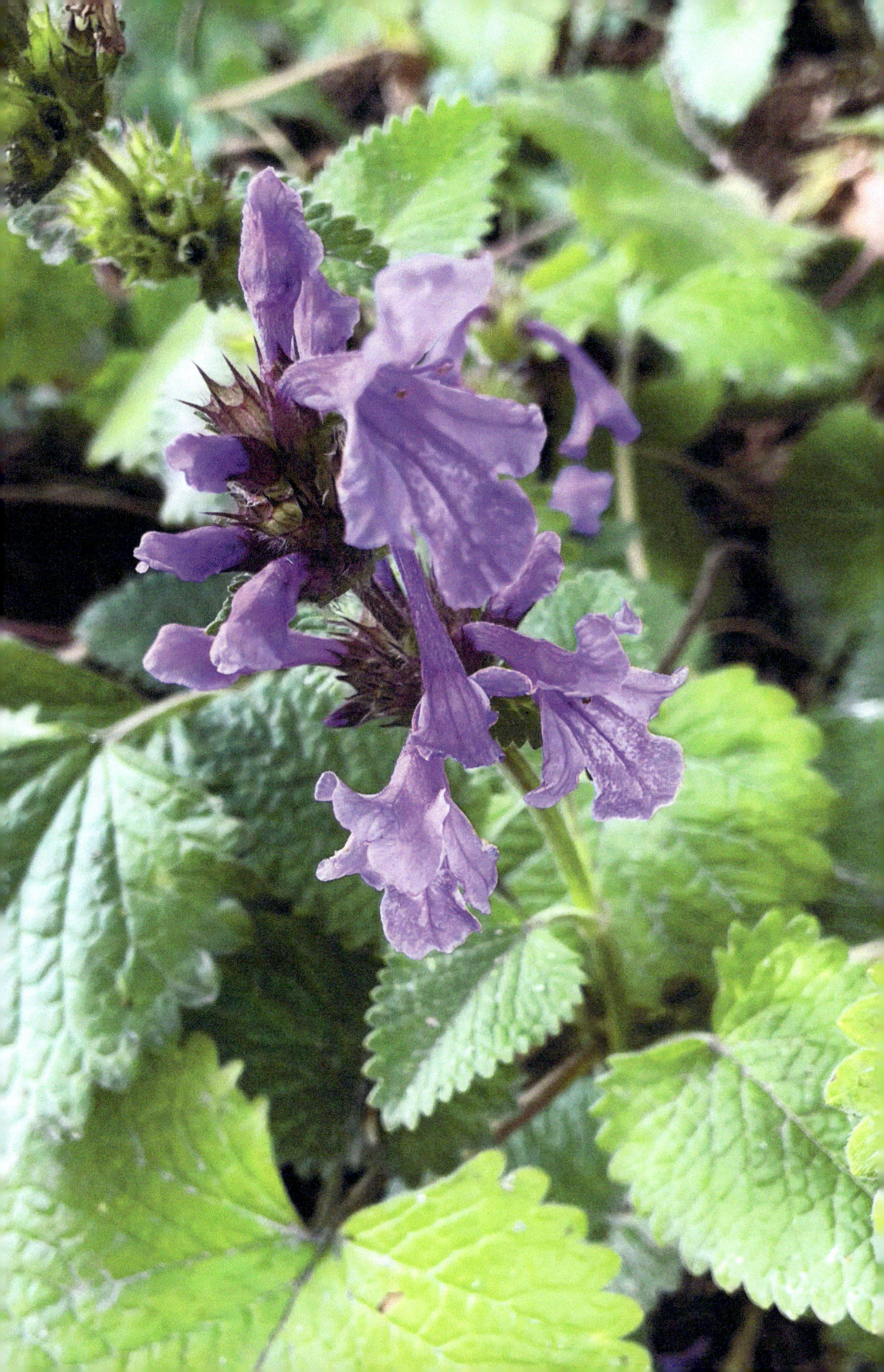

rate and oxygen saturation occurred. The most pronounced effect was noted in patients with benign obstructive jaundice.

Relaxant and analgesic
The same texts provide confirmation of the statements on headaches in Gerard, Culpeper and the *Medicina Britannica*; Betony, it is said, 'relaxes skeletal muscle and has a tropism for the muscles of the upper back, shoulders, and neck'. It is therefore useful in the treatment of headaches secondary to muscle tension and/or hypertension that is worsened by anxiety.

Antioxidant
In 2013, Betony demonstrated significant antioxidant properties against free-radical cell damage. This is thought to be a consequence of the strong antioxidant activity of the flavonoids and the phenolic glycosides. which are believed to contribute to the lowering of blood pressure.

Anti-inflammatory
In 2012, extracts of the plant parts showed significant anti-inflammatory activity in rats, similar in strength to diclofenac. In 2017, this anti-inflammatory effect was confirmed by Paun et al., and assigned to the presence of ursolic acid, caffeic acid, rosmarinic acid, quercetin and also anthocyanidins (genistin). This again supports its use in the treatment of headaches and Gerard's description that it 'hath great virtue to heal the body, being hurt within by bruising or such like'.

Amenorrhoeal
An encouraging study in 2013 involved Betony being evaluated in the treatment of abnormal uterine bleeding caused by polycystic ovary syndrome (PCOS). A randomised clinical trial of 66 women aged 15–45 years were assigned to either medroxyprogesterone (a progestin medication) or Betony for three months. Results showed that while decrease in prevalence rate was similar, the side effects for Betony were less serious as compared to medroxyprogesterone, and Betony may therefore be considered as an alternative in treating abnormal uterine bleeding arising from PCOS. Here we also find confirmation for Hildegard of Bingen's recommended use for Betony.

TOPICAL USES

A poultice made from the herb can be applied to heal wounds and bruises on the skin. Betony's anti-inflammatory properties help ease the inflammation of the skin caused by eczema as well as other skin conditions.

DOSAGE

Tisane – 1–2tsp/5–10g 3 times per day.
Tincture – 1:5 45% – 2–6ml – 20 drops = 1ml/1tsp = 5ml.

PRECAUTIONS

Not suitable for children or those who are pregnant or lactating.

Betony recipes

Medicinal recipes

Betony tisane

Pour 250ml boiling water over 2 tsp/10g of the dried leaf and allow to steep for 10–15 minutes. Use for headaches, lack of energy, anxiety and digestive ailments.

Betony infused tincture – 1:5 45%

If you are using 40% alcohol, ie vodka, make a simple tincture by covering 1 part herb to 5 parts fluid.

If you are using Everclear or other 100% proof, use the following method for a specific tincture:

- 100g dried Betony
- 225ml alcohol
- 275ml water

Cover 50g dried Betony with 225ml of the alcohol. Then steep/infuse another 50g of dried Betony in 275ml of water for 15 minutes. Strain thoroughly and top up if the water is less than 275ml. Add the infusion to the alcohol mix and leave for 14 days before straining. Use for diarrhoea, 4ml per day and also for headaches and bleeding from PCOS.

For headaches

The dried herb may also be smoked as tobacco, combined with Eyebright and Coltsfoot, for relieving headache or combined with lavender.

For relaxation

- 1 part Betony
- 1 part Vervain
- 2 parts Lemon Balm

Combine and use 1tsp per cup of boiled water and drink 3 times per day

An everyday tea substitute

- 1 part Raspberry leaf
- 1 part Agrimony
- 1 part Betony

Combine and use 1tsp per cup of boiled water and drink 3 times per day.

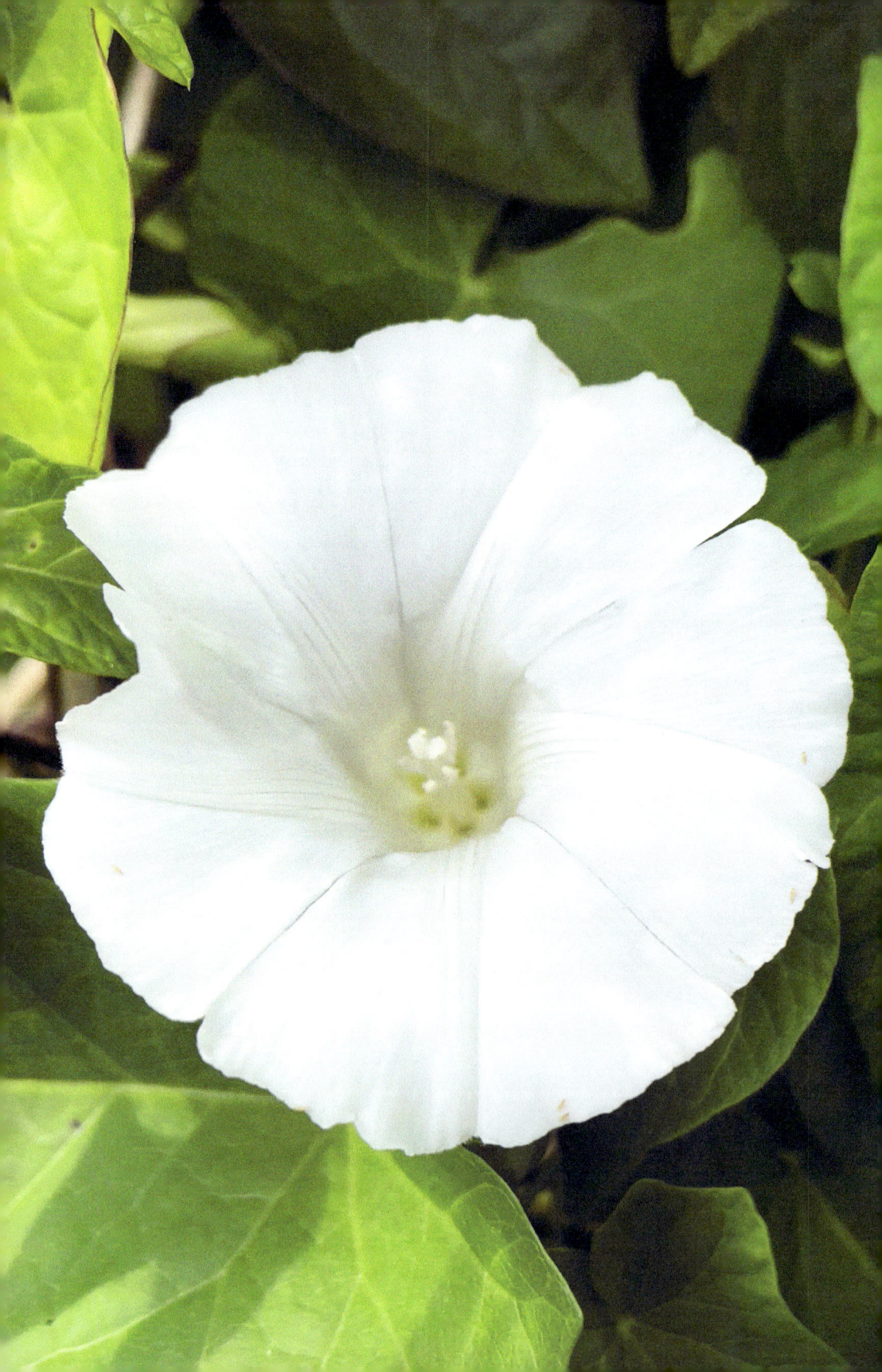

BINDWEED
Calystegia sepium/arvensis

Calystegia are plants in the *Convolvulaceae* family, commonly known as Bindweeds or the far more attractive name Morning glories. Several species of *Calystegia* are found in the UK, such as Hedge bindweed (*Calystegia sepium*) and Large bindweed (*Calystegia sylvatica*), and are known for their vigorous growth habit and twining vines.

HISTORICAL USES

In his *De Materia Medica* the ancient Greek physician Dioscorides is said to have prescribed Bindweed to heal wounds and stop internal bleeding.

Medieval herbalism, including Nicholas Culpeper's findings, cited it as a laxative, but also as treatment for spider bites, to delay menstruation, as a brain tonic to promote intellect and as a tranquilliser to help with insomnia, confusion, fits, nervous disorders, blood impurity and venereal disease. Culpeper said '… *the juice of the leaves, being drunk, do loosen and open the belly, and being pounded and laid to the grieved place, dissolveth wasteth and consumeth hard swellings.*'

ETYMOLOGY OF COMMON NAME
Taken directly from the plant's behaviour to bind itself to others.

PLANT LORE
Bindweed can be used like twine and was employed in handfastings.
It was also believed that fairies used the flowers as trumpets or to fashion delicate clothing. Seeing bindweed flowers was sometimes considered a sign that fairies were nearby.

USE
The flowers.

EDIBILITY
Not edible.

HARVEST
When in bloom.

MEDICINAL PROPERTIES
Laxative, purgative, antidiabetic, antibacterial, anticancerogenic, neuroprotective and tranquilliser.

MODERN RESEARCH

The use of the Bindweeds as a laxative and purgative, as Culpeper says, are a result of the anthraquinones they contain. However, in smaller doses Bindweed has shown some promising medicinal properties in other areas as follows:

Antidiabetic

In the early 1990s, calystegine, a naturally occurring alkaloid, was isolated from Bindweeds. Calystegines are known to act as glycosidase inhibitors, and a 2014 study showed that Bindweed could become a potential for the treatment of diabetes when it was confirmed to have a significant hypoglycaemic and hypolipidemic effect in hyperglycaemic rats.

Antibacterial

In Cameroon, medicinal plants (one of which is Bindweed) are traditionally used for the treatment of urinary tract infections. In 2017, a study was undertaken to evaluate the antibacterial activity of Bindweed and its potential for a collaborative effect with amoxicillin. Bindweed contains several bioactive compounds, including alkaloids, flavonoids and phenolic acids, which are known to have antimicrobial activities. The results confirmed that all extracts exhibited antibacterial activities, which validated the traditional use of these plants in the treatment of UTIs.

Anticancerogenic

In 2019, during the ongoing search for anticancer properties in plant extracts, different plants were tested to find the optimum extract that induce the death of cancer cells. One of these extracts was the methanolic extract of Bindweed leaf. Results indicated that it created a strong cytotoxic effect on cancer cells when compared to the standard drugs. In 2022, the plant was studied again, and two new resin glycosides were isolated and found to possess inhibitory effects on tumours, meaning they might in fact be the lead compound of future antitumour agents.

Neuroprotective and tranquilliser

While I have not found any studies that confirm Culpeper's use of Bindweed as a brain tonic to promote intellect or as a tranquilliser to help with insomnia, confusion, fits or nervous disorders, calystegines can have significant effects on the central nervous system. They are known to act as anticholinergics, which can produce sedative effects and interact with neurotransmitter systems, particularly acetylcholine. When acetylcholine receptors are inhibited this can influence cognition and mood. However, this interaction can also lead to toxicity, so the use of Bindweed is not recommended.

TOPICAL USES

I have not been able to find any recent studies to verify the use of Bindweed by Dioscorides to heal wounds. However, some traditional herbalists have used bindweed extracts topically to soothe skin irritations and alleviate symptoms of conditions such as eczema, dermatitis and minor burns. As can be seen from the above, Bindweed may possess antibacterial properties, and the tannins would of course be astringent. However, the alkaloids it contains could be an irritant, so caution is advised.

DOSAGE

Tisane – 1–2tsp 3 times per day.

PRECAUTIONS

The plant is rarely used anymore owing to its strong intestinal effects. Bindweeds can be toxic if ingested in large quantities and may cause skin irritation in some individuals. Not suitable for children or those who are pregnant or lactating.

Bindweed recipes

Medicinal recipes

Bindweed tisane

Pour 250ml boiling water over 1tsp/5g of dried Bindweed leaf and allow to steep for 10-15 minutes. Use for UTIs, as a laxative and a mild sedative. Proceed with caution owing to the possibility of toxicity.

Bindweed compress

- Fresh bindweed leaves
- Warm water
- Clean cloth or bandage

Crush the bindweed leaves and soak them in warm water for a few minutes, then place them on a clean cloth or bandage. Apply the compress to the affected area for 15-20 minutes to reduce inflammation and pain, but apply a patch test first to monitor reactions.

Bindweed poultice

- Fresh bindweed leaves
- Clean cloth or bandage

Crush the leaves into a paste using a mortar and pestle. Apply the paste directly to the affected area of the skin. Cover with a clean cloth or bandage. Leave for 20-30 minutes, then remove and rinse the area with water. Use for its anti-inflammatory properties to treat skin conditions or wounds, but apply a patch test first to monitor reactions.

Bindweed infused oil

- Fresh bindweed leaves and flowers
- Olive oil or another carrier oil

Fill a glass jar with fresh bindweed leaves and flowers, then pour the oil of your choice (olive oil, grapeseed oil, etc.) over the leaves and flowers until they are fully submerged. Seal the jar and place it in a sunny spot for 2-3 weeks, shaking it daily, then strain the oil through a cheesecloth or fine mesh strainer. Store the infused oil in a dark glass bottle in a cool place and use topically for skin conditions like eczema or psoriasis.

BISTORT
Bistorta officinalis

Bistorta officinalis, commonly known as Bistort, is a plant native to the UK in the *Polygonaceae* family. It is commonly found in damp or wet habitats, such as marshes, and stream banks.

HISTORICAL USES

John Gerard (1545–1612) told us in his *Herball* that *'the juice of Bistort put into the nose prevaileth much against the disease called polyps, against the biting of serpents or any venomous beast, being drunk in wine or the water of Angelica. The root boiled in wine and drunk, stoppeth the lask and bloody flux; it stayeth also the overmuch flowing of women's monthly sicknesses. The root taken as aforesaid stayeth vomiting, and healeth the inflammation and soreness of the mouth and throat: it likewise fasteneth loose teeth, being holden in the mouth for a certain space, and at sundry times.*

Nicholas Culpeper in his *Herbal* concurred by saying that *'the root in powder taken in drink expelleth the venom of the plague, the smallpox, measles, purples or any other infectious disease, driving it out by sweating.'*

The Dutch botanist and physician Herman Boerhaave (1668–1738) recommended a decoction of Bistort, or the tincture, for *'fixing of loose teeth, diabetes, a too abundant female relief, in passing of blood by any outlet, vomiting, diarrhoea,*

ETYMOLOGY OF COMMON NAME
Latin *bistorta*, from *bis*, 'twice', and *torta*, 'twisted', in reference to its twisting roots.

PLANT LORE
Burning Bistort is said to increase psychic powers, and carrying some of it was believed to help a woman conceive.

USE
The root and leaves.

EDIBILITY
The leaves, seed and roots are edible raw. The leaves are best used raw in salads when young as they do become a little chewy as they age

HARVEST
In spring for the leaves and autumn for the root.

MEDICINAL PROPERTIES
Astringent, anti-inflammatory and antimicrobial.

ACTIVE CONSTITUENTS
Tannins, flavonoids, polygonosides, anthraquinones, phenolic acids, essential oils.

and to prevent miscarriages ... bistort and tormentil root have an equal claim to astringency, and therefore equal virtues.'

Bistort is used in traditional Chinese medicine as a remedy for smallpox, measles and pimples plus any diseases with bleeding as a symptom.

MODERN RESEARCH

Bistort is also known as Adderwort and Snakeweed for its entwined roots. Modern research confirms the following properties:

Astringent

The root of Bistort is one of the strongest astringent medicines in the vegetable kingdom. It is highly haemostatic and, as the above have all indicated, may be used on both external or internal bleeds or wherever astringency is required. Most studies have confirmed the historical uses of Bistort and its effectiveness in the treatment of jaundice, irritable bowel syndrome, peptic ulcers, ulcerative colitis, worm infestations, bleeding haemorrhoids, cystitis and haematuria.

Anti-inflammatory

Further studies have shown that an ethanolic extract of Bistort root showed a strong anti-inflammatory effect, which is beneficial when used as a gargle for mouth and throat infections. This would also be why Gerard recommends it for nasal polyps. In dental practice it can be used to treat oral inflammation, for the treatment of catarrhal stomatitis, gingivitis, periodontal disease and other oral diseases, and for treating chronic wounds and boils. Gingivitis may well be the reason for loose teeth mentioned by Boerhaave, and here we can see why it would have helped with this condition.

Antimicrobial

A 2020 study investigated the antimicrobial activity of an infusion of Bistort root and found that the infusion contained mainly galloyl glucose derivatives, procyanidins and chlorogenic acid, which displayed antimicrobial activity against skin pathogens. A further 2020 study found that Bistort exhibited anti-virulence activity against *Pseudomonas aeruginosa*, giving it the potential to become a part of medical practice for the treatment of bacterial infections.

TOPICAL USES

For all of the reasons above, Bistort makes a good remedy for skin infection, skin eruptions, measles and burns.

DOSAGE

Root decoction – 1tsp/5g, half a cup, 3 times per day.
Tisane – 1–3ml (20–30 drops) in water.
Tincture – 1:5 25% – 1–3ml, 3 times per day – 20 drops = 1ml/1tsp = 5ml.

PRECAUTIONS

No health hazards or side effects are known in conjunction with the proper administration of designated therapeutic dosages. Not suitable for children or those who are pregnant or lactating.

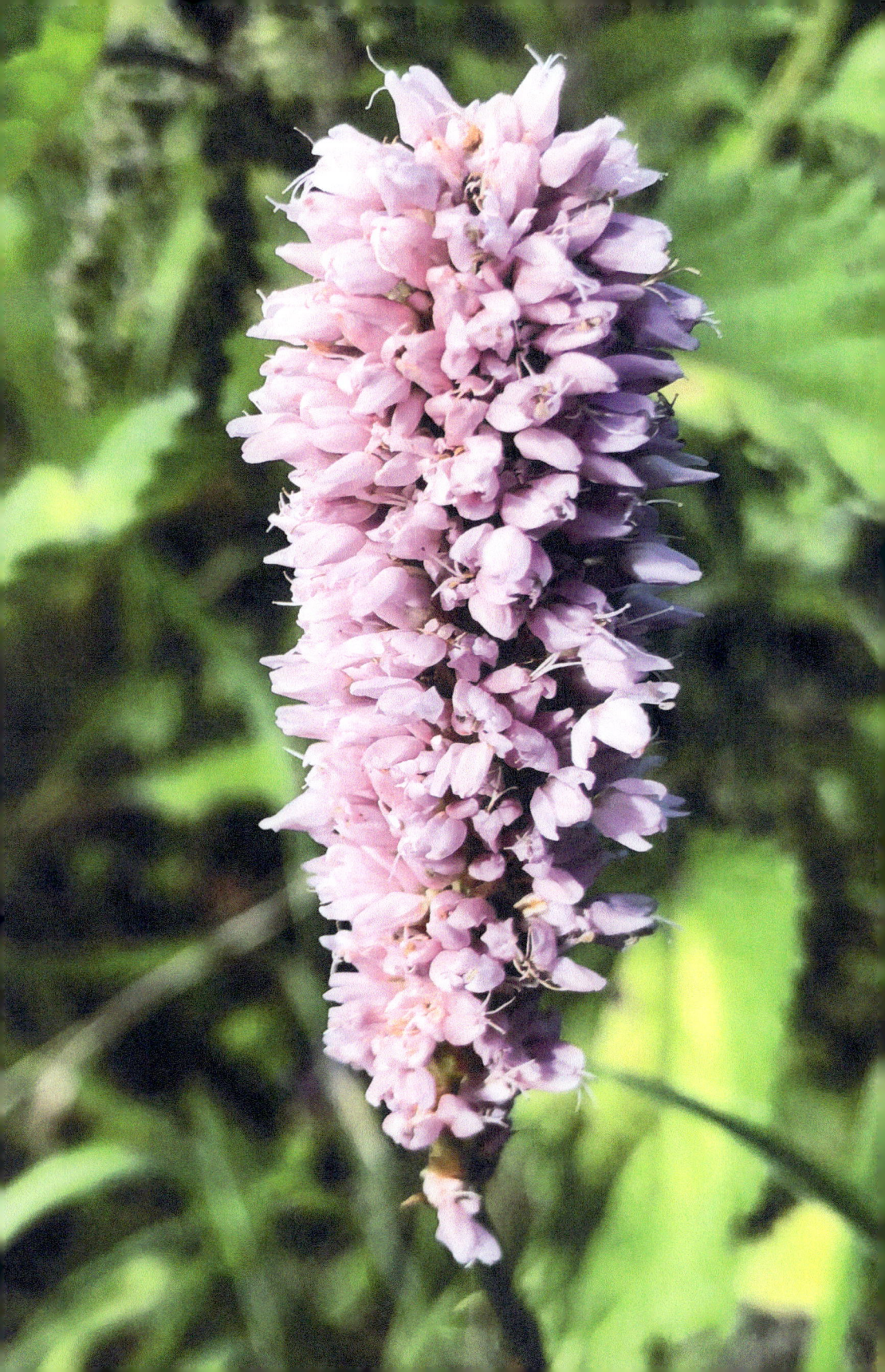

Bistort recipes

Medicinal recipes

Bistort leaf tisane

Pour 250ml boiling water over 1tsp/5g of the dried leaf and allow to steep for 10-15 minutes. Use as a gargle for mouth ulcers and sore throats.

Bistort root decoction

Boil 1-2g roots in water for 10 minutes. Strain, cool and drink up to 3 times per day for inflammations in the throat or to arrest an internal bleed.

Bistort decocted tincture – 1:5 25%

If you are using 40% alcohol, ie vodka, you will need to dilute this at the ratio of 60ml water to every 100ml of vodka to make a 25% medium and then cover one part herb to 5 parts fluid.

If you are using Everclear or other 100% proof, use the following method for a specific tincture:

- 100g Bistort root
- 125ml alcohol
- 375ml water

Take 100g of powdered root and split into two parts of 50g each. Place 50g in 125ml alcohol and 50g in 375ml of water. Bring the water to a gentle boil, reduce heat and simmer for 20-40 minutes. Remove from heat and allow to cool a bit. Strain thoroughly and top up if the water is less than 375ml. Add the decoction to the dried Bistort and alcohol mix, and leave for 14 days before straining. Use for cystitis, ulcers, colitis, haemorrhoids, etc.

For haemorrhoids

- 1 part Marshmallow root powder
- 1 part Bistort root powder
- 1 part Cranesbill root powder

Simmer the ingredients gently for an hour with 100g coconut oil. Strain and allow to cool gradually before applying. This is equally good for chapped hands, sore lips, etc.

BLACK HOREHOUND
Ballota nigra

Ballota nigra, commonly known as Black horehound, is a native plant in the Mint family, the *Lamiaceae*, and is found in various habitats, including meadows, woodland edges and hedgerows. It has been used historically to flavour beverages and liqueurs as well as to treat various ailments, such as indigestion, nausea and flatulence.

HISTORICAL USES

In describing the virtues of Black horehound in his *Herball*, Gerard took his lead from Dioscorides, saying '*Being stamped with salt and applied, it cureth the biting of a mad dog, against which it is of great efficacy. The leaves roasted in hot embers do wane and consume away hard lumps or knots in or about the fundament. It also cleanseth foul and filthy ulcers, as the same author teacheth.*'

Culpeper's Herbal recommended Black horehound as a remedy against '*hysteric and hypochondriac affections ... It is an intense bitter, which bespeaks it to be a strengthener of weak stomachs; it is endowed with the properties of a balsam, and is a powerful alterative, capable of opening obstructions of any kind; it is a promoter of the menses; some praise it very much as a pectoral in coughs and shortness of breath; but it is necessary to observe some caution, viz, that it ought only to be

ETYMOLOGY OF COMMON NAME
Latin *bistorta*, from *bis*, 'twice', and *torta*, 'twisted', in reference to its twisting roots.

PLANT LORE
Burning Bistort is said to increase psychic powers, and carrying some of it was believed to help a woman conceive.

USE
The root and leaves.

EDIBILITY
The leaves, seed and roots are edible raw. The leaves are best used raw in salads when young as they do become a little chewy as they age.

HARVEST
In spring for the leaves and autumn for the root.

MEDICINAL PROPERTIES
Astringent, anti-inflammatory and antimicrobial.

ACTIVE CONSTITUENTS
Tannins, flavonoids, polygonosides, anthraquinones, phenolic acids, essential oils.

administered to gross phlegmatic people, and not to thin plethoric persons. The powder is good to kill worms.'

Physician William Meyrick said of it in 1790:

This, is one of those neglected English herbs which are possessed of great virtues, though they are but little known, and still less regarded. It is superior to most things as a remedy in hysteria, and for low spirits.

In his 1897 second edition of the book *Herbal Simples* William Fernie wrote *'If its leaves are applied externally as a poultice, they will relieve the pain of gout, and will mollify angry boils.'*

MODERN RESEARCH

Black horehound is also known as 'Stinking horehound', and not without cause, because it smells bad! The whole plant is used in repellents against insects, and its diterpene compounds are well known for insecticide and antifeedant activities (Savona et al., 1977). However, it has a long history of herbal use, as can be seen above and has been confirmed as follows:

Anxiolytic

Confirmation of it as a remedy for the 'hysteric and hypochondriac affections' described by Culpeper and for 'hysteria, and for low spirits' described by Meyrick came in 1996 in a study that reported antidepressant activity in rats. This was followed by a clinical study in which patients with anxiety disorder and symptoms of depression and sleep disorders, were administered liquid extract of Black horehound for 90 days. After 60 days, 65% of patients showed improvement, and after 90 days 73% of patients reported a relief in symptoms. Patients with sleep disorders experienced particularly remarkable improvement, and of 10 patients taking benzodiazepines prior to the study, 3 discontinued and 4 reduced their dose by half.

It is proven that phenylpropanoids from the plant, a class of organic compounds from the amino acid phenylalanine, show a binding affinity to morphine, dopamine and benzodiazepine receptors in the body. The binding affinity of these phenylpropanoids is the likely source of these anxiolytic and sedative properties.

Antioxidant

Many studies have shown that high intake of antioxidants in the diet protects lung, joint and cardiac function, while resulting in a lower prevalence of chronic disorders. Black horehound has been shown to have powerful antioxidant properties, which may be the reason Culpeper describes it as 'a powerful alterative, and capable of opening obstructions of any kind'. Its ability to heal joint function may be the reason that Fernie recommended its use in gout.

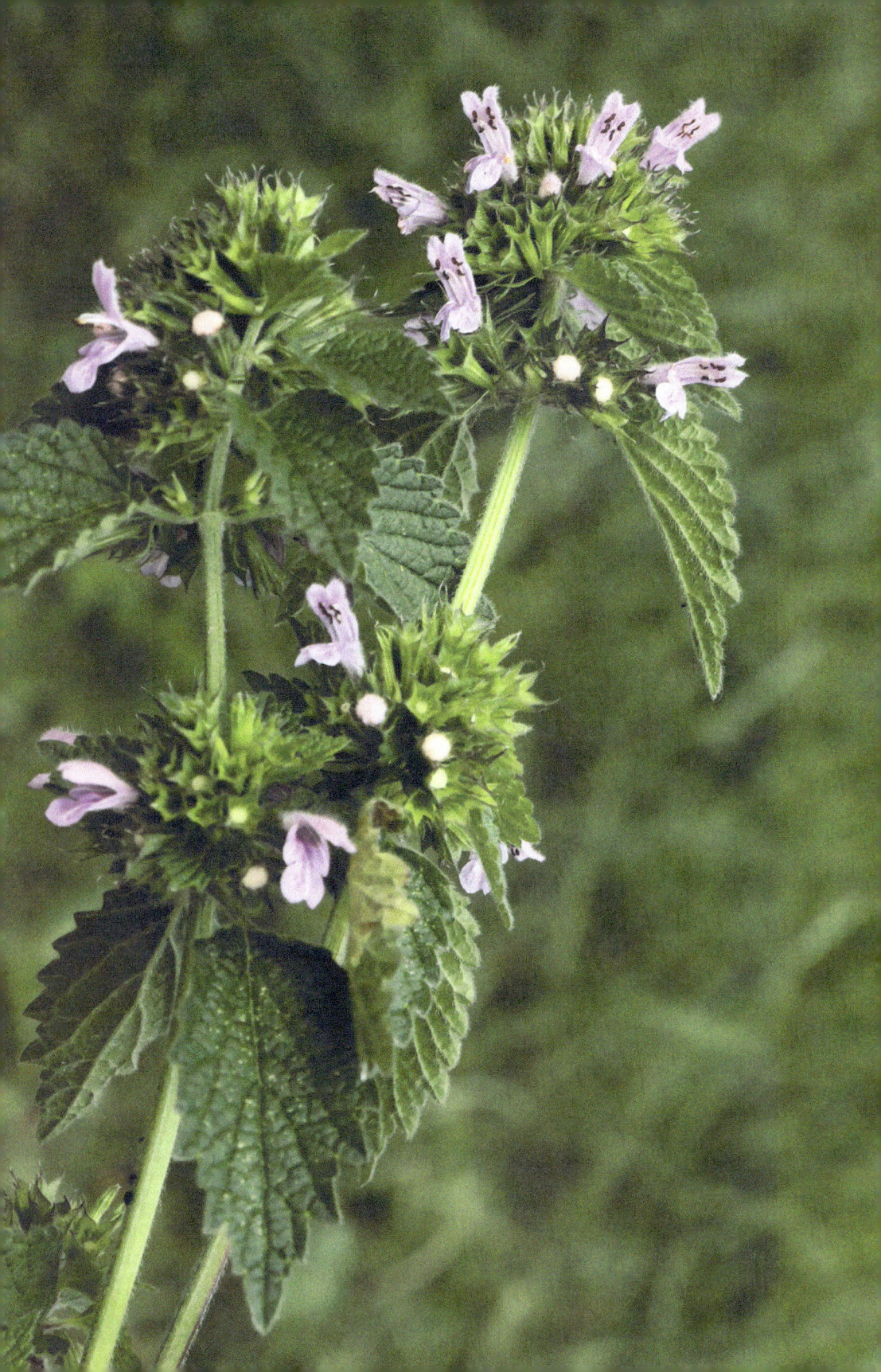

Antidiabetic

In a 2007 study, Horehound was seen to cause a reduction in blood glucose levels in albino rats. It is proposed that it has an insulin-stimulating effect and could be very useful for treating diabetes where control of the blood glucose level is the most important treatment.

Anti-dyslipidaemic

A study has also shown that Horehound can decrease the total cholesterol with no changes in triglycerides levels. LDL cholesterol increases the risk of cardiovascular disease, so its lowering is a positive factor in the treatment of patients with metabolic syndrome, coronary heart disease and stroke etc.

Anti-inflammatory

The anti-inflammatory properties seen by the historical writers were confirmed in a 2014 animal studies, with a recorded inflammatory decline of 95.7% (Ullah et al., 2014). While the precise mechanism of the activity is not known, phenylpropanoids are known for their anti-inflammatory activities, as are flavonoids and triterpenes, and all are found in Black horehound. They can inhibit the production of pro-inflammatory cytokines and enzymes and reduce oxidative stress, which is often associated with inflammation.

Antimicrobial

Horehound has also been suggested as an alternative to antibiotics in studies where it was reported that it inhibited methicillin-resistant *Staphylococcus aureus* (MRSA). Other research has indicated that Horehound has anti-bacterial activity against *Escherichia coli*, *Staphylococcus aureus*, *Proteus mirabilis*, *Klebsiella pneumoniae*, *Enterococcus faecalis*, *Salmonella typhi*, *Bacillus mycoides*, *Bacillus subtilis*, *Micrococcus lysodeikticus* and *Candida albicans*.

Anticancerogenic

Horehound has also been investigated for anticancer activities. Ballotinone and ballonigrin, the natural compounds of the plant, have been found to have binding activity against the proteins that play a major role in the start of cervical cancer. The binding of ballotine and ballonigrin to these proteins could therefore play an important role in prevention of this cancer.

In 2020 a study on Horehound's anticancer activity against prostate cancer was investigated. Prostate cancer cells were treated with different concentrations of Horehound and results found that the ethanolic leaf extract increased the level of tumour suppressor proteins significantly.

TOPICAL USES

An Iranian study from 2014 proved that an extract from Horehound had a considerable tyrosinase inhibitory activity. Because tyrosinase is an enzyme that plays a key role in melanin biosynthesis, this extract can be helpful in the treatment of melasma, solar lentigo and other anomalous skin pigmentations.

DOSAGE

Tisane – 1tsp/5g. Drink half a cup, 3 times per day.
Tincture – 1:10 45%. 1–2ml daily – 20 drops = 1ml/1tsp = 5ml.

PRECAUTIONS

Black horehound contains chemicals that affect the brain and there is some concern that it might affect treatment for Parkinson's disease, schizophrenia and psychotic disorders. Not suitable for children or those who are pregnant or lactating.

Black horehound recipes

Medicinal recipes

Black horehound tisane

Pour 250ml boiling water over 1tsp/5g of the dried leaf and allow to steep for 10-15 minutes. Sweeten with honey and use to help relieve digestive spasms, gout, nausea and vomiting.

Black horehound infused tincture: 1:10 45%

If you are using 40% alcohol, ie vodka, cover one part herb to 10 parts fluid.

If you are using Everclear or other 100% proof, use the following method for a specific tincture:

- 100g dried leaves
- 450ml alcohol
- 550ml water

Take 100g of dried leaves and split into two parts of 50g each. Place 50g in 450ml alcohol and 50g in 550ml of boiled water. Infuse in the water for 10 minutes, then strain and top up if the water is less than 550ml. Add the infusion to the alcohol mix and leave for 14 days before straining. Use to help relieve anxiety, depression, digestive distress and vomiting. However, please note the precautions in the section above.

Black horehound syrup

- 500ml tisane
- 500g sugar

Warm your tisane over a low heat and bring to a simmer. Then cover partially and reduce the liquid down to half its original volume, ie 250ml. Add the sugar and stir constantly, but do not let the mix boil. Remove the syrup from the heat and cool. Syrups keep for up to two years unopened. After opening, store in the refrigerator and use within 1 month. Take a dessertspoon 1 to 3 times a day to help relieve digestive spasms, nausea and vomiting.

Black horehound parasite pessary

- 60ml cocoa butter
- 60ml coconut oil
- 2tbsp powdered dried herb

Combine the cocoa butter and coconut oil in a small saucepan. Add the powdered herb to the saucepan while the cocoa butter and coconut oil are still melted. Stir well to combine. Pour the suppository mixture into clean suppository moulds. Refrigerate the suppositories until they are firm or until ready to use. If stored properly, suppositories will typically last at least several months.

BUGLE
Ajuga reptans

Ajuga reptans, also known as Carpet bugle, is a member of the mint family, *Lamiaceae*. In traditional herbal medicine, certain parts of Bugle have been used, particularly for their astringent properties.

HISTORICAL USES

John Gerard said of Bugle in his *Herball*:

The decoction of Bugle drunken, dissolveth clotted or congealed blood within the body, healeth and maketh sound all wounds of the body, both inward and outward, openeth the stoppings of the liver and gall, and is good against the jaundice and fevers of long continuance. Bugula is excellent in curing wounds and scratches, and the juice cureth the wounds, ulcers and sores of the secret parts, or the herb bruised and laid thereon.

One of Nicholas Culpeper's great quotes is of Bugle, *'If the virtues of it make you fall in love with it (as they will if you be wise) keep a syrup of it to take inwardly, and an ointment and plaster of it to use outwardly, always by you.'*

He went on to agree with Gerard, saying that *'The decoction of the leaves and flowers in wine dissolveth the congealed blood in those that are bruised inwardly by a fall and is very effectual for any inward*

ETYMOLOGY OF COMMON NAME
The plant is believed to be so named for its bugle-shaped flowers.

PLANT LORE
Bugle is often associated with healing and recovery in folklore. It has a reputation as a 'carpenter's herb', which stems from its use in treating wounds and injuries, reflecting its strong association with physical healing.

USE
All parts.

EDIBILITY
The young leaves are eaten raw or cooked and the root is said to be edible but astringent.

HARVEST
In late spring just before it comes into flower.

MEDICINAL PROPERTIES
Antimicrobial, anti-inflammatory, anticancerogenic, astringent and vulnerary.

ACTIVE CONSTITUENTS
Iridoid glycosides, flavonoids, phenolic acids, triterpenoids, essential oils.

wounds, thrusts or stabs in the body or bowels; it is an especial help in wound drinks and for those that are liver-grown, as they call it. It is wonderful in curing all ulcers and sores, gangrenes and fistulas, if the leaves, bruised and applied or their juice be used to wash and bathe the place and the same made into lotion and some honey and gum added, cureth the worse sores. Being also taken inwardly or outwardly applied, it helpeth those that have broken any bone or have any member out of joint.'

MODERN RESEARCH

Bugle should not be confused with Bugleweed, *Lycopus virginicus*, which is native to the US and also from the Mint family. Modern research has confirmed the following properties of the British native Bugle:

Astringent and vulnerary

As both Gerard and Culpeper suggest, Bugle can be used for arresting internal bleeds and treating wounds, but from the tannins it contains is also useful for treating diarrhoea and as a gargle for a sore throat.

Anti-inflammatory and antimicrobial

Applying Bugle topically can encourage healing by means of its antioxidant, anti-inflammatory and antimicrobial compounds. A 2017 study confirmed that Bugle contains high amounts of polyphenols and iridoids, which are important antioxidant and antimicrobial agents.

In 2019 further antimicrobial testing revealed that Bugle presented potent activity against *Aspergillus niger* and Candida *albicans*. In this study, the anti-inflammatory effect was found to be comparable with the NSAID (nonsteroidal anti-inflammatory drug) diclofenac.

Anticancerogenic

A further study in 2020 found that a methanolic extract of Bugle was able to reduce the reactive oxygen species levels in cancer cell lines, such as malignant melanoma, cervical cancer and lung adenocarcinoma. The effect of this is that production of the cancerous cells is suppressed.

TOPICAL USES

Externally it can be applied for bruising and all kinds of external sores and swellings. It is widely used in the treatment of mouth ulcers.

DOSAGE

Tisane – 50–100g flowers in 1l water, several times per day.

PRECAUTIONS

Not suitable for children or those who are pregnant or lactating.

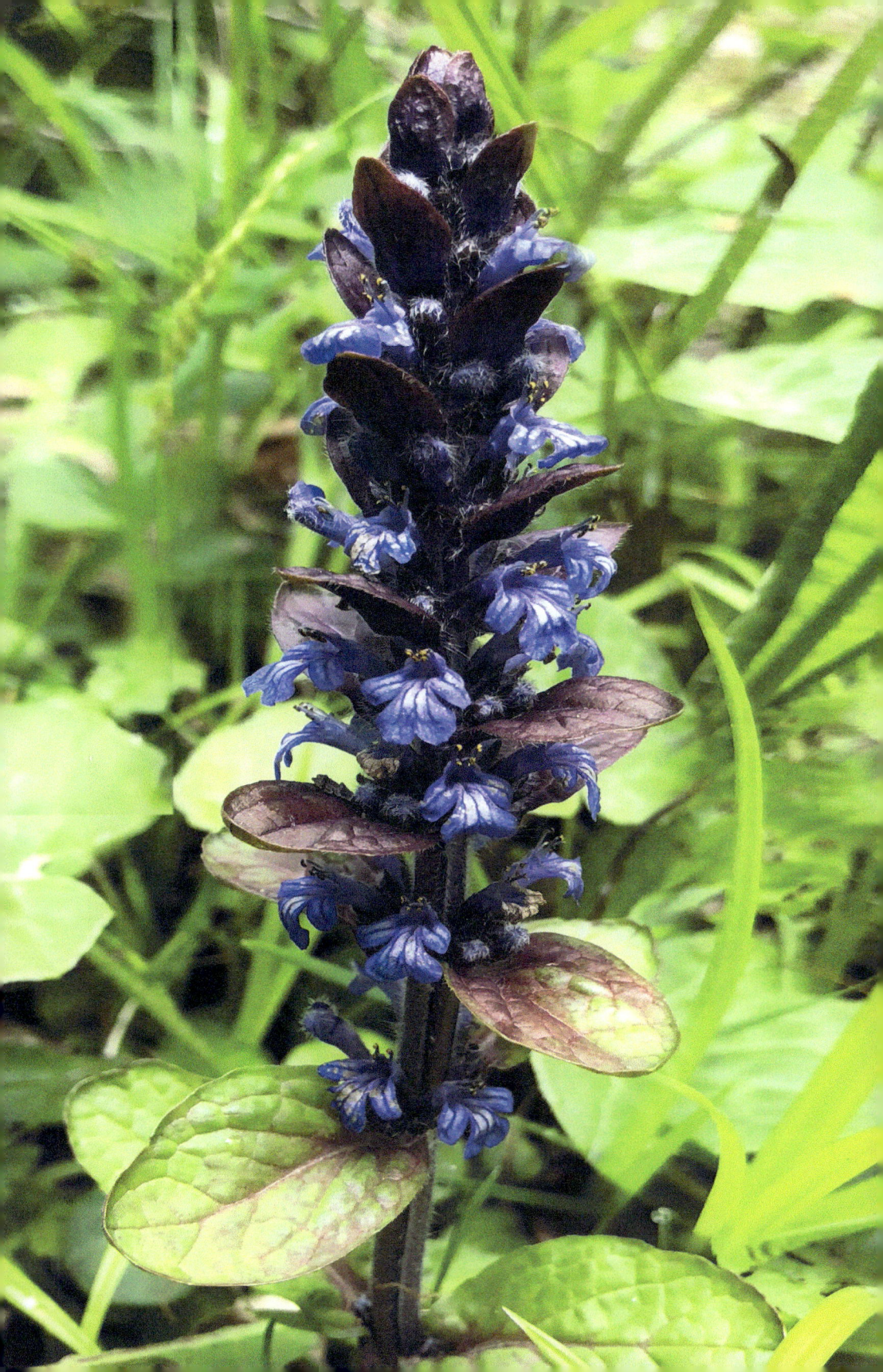

Bugle recipes

Medicinal recipes

Bugle tisane

Pour 500ml boiling water over 25-50g of the dried herb and allow to steep for 10-15 minutes. Drink throughout the day for internal injuries, ulcers and as a mouthwash. Can also be used externally to wash out wounds.

Bugle syrup

- 500ml tisane
- 500g sugar
- 25ml tincture, optional (preservative)

Warm your tisane over a low heat and bring to a simmer. Then cover partially and reduce the liquid down to half its original volume, ie. 250ml. Add the sugar and stir constantly, but do not let the mix boil. Remove the syrup from the heat and add the tinctures at a ratio of 5%. Syrups keep for up to two years unopened. After opening, store in the refrigerator and use within 1 month. A general dosage is a dessertspoon taken 1 to 3 times for internal ulcers, diarrhoea and sore throats.

Bugle infused oil

- 100g dried and powdered plant
- 2 tbsp alcohol, such as Everclear
- 1l grapeseed oil

Place the herbs in a jar with the alcohol and allow to steep for 10 minutes before adding the oil. Leave for 4 weeks and then strain. Make into a salve by using a 1:3 ratio of melted beeswax to oil. Use as an anti-inflammatory and healer.

BURDOCK
Arctium lappa/minus

In the UK, there are two main species of Burdock commonly found: Greater burdock (*Arctium lappa*), and Lesser burdock (*Arctium minus*). Both are members of the *Asteraceae* family and are often found in waste areas, along roadsides and in disturbed habitats. Both species have a long history of medicinal and culinary use, particularly the roots.

HISTORICAL USES

Historically, the Japanese people called burdock root Gobo and used it for constipation, syphilis, mercury poisoning, paralysis, to stimulate blood circulation and to induce perspiration. They considered the leaves good for external elimination of pain over broken bones, for skin burns and for rash. The seeds were used to eliminate toxins, to control fever and as a diuretic. Today, the average Japanese consumer still buys Gobo leaves as a source of strength and endurance.

Meanwhile, the Pilgrims left records indicating that Burdock was one of the herbs they carefully safeguarded on their journey to the New World. There they found that Native Americans were already using a local species, and medicine men of several North American tribes drank a bitter brew of

ETYMOLOGY OF COMMON NAME
From *bur*, the prickly seed vessel, and *dock*, the name for various tall, coarse weeds or herbs.

PLANT LORE
In some European folktales, burdock is associated with fairies. It was believed that fairies used burdock leaves as shelter and the burrs as tools or weapons. Seeing burdock growing near one's home was considered a sign of fairy activity and good fortune.

USE
Root, leaves and seeds

EDIBILITY
The root was traditionally used to flavour the drink dandelion and burdock. Immature stalks can be harvested in late spring, before flowers appear and resemble artichoke in taste.

HARVEST
The root and seed in autumn and the leaves when young.

MEDICINAL PROPERTIES
Anti-inflammatory, vulnerary, antioxidant, detoxifier, antibacterial, anticancerogenic and antibacterial.

ACTIVE CONSTITUENTS
Inulin, polyphenols, sesquiterpene lactones, polysaccharides, tannins, essential oils, phenolic acids.

Burdock to concentrate better and to prolong the image of love in their minds.

John Gerard told us in his *Herball* that 'The roots being taken with the kernels of pine-apples, as Dioscorides witnesseth, are good for them that spit blood and corrupt matter, while Apuleius saith that the same being stamped with a little salt, and applied to the biting of a mad dog, cureth the same, and so speedily setteth free the sick man. He also teacheth that the juice of the leaves given to drink with honey, procureth urine, and taketh away the pains of the bladder; and that the same drunk with old wine doth wonderfully help against the bitings of serpents ... The root stamped and strained with a good draught of Ale is a most approved medicine for a windy or cold stomach.'

Nicholas Culpeper advised in his *Herbal* that '*Burdock leaves are cooling and moderately drying, whereby good for old ulcers and sores ... the root beaten with a little salt and laid on the place suddenly easeth the pain thereof ... the seed being drunk in wine 40 days together doth wonderfully help the sciatica: the leaves bruised with the white of an egg and applied to any place burnt with fire, taketh out the fire, gives sudden ease and heals it up afterwards ... The seed is much commended to break the stone and is often used with other seeds and things for that purpose.*'

In *Fray's Golden Recipes for the Use of All Ages* (1897) Burdock was lauded as follows:

> *The value of this plant cannot be too much known for its direct action on the blood, whether for scurvy, skin eruptions, leprosy, scrofula, venereal, ulcers, kidney disease, convulsions, fits, etc. It is invaluable.*

MODERN RESEARCH

Both Burdock species are wonderful detoxifiers and can also be used interchangeably as follows:

Anti-inflammatory and vulnerary

Burdock contains the compounds arctigenin and lignans, which have been studied for their anti-inflammatory properties, which is no doubt why Culpeper was seeing the effects referred to above in relation to pain.

A 2021 case study using an Amish burns and wound ointment demonstrated an alternative therapy to negative pressure wound therapy and skin grafting. Burdock leaves were coated with an ointment that contained honey, Aloe vera gel, lanolin, wheatgerm, olive oil, beeswax, Marshmallow root, Lobelia, Comfrey, White oak bark, Myrrh, Wormwood and vegetable glycerine. This was applied to the patient's arm and subsequently wrapped loosely in mesh. The Burdock leaves in this case were to replace conventional dressings because they do not stick to the wound, which allows for decreased pain. The patient was then

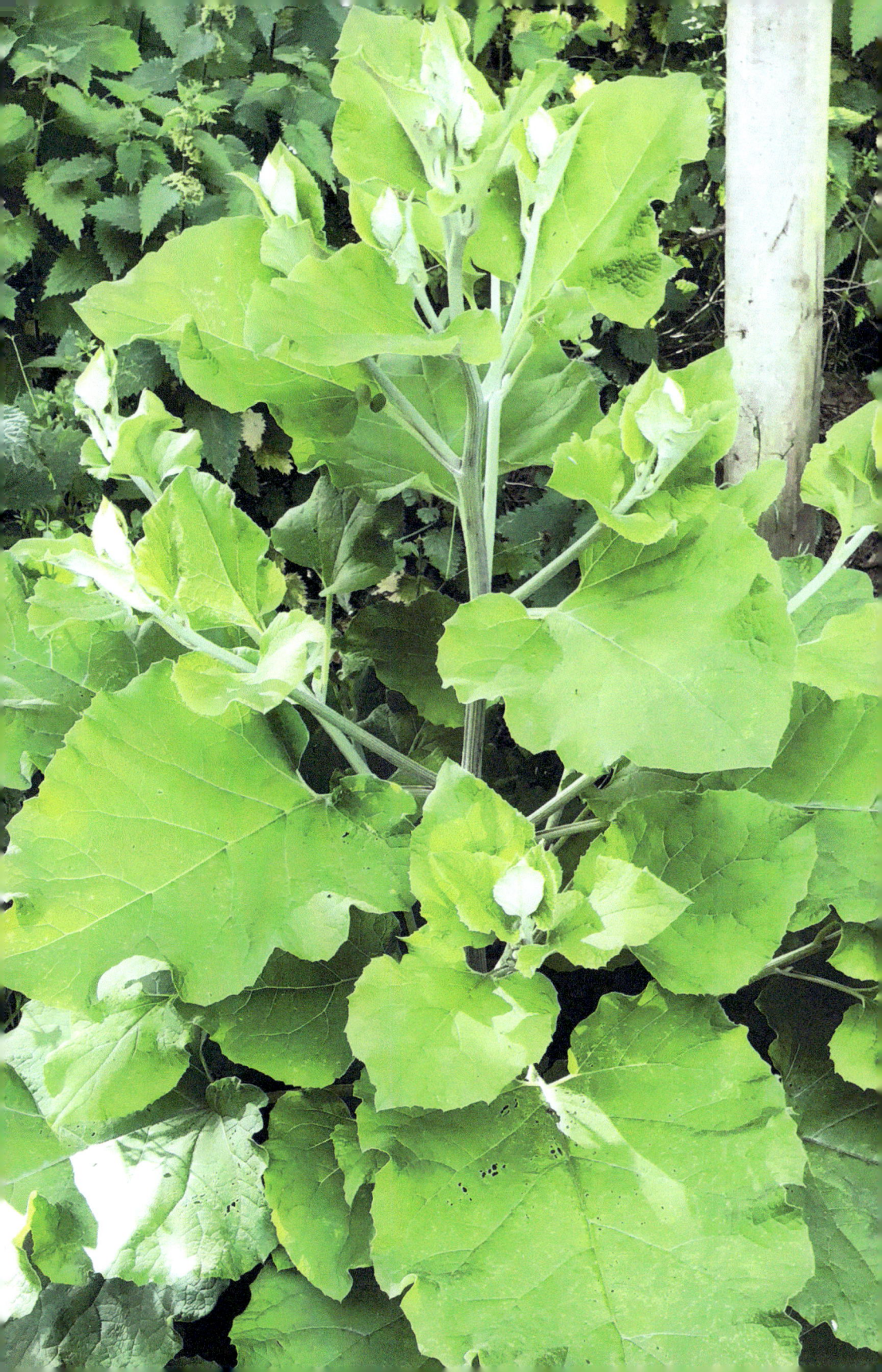

discharged home where dressing changes occurred once a day. Upon follow up one week after discharge, the wound demonstrated healthy granulation of the tissue with no erythema, pus or increased warmth and continued to heal well. This approach was deemed effective in healing the wound, albeit slightly slower than conventional therapy, and resulted in less pain owing to dressing changes, but may also be because, as Culpeper says, 'Burdock leaves are cooling and moderately drying, whereby good for old ulcers and sores.'

Antioxidant and detoxifier

Burdock is an alterative, which means that it acts in a gentle and tonifying way to *'improve the quality of the blood, increase the appetite, promote digestion, and accelerate the processes of elimination'* (Felter, 1922, p82). This again would be why the historical effects by Fray, Culpeper and Gerard were seen. The arctigenin and lignans that it contains are believed to support liver health, by eliminating toxins from the body. The active ingredients of the root – phenolic acids, quercetin and luteolin – may also help 'detoxify' blood and promote blood circulation to the skin surface, improving the skin quality/texture and curing conditions like eczema.

Anticancerogenic

Burdock has for decades been used as a complementary therapy among breast cancer survivors (Mills et al., 2003), and it has also shown antitumour effects on pancreatic cancer cell lines (Matsumoto et al., 2006) as well as causing necrosis in solid tumours in mice (Dombrádi and Földeák, 1965). The polyphenols and flavonoids in the root such as quercetin have synergistic effects with certain chemotherapeutic drugs, such as cisplatin (Scambia et al., 1990) while the arctigenin in the seeds has shown the ability to remove the tumour cells with low nutrients.

In 2019, a study using Burdock hydroalcoholic extract confirmed that it reduced tumour growth and enhanced survival of mice, while in a 2020 study, arctigenin was found to inhibit production of cytokines, proteins that promote inflammation, in breast cancer cells. Another study, in 2020, then found the same cytotoxic results in leukaemia and multiple myeloma, this time using a combination of Thyme and Burdock, which both induced cell cycle arrest and ferroptosis (cell death). Both could therefore be considered as potential herbal drug candidates to arrest cancer cell proliferation.

Antimicrobial

The roots of Burdock have demonstrated activity against gram-negative organisms such as *Escherichia coli* and *Pseudomonas aeruginosa* as well as against the gram-positive organism

Staphylococcus aureus. Similarly, it has shown activity against the fungi species *Microsporum gypseum*, *Trichophyton* spp. and *Epidermophyton floccosum*, all causes of fungal infections (Reisch et al., 1967; Pereira et al., 2005; Gentil et al., 2006). These actions were lost when the roots were dried, however.

Studies have also found that Burdock has antibacterial qualities that are particularly useful for killing biofilms – a cluster of microbes that stick to either living or non-living surfaces. A 2015 study found that a methanol extract of Burdock was able to inhibit this biofilm and suggested it could be useful to treat biofilm-related urinary tract infections. Research published in 2017 proposed that the chlorogenic acid in Burdock is probably responsible for its diverse antipathogenic potential.

TOPICAL USES

A 2020 study on Burdock obtained promising results regarding anti-acne properties. One of the peptides was found to have possible antibiotic, anti-oxidative and anti-seborrheic properties. In his 1936 book *Herbal Manual* Harold Ward wrote of Burdock, '*An excellent lotion may be made by infusing the leaves in the proportion of 1 ounce to 1 pint of water.*'

DOSAGE

Leaf tisane – 1 cup/250ml, 3 times per day.
Root decoction – ½ cup, 3 times per day.
Root/Seed tincture – 1:5 25% 8–12ml, 3 times per day – 20 drops = 1ml/1tsp = 5ml.

PRECAUTIONS

Not suitable for children or those who are pregnant or lactating.

Burdock recipes

Medicinal recipes

Burdock leaf tisane

Pour 250ml boiling water over 1tsp/5g of the dried leaf and allow to steep for 10-15 minutes. Use as a spring tonic and detox.

Burdock root decoction

- 1tsp/5g Burdock root
- 250ml water

If you are using fresh root, grate it, dry and roast in the oven for 10 minutes or until golden brown. Place a teaspoonful of the root in a pan with the water and bring to a slow boil for 10-15 minutes. Use for detoxification, high blood pressure, liver toxicity, gout, chronic inflammation, constipation and oedema. Persistence with low doses is more favourable than larger, over short periods.

Burdock root decocted tincture: 1:5 25%

If you are using 40% alcohol, ie vodka, you will need to dilute this at the ratio of 60ml water to every 100ml of vodka to make a 25% medium and then cover one part herb to 5 parts fluid.

If you are using Everclear or other 100% proof, follow this method for a specific tincture:

- 100g dried Burdock root
- 125ml alcohol
- 375ml water

Take 100g of powdered root and split into two parts of 50g each. Place 50g in 125ml alcohol and 50g in 375ml of water. Bring the water to a gentle boil, reduce heat and simmer for 20-40 minutes. Remove from heat and strain thoroughly, topping up if the water is less than 375ml. Add the decoction to the alcohol mix and leave for 14 days before straining. Use as an alternative to decoction.

Burdock acne lotion

In his 1936 Herbal Manual Harold Ward explained, *'An excellent lotion may be made by infusing the leaves in the proportion of 1 ounce to 1 pint of water.'* However, I made a coconut oil-based ointment for someone with acne as follows:

- 1 part Burdock root
- 1 part Hoary willowherb
- 1 part Hops
- 2 tbsp alcohol, such as Everclear

Place the herbs in a jar with the alcohol, muddle and allow to steep for 10 minutes before adding the oil. Infuse in coconut oil in a warm oven (75-100°) for 3-4 hours. Once infused, strain and keep in the fridge between use. If you have the decocted tincture above you can add this at a ratio of 20% tincture while the oil is cooling. This will also help preserve the blend.

BURNET
Sanguisorba spp

The two *Sanguisorba* species native to the UK are Great burnet (*Sanguisorba officinalis*), commonly found in damp meadows, grasslands and marshy areas, and Salad burnet (*Sanguisorba minor*), which prefers dry grasslands, open woodlands and rocky habitats.

HISTORICAL USES

Burnet was formerly in high repute as a vulnerary herb, hence its Latin name *sanguis*, meaning blood, and *sorbeo*, to staunch. Owing to its astringency it was traditionally used in instances of diarrhoea and dysentery.

John Gerard said of it in his *Herball*, '*the leaves steeped in wine and drunken comfort the heart and make it merry and are good against the trembling and shaking thereof.*' It was used in such quantity that it was formerly known as 'toper's plant'.

Nicholas Culpepper's *Herbal* wrote of 'The Great Wild Burnet', '*This is a most precious herb, little inferior to Betony ... it is a friend to the heart, liver, and other principal parts of a man's body. Two or three of the stalks, with leaves put into a cup of wine, especially claret, are known to quicken the spirits, refresh and cheer the heart, and drive away melancholy: It is a special help to defend the heart from noisome vapours, and from infection of the pestilence, the juice thereof being*

ETYMOLOGY OF COMMON NAME
Middle English for 'brown cloth' or 'plants with brown flowers'.

PLANT LORE
The Latin name *sanguis* means blood and *sorbeo* is to soak up.

USE
All parts.

EDIBILITY
Young Burnet leaves are used as an ingredient in salads, dressings and sauces, having a flavour described as 'mildly cucumber'. Typically, the youngest leaves are used, as they tend to become bitter with age.

HARVEST
Leaves in spring and root in autumn.

MEDICINAL PROPERTIES
Astringent, antioxidant, anti-inflammatory, antimicrobial.

ACTIVE CONSTITUENTS
Flavonoids, tannins, triterpene gycosides, tormentolic acid, sterols.

taken in some drink, and the party laid to sweat thereupon.'

MODERN RESEARCH

Great burnet and Salad burnet can be used interchangeably as follows:

Astringent

As the above writers mention, Burnet's primary use was as a vulnerary. Its roots have haemostatic, pain relieving and astringent properties, and have been used in traditional Chinese medicine for the treatment of burns, scalds, inflammation and internal haemorrhage (Liu et al., 2004).

Antiviral

A 2013 study demonstrated that Burnet blocks certain strains of HIV-1 and exhibits potency against strains resistant to specific drugs by targeting protease activities. These findings provide evidence for the potential use of Burnet in the prevention and treatment of HIV-1 infection.

Anticancerogenic

Burnet root contains triterpenoid saponins and tannins, which have been revealed to possess anticancer effects by inducing apoptosis (programmed cell death) and cell cycle arrest. These qualities might indicate potential roles in clinical applications for the treatment of inflammatory diseases, bleeding disorders and cancer.

Anti-inflammatory

A 2020 study in mice indicates that active components in Burnet improve colitis by providing intestinal anti-inflammatory profiles via promotion of Atg7-dependent autophagy. Put simply, it raises proteins that clear out damaged cells and suppresses intestinal inflammation, which could prove useful in treating irritable bowel disease.

Stimulant

In 2021, somewhat backing up Gerard and Culpeper's findings that it quickens the spirits, refreshes and cheers the heart, and drives away melancholy, research showed that Burnet root can enhance performance. Both long-duration and high-intensity physical activity lead to the accumulation of lactate and subsequently induce a pH imbalance, which generates many free radicals, resulting in damage to muscles. Burnet suppresses the activity and expression of lactate dehydrogenase (LDHA), and in studies has enhanced the physical performance in the mouse by approximately 40%. The compounds, such as saponins, vitamin C and chrysanthemin, were reported to be responsible for this enhanced physical performance. In addition, among the compounds of the roots, gallic acid and catechin were reported as agents for improving physical performance and enhancing abdominal fat loss, respectively.

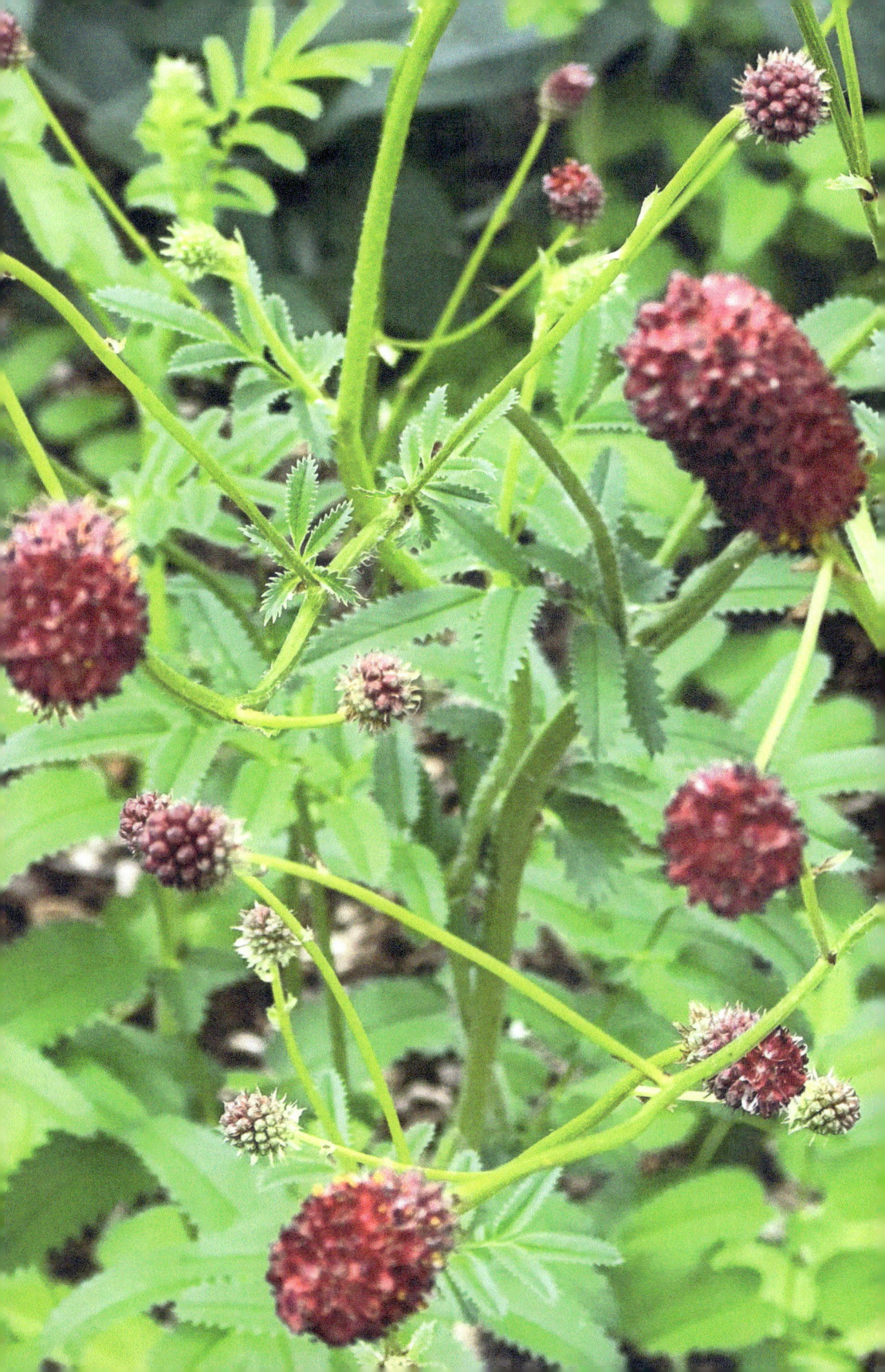

TOPICAL USE

It is also used externally as an ointment or lotion for treating wounds, burns, haemorrhoids and eczema.

DOSAGE

Tisane – 2tsp/10g. Half a cup, 3 times per day.
Tincture – 1:5 25% 2–8ml, 3 times per day – 20 drops = 1ml/1tsp = 5ml.

PRECAUTIONS

It is conceivable that an overdose of the drug would trigger intestinal colic.

Burnet recipes

Medicinal recipes

Burnet tisane

Pour 250ml boiling water over 1 tsp/5g of the dried leaf and flower, and allow to steep for 10–15 minutes. Use for diarrhoea and irritable bowel disease. It can also be used as an external wash for eczema.

Burnet root decoction

Boil 10–15g of dried root, flowers and leaves in 300–400ml of water for 20 minutes. Use for fatigue and as a boost prior to physical exercise.

Burnet infused tincture: 1:5 25%

If you are using 40% alcohol, ie vodka, you will need to dilute this at the ratio of 60ml water to every 100ml of vodka to make a 25% medium and then cover 1 part herb to 5 parts fluid.

If you are using Everclear or other 100% proof, use the following method for a specific tincture:

- 100g dried Burnet
- 125ml alcohol
- 375ml water

Take 100g of chopped herb and split into two parts of 50g each. Place 50g in 125ml alcohol. Take the other 50g part and place in 375ml of boiling water and allow to steep for 10 minutes. Strain thoroughly and top up if the water is less than 375ml. Add to the dried Burnet and alcohol mix, and leave for 14 days before straining. Use for irritable bowel syndrome and ulcerative colitis.

BUTTERCUP
Ranunculus spp.

In the UK, several species of *Ranunculus*, commonly known as Buttercups, can be found. These include Meadow buttercup (*Ranunculus acris*) and Bulbous buttercup (*Ranunculus bulbosus*), which grow in grasslands, woodlands, and disturbed areas, and Creeping buttercup (*Ranunculus repens*), which prefers wetter habitats such as marshes, ditches and riverbanks.

HISTORICAL USES

When fresh, Buttercups contain protoanemonine, which causes blister formation and cauterisations that are difficult to heal. Beggars in times past used Buttercups to cause and keep open their sores in order to obtain sympathy.

John Gerard called these plants 'Crowfeet' in his *Herball* owing to the shapes of the leaves, and wrote, '*Many do tie a little of the herbe stamped with salt unto any of the fingers, against the pain of the teeth; which medicine seldome faileth; for it causeth greater paine in the finger than was in the tooth, by the meanes whereof the greater paine taketh away the lesser.*'

Nicholas Culpeper referred to them as 'Butterflowers', and wrote, '*This fiery and hot-spirited herb of Mars is no way fit to be given inwardly, but an ointment of the leaves of flowers will draw a blister*

ETYMOLOGY OF COMMON NAME
From the mistaken notion that this flower gives butter a yellow colour through the cows feeding on it (this is not the case).

PLANT LORE
Buttercups were sometimes used in weather forecasting. It was believed that the flowers could predict rain: if they closed their petals, rain was imminent.

USE
The aerial parts.

EDIBILITY
Not edible – all parts of the plant are poisonous until dried.

HARVEST
In spring.

MEDICINAL PROPERTIES
Analgesic, anticancerogenic, antimicrobial and anti-inflammatory.

ACTIVE CONSTITUENTS
Protoanemonin, saponins, flavonoids, triterpenoid saponins, alkaloids, essential oils, oxalates.

and may be so fitly applied to the nape of the neck, to draw back rheum from the eyes. The herb being bruised, and mixed with a little mustard, draws a blister as well and as perfectly as cantharides [Spanish fly], and with far less danger to the vessels of urine, which cantharides naturally delight to wrong. I knew the herb once applied to a pestilential rising that was fallen down, and it saved life even beyond hope; it was klgood keeping an ointment and plaister of it, if it were but for that.'

In his 1897, second edition of the book *Herbal Simples* William Fernie stated, '*The juice of the common Buttercup (Bulbosus), known sometimes as 'St Anthony's turnip', if applied to the nostrils, will provoke sneezing, and will relieve passive headache in this way. The leaves have been applied as a blister to the wrists in rheumatism, and when infused in boiling water as a poultice over the pit of the stomach as a counter-irritant. For sciatica the tincture of the bulbous buttercup has proved very helpful.*'

Fernie added, '*the fresh leaves of the Crowfoot (Ranunculus acris) formed a part of the famous cancer cure of Mr Plunkett in 1794. This cure comprised Crowfoot leaves, freshly gathered, and dog's-foot fennel leaves, of each an ounce, with one drachm of white arsenic levigated, and with five scruples of flowers of sulphur, all beaten together into a paste, and dried by the sun in balls, which were then powdered, and being mixed with yolk of egg, were applied on pieces of pig's bladder.*'

MODERN RESEARCH

There are over 600 species of *Ranunculus*, so the focus here is on the three mentioned previously that are commonly found. Research has found the following properties attributed to these:

Antimicrobial

In 1993, the antimicrobial properties of the Bulbous buttercup were investigated. The plant showed marked inhibitory effects and broad-spectrum activity against aerobic and anaerobic multi-resistant pathogenic strains, owing to the protoanemonin it contains. This is similar to studies that have taken place on Anemone, which also contains these properties. Combinations of protoanemonin and antibiotics were also investigated in 22 combinations, of which 20 were found to be partially synergistic, with one case of total synergism. This striking result was obtained with the combination of protoanemonin and cefamandole antibiotic against a pathogenic strain of *Staphylococcus aureus*, a common cause of skin infections.

Antioxidant

A 2014 study showed that extracts of Bulbous buttercup possess antiradical activity and could be used as a natural antioxidant ingredient in the food and drug industries.

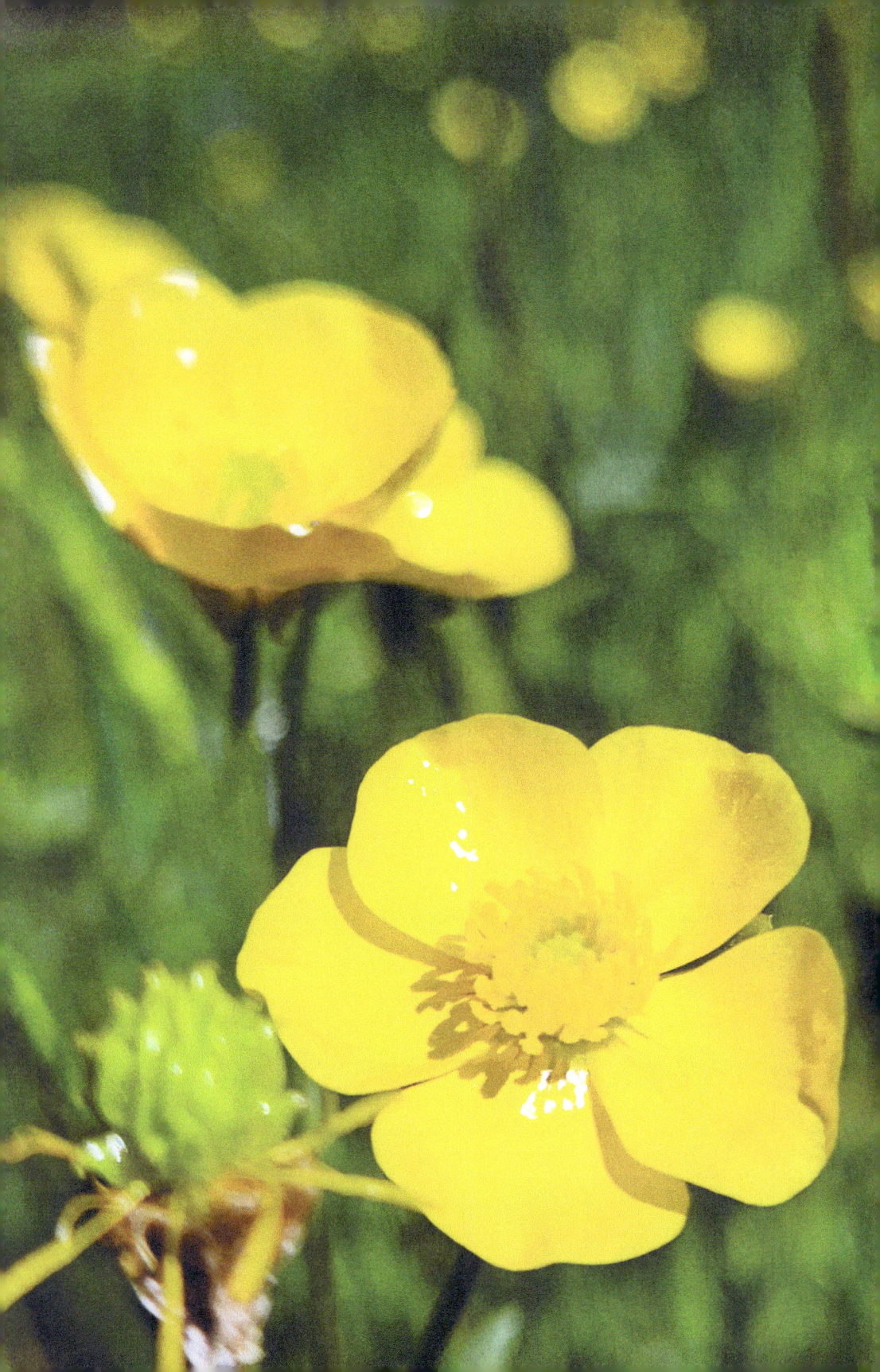

Anticancerogenic

In Mongolian medical literature there are reports that Creeping buttercup has been used since ancient times to treat various disorders. Studies in 2022 aimed to verify these uses, finding that saponins and protoanemonin contained in the extract of Creeping buttercup inhibited the growth of gastric tumours and cells, while phenolic compounds inhibited the growth of colon and rectal tumour cells. These findings lend some credence to the cancer remedy recommended by Fernie.

Anti-inflammatory

Anemonin and ranunculin are potent anti-inflammatory compounds that are abundant in Buttercups. The compound β-sitosterol has also now been isolated from them. The results from a 2020 study illustrated that β-sitosterol treatment reduces the expression of inflammatory mediators. These findings support Fernie's use of Buttercup for rheumatism and sciatica.

TOPICAL USES

While Culpeper extolled the virtues of Buttercup as a topical ointment, he used it to draw the humours via blistering. A 2012 study, however, found that Creeping buttercup has anti-haemorrhagic properties, and when applied directly to the skin, the anti-inflammatory actions help to ease the symptoms and pain associated with stiffness and joint pain.

DOSAGE

External only.

PRECAUTIONS

The administration of the plant during pregnancy is absolutely contraindicated. Extended skin contact with the freshly harvested, bruised plant can lead to blister formation and cauterisations that are difficult to heal owing to the protoanemonine. If taken internally, severe irritation to the gastrointestinal tract, combined with colic and diarrhoea, as well as irritation of the urinary drainage passages, are possible. Not suitable for children or those who are pregnant or lactating.

Buttercup recipes

Medicinal recipes

NB: Buttercup must be dried before use to remove toxins.

Buttercup cold infusion

Add 200ml of boiling water to 1tsp of dried herb and leave overnight, before filtering. Use 2 to 3 times per day in compresses by soaking a cloth in the infusion and applying to stiff and aching joints to help to ease the symptoms and pain.

Buttercup compress

Soak a cloth in a tisane of the dried herb and use to soothe mild skin infections.

Buttercup poultice

- 1tsp *dried* herb moistened with a little water
- 2tsp coconut oil
- cheesecloth or cotton bandage

Finely chop the plant and add heated coconut oil to make a paste. Allow to cool slightly and spread the paste evenly over the desired area, then wrap with the cloth or bandage. Use for rheumatism and joint pain.

Topical application for warts

- Fresh Buttercup leaves and flowers.

Crush the leaves and flowers to extract the juice. Apply a small amount of the juice directly to the wart once daily. Avoid contact with healthy skin, as the juice can cause irritation.

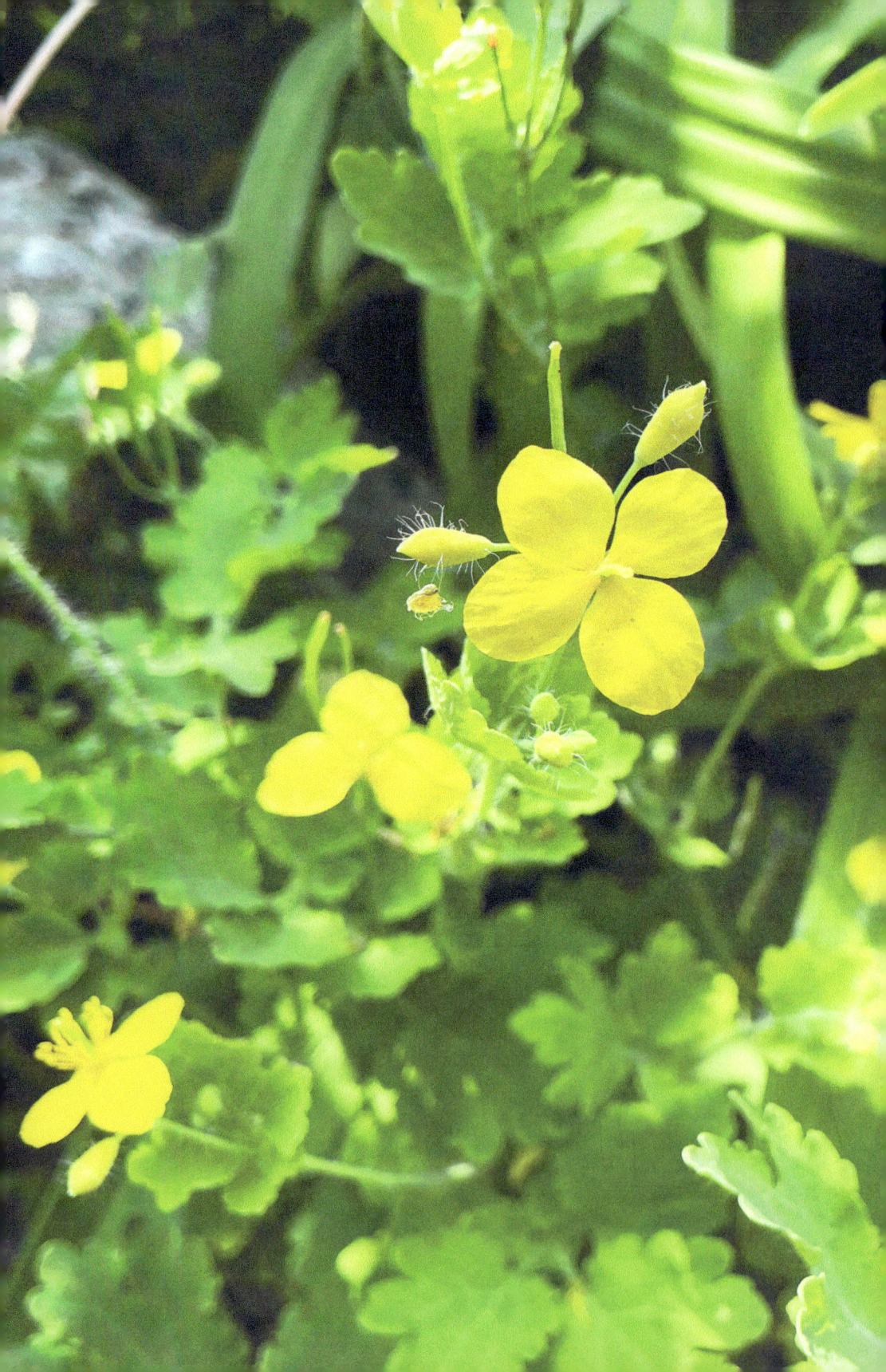

CELANDINE (GREATER)
Chelidonium majus

Chelidonium majus, commonly known as Greater celandine or Tetterwort, is a member of the Poppy family, *Papaveraceae*. It is commonly found in woodland edges and hedgerows. While Greater celandine has been used medicinally for centuries, it contains toxic compounds, including alkaloids such as chelidonine and sanguinarine, which when ingested in large amounts can cause poisoning.

HISTORICAL USES

This is a herb with a long history of use stretching back to ancient times. Dioscorides in *De Materia Medica* said celandine soaked in wine together with anise fruits was helpful in treating jaundice and dermatologic disorders such as herpes, while, chewing on a root relieved toothache (Osbaldeston and Wood, 2000). Pliny advised a kind of eye lotion, which takes its name, *chelidonia*, from the name of the plant (Jones, 1966).

In *Physica*, Hildegard of Bingen (1098–1179) recommended Greater celandine juice to enhance sight, and when mixed with tallow as a cure for skin ulcers.

Albertus Magnus, a medieval philosopher in the thirteenth century AD, wrote, '*No less extraordinary is the property*

ETYMOLOGY OF COMMON NAME
From the Middle English/Old French *celidoine*, and based on the Greek *khelidōn*, for 'swallow' (the flowering of the plant being associated with the arrival of migrating swallows).

PLANT LORE
Celandine was believed to have sprung from the blood of Prometheus, the Titan, who brought fire to humanity, linking it to themes of healing and transformation. Witches carried it in a bag around their necks to avoid being detected or imprisoned.

USE
All parts.

EDIBILITY
Not edible

HARVEST
Celandine herb is gathered during flowering season while the root is harvested in autumn.

MEDICINAL PROPERTIES
Anti-inflammatory, ophthalmic purgative and antimicrobial, anticancerogenic and antidiabetic.

ACTIVE CONSTITUENTS
Alkaloids, flavonoids, phenolic acids, saponins, essential oils, resins, carotenoids.

LEFT: GREATER CELANDINE

of the herb Celandine; which, it is said, if any man shall have this herb, with the heart of a Mole, he shall overcome all his enemies, all matters in suit, and shall put away all debate' (Best and Brightman, 1999).

John Gerard wrote in his *Herball*, 'The juice is good to sharpen the sight, for it cleanseth and consumeth away slimy things that cleave about the ball of the eye, and hinder the sight, and especially being boiled with honey in a brazen vessel, as Dioscorides teacheth. The root cureth the yellow jaundice, which cometh of the stopping of the gall, especially when there is no ague adjoined with it, for it openeth and delivereth the gall and liver from stoppings. The root being chewed, is good against the toothache.'

In his *Herbal*, Nicholas Culpeper called this one of the best cures for the eyes, 'The juice dropped into the eyes, cleanses them from films and cloudiness which darken the sight. The herb or root boiled in wine, and drank, with a few aniseeds opens obstructions of the liver and gall, helps the yellow jaundice, the dropsy and the itch, and those that have old sores in their legs, or other parts of the body will quickly heal them; and rubbed often upon warts, will take them away.'

In his 1897 (second edition) *Herbal Simples*, William Fernie wrote, 'Queen Elizabeth in the forty-sixth year of her age was attacked with such a grievous toothache that she could obtain no rest by night or day because of the torture she endured. The lords of her council decided on sending for an "outlandish physician" named Penatus, who was famous for curing this agonising pain. He suggested that the Chelidonius major – *our greater Celandine* – should be put into the tooth, and stopped with wax, which would so loosen the tooth that in a short time it might be pulled out with the fingers.'

Harold Ward's *Herbal Manual* of 1936 added, 'The infusion is taken in wineglassful doses three times daily, as part of the treatment for jaundice, eczema, and scrofulous diseases. This infusion is also helpful when applied directly to abrasions and bruises, and the fresh juice makes a useful application for corns and warts.'

MODERN RESEARCH

Greater celandine root, as mentioned, contains chelidonin and sanguinarin, which are widely used in toothpaste and mouthwash for the prevention/treatment of gingivitis and other inflammatory conditions. This gives credence to the historical treatment described by Fernie above. The other properties found are as follows:

Purgative

The above authors are right to say that Celandine opens the liver and gall as it has properties that help to purge bile and/or enhance healing. Two studies have confirmed this in liver diseases (Vahlensieck, 1995) and (Paul and Das, 2013).

Antimicrobial

The antimicrobial activity of Celandine is attributed mostly to its alkaloids and flavonoids (Zuo et al., 2008). Its effectiveness has been demonstrated against *Candida pseudotropicalis, Microsporum gypseum, Microsporum canis, Trichophyton mentagrophytes, Epidermophyton occosum and Streptococcus mutans* (Cheng et al., 2006), known as causes of ringworm, athlete's foot and *Candida* infections.

A chloroform extract has been shown to decrease the viability of adenoviruses responsible for diseases of the upper respiratory tract and conjunctiva in humans (Kéry et al., 1987), while the glycosaminoglycan present in the plant's sap and the alkaloids chelidonine, chelerythrine, sanguinarine, coptisine and berberine have shown that they were able to inhibit the development of HIV-1 by decreasing the activity of the virus (Tan et al., 1991; Gerenčer et al., 2006).

Ophthalmic

The foremost medicinal use of Celandine, described by the historical authors, was treating visual impairment and eye diseases. Wdowiak (2015) reports that in 18th-century Ukraine, drops of celandine juice mixed with vodka were put into eyes; also, in the small town of Giby, Celandine pollen was used against eye infections (Kujawska et al., 2017). The rationale for the above is no doubt the antimicrobial and anti-inflammatory effects seen from the plant, but, given the presence of alkaloids, there is a risk of severe irritation to the skin and mucous membranes.

Anti-inflammatory

The anti-inflammatory activity of the plant has been shown to work by significantly suppressing the progression of arthritis in mice, and has shown potential immunomodulatory activity in clinical studies where tinctures improved immunity and promoted a reduction of recurrences in children with chronic tonsillitis.

Anticancerogenic

Several studies suggest that Ukrain™ (an anticancer drug whose major components are Celandine alkaloids such as chelerythrine) exerts cytotoxic effects on cancer cells without negative effects on normal cells. Animal studies have shown inhibitory activity on stomach cancers, and some clinical studies suggest beneficial effects in the treatment of patients suffering from bladder, breast, pancreatic, rectal and colorectal cancer, with less adverse reactions seen as compared with conventional drugs.

Antidiabetic

A 2015 study of chelerythrine also found that while the traditional antidiabetic drugs result in adverse effects, including obesity and weight gain, as well as fluid retention and cardiovascular risk, chelerythrine works in a similar way but without the side effects, making it a promising pharmacological agent for further development in the clinical treatment of insulin resistance.

TOPICAL USE

We have seen above that the plant is an effective antifungal, and the yellow milky sap has been used in folk medicine for the treatment of viral warts for years. A 2021 study then revealed that nanofibrous meshes containing Celandine extract displayed characteristics similar to natural skin and could therefore be beneficial in aiding the healing process. Additionally, the meshes inhibited *Staphylococcus aureus* and *Pseudomonas aeruginosa* growth without causing any effect on normal skin cells, which suggests promising suitability for the prevention and treatment of bacterial wound infections.

DOSAGE

Tisane – ¼ tsp/1.25g. Drink half a cup, 2 times per day.
Tincture – 1:10 45% 2–4ml, 3 times per day – 20 drops = 1ml/1tsp = 5ml.

Greater celandine is a restricted herb with a maximum weekly dose of (tinctures) 50ml, but herbalists use as little as 10ml per week for successful results. The weekly maximum dose of the fresh extract is 10ml.

PRECAUTIONS

Based on the reported undesirable effects of the plant, including cases of liver damage, the European Medicines Agency (2011) assessed that special precautions are necessary, especially in people suffering from liver diseases or taking liver-damaging drugs. Not suitable for children or those who are pregnant or lactating.

Greater celandine recipes

Medicinal recipes

Celandine leaf tisane

Pour 250ml boiling water over ¼tsp/1.25g of the dried herb and allow to steep for 10–15 minutes. Use for upper respiratory infections and as a bile stimulant.

Celandine decocted tincture: 1:10 45%

If you are using 40% alcohol, ie vodka, cover 1 part herb to 10 parts fluid.

If you are using Everclear or other 100% proof, use the following method for a specific tincture:

- 100g dried Celandine
- 450ml alcohol
- 550ml water

Take the whole aerial herb any time during a hot dry spell in summer. Wearing gloves, cut the stems into 4–5cm sections and dry thoroughly. Take 100g of herb and split into two parts of 50g each. Place 50g in 450ml alcohol and 50g in 550ml of water. Bring the water to a gentle boil, reduce heat and simmer for 20 minutes. Remove from heat and allow to cool a bit. Strain thoroughly and top up if the water is less than 550ml. Add the decoction to the alcohol mix and leave for 14 days before straining. Use for the treatment of tonsillitis, gastroenteritis and as an anti-inflammatory for rheumatism.

Topical wound ointment

Follow the steps above to make a tincture. Keep your tincture to one side and then take:

- 100g dried plant
- 2tbsp alcohol, such as Everclear
- 1l grapeseed oil

Place the herbs in a jar with the alcohol and allow to steep for 10 minutes before adding the oil. Leave for 4 weeks and then strain. Make into a salve by using 80ml oil and 20ml tincture, then use a 1:4 ratio of melted beeswax to your tincture/oil mix, ie 1 part wax to 3 parts liquid. Melt the wax pellets in the oil in a double boiler or bain-marie. Remove from the heat and slowly add your tincture. Allow to cool and set completely before using for the external treatment of wounds and fungal infections.

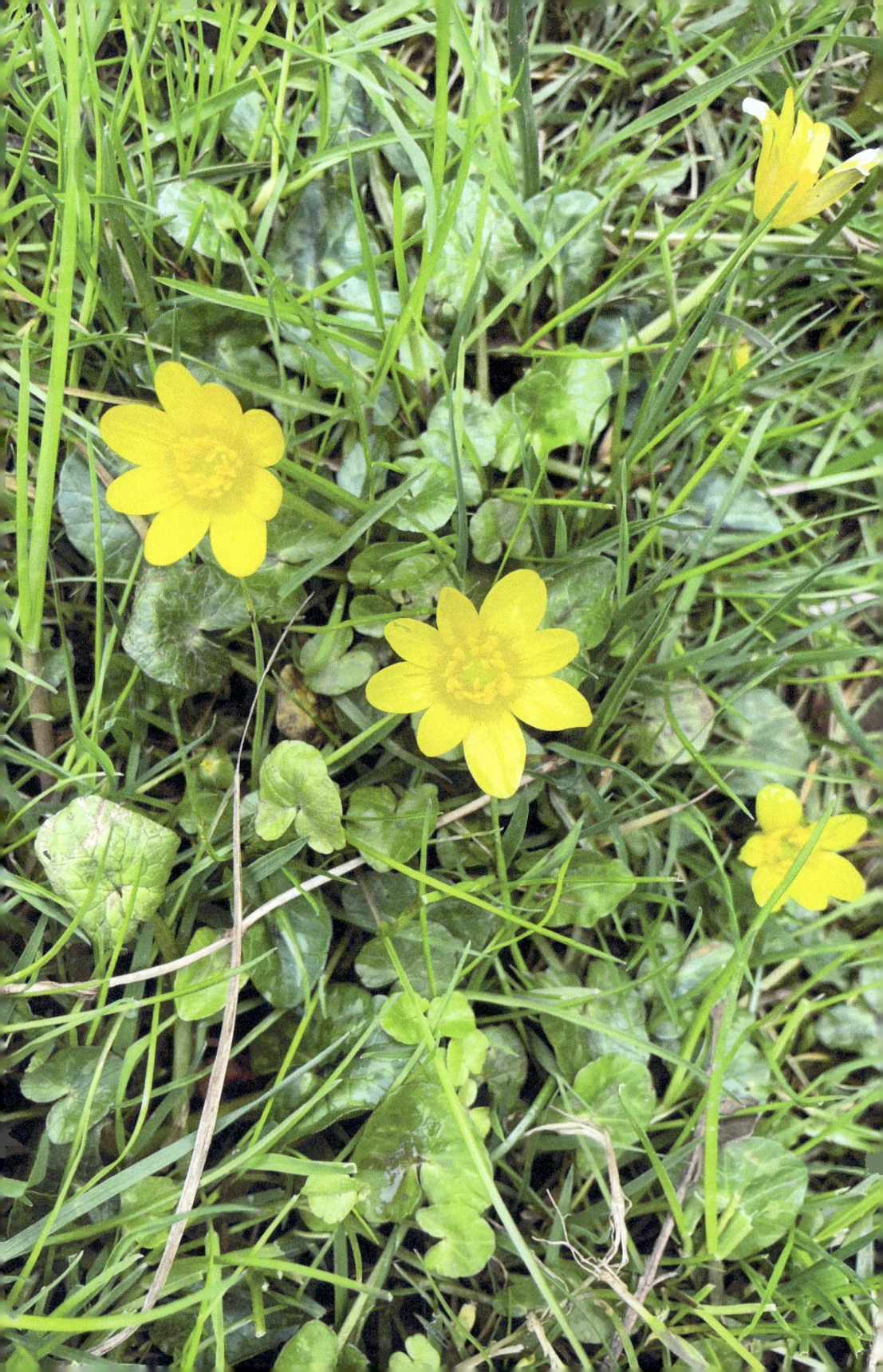

CELANDINE (LESSER)
Ranunculus ficaria

Despite sharing the common name Celandine, the Greater and Lesser celandines are not related. Greater celandine belongs to the Poppy family while *Ranunculus ficaria*, commonly known as Lesser celandine, is a member of the Buttercup family, *Ranunculaceae*. It is one of the first spring flowers to emerge and is commonly found in woodlands, hedgerows, meadows and along stream banks. All parts of the Lesser celandine plant contain toxic substances, including protoanemonin and ranunculin, which can cause irritation and blistering of the skin and mucous membranes. Despite this toxicity, however, Lesser Celandine was used for various purposes in folk medicine.

HISTORICAL USES

According to John Gerard, Galen and Dioscorides affirmed the use of Lesser celandine to '*exulcerateth or blistereth the skin ... the juice of the roots mixed with honey, and drawn up into the nostils, purgeth the head of foul and filthy humours. The later age use the roots and grains for the piles, which being often bathed with the juice mixed with wine or with the sick man's urine, are drawn together and dried up, and the pain quite taken away.*'

ETYMOLOGY OF COMMON NAME
Also from the Middle English/Old French *celidoine*. The smaller of the Celandines was named according to its small size but has a similar flowering time to the Greater variety.

PLANT LORE
Lesser celandine is one of the first flowers to bloom in early spring, often appearing when the weather begins to warm. It symbolises happiness, optimism and the awakening of nature.

USE
All parts.

EDIBILITY
Must be cooked before consumption.

HARVEST
During flowering season.

MEDICINAL PROPERTIES
Anti-inflammatory, antimicrobial and analgesic.

ACTIVE CONSTITUENTS
Alkaloids, flavonoids, tannins, phenolic compounds, mucilage, essential oils, oxalates.

LEFT: LESSER CELANDINE

Nicholas Culpeper agreed in his *Herbal*, saying, '*It is certain by good experience that the decoction of the leaves and root doth wonderfully help piles and haemorrhoides, also kernels by the ears and throat, called the king's evil, or any other hard wens or tumours.*'

MODERN RESEARCH

Also known as Pilewort, this plant, like its relatives the Anemone and Buttercup, contains protoanemonin, a mild toxin, which turns to non-toxic anemonin via the process of heating or drying, and has the following properties:

Anti-inflammatory and analgesic

As the above authors have stated, Lesser celandine is administered externally in the form of ointment or herbal tea for the treatment of haemorrhoids, by stimulating blood circulation. Infusions or decoctions of the leaves and roots of Lesser celandine have also been known to also have trophic and anti-inflammatory effects in varicose veins and skin disorders.

Antimicrobial

In a 2021 study, the antimicrobial and antioxidant effects of Lesser celandine were investigated, and it was found that both effects were present and increased depending on the concentration used. The result of this is that Lesser celandine can potentially be effective as an antioxidant and antimicrobial agent in the same way as Buttercup.

TOPICAL USE

Its most obvious use, given the name Pilewort, is as an ointment for haemorrhoids. It can also be ground up and added to baths to treat haemorrhoids, warts and scratches.

DOSAGE

External only.

PRECAUTIONS

Eating the fresh plant can cause side effects such as severe irritation of the stomach and intestines. Always dry the plant before use. Not suitable for children or those who are pregnant or lactating.

Lesser celandine recipes

Medicinal recipes

Lesser celandine poultice

- 1 whole plant, dried
- 3tsp coconut oil
- cheesecloth or cotton bandage

Finely chop the plant and add the coconut oil to make a paste. Spread the paste evenly over the desired area and wrap with the cloth or bandage. Use to shrink haemorrhoids or soothe varicose veins.

Lesser celandine bath

- 1 whole plant, dried
- 1l water

Steep the herb in the water for 15 minutes, then strain and add to the bathwater to soothe haemorrhoids and varicose veins, and to ease skin infections.

Lesser celandine balm

- 100g dried plant
- 2tbsp alcohol, such as Everclear
- 1l grapeseed oil

Place the herbs in a jar with the alcohol and allow to steep for 10 minutes before adding the oil. Leave for 4 weeks and then strain. Make into a balm by using a 1:3 ratio of melted beeswax to your oil mix, ie. 1 part wax to 3 parts liquid. Melt the wax pellets in the oil in a double boiler or bain-marie. Remove from the heat and allow to cool and set completely before using for the external treatment of haemorrhoids and varicose veins.

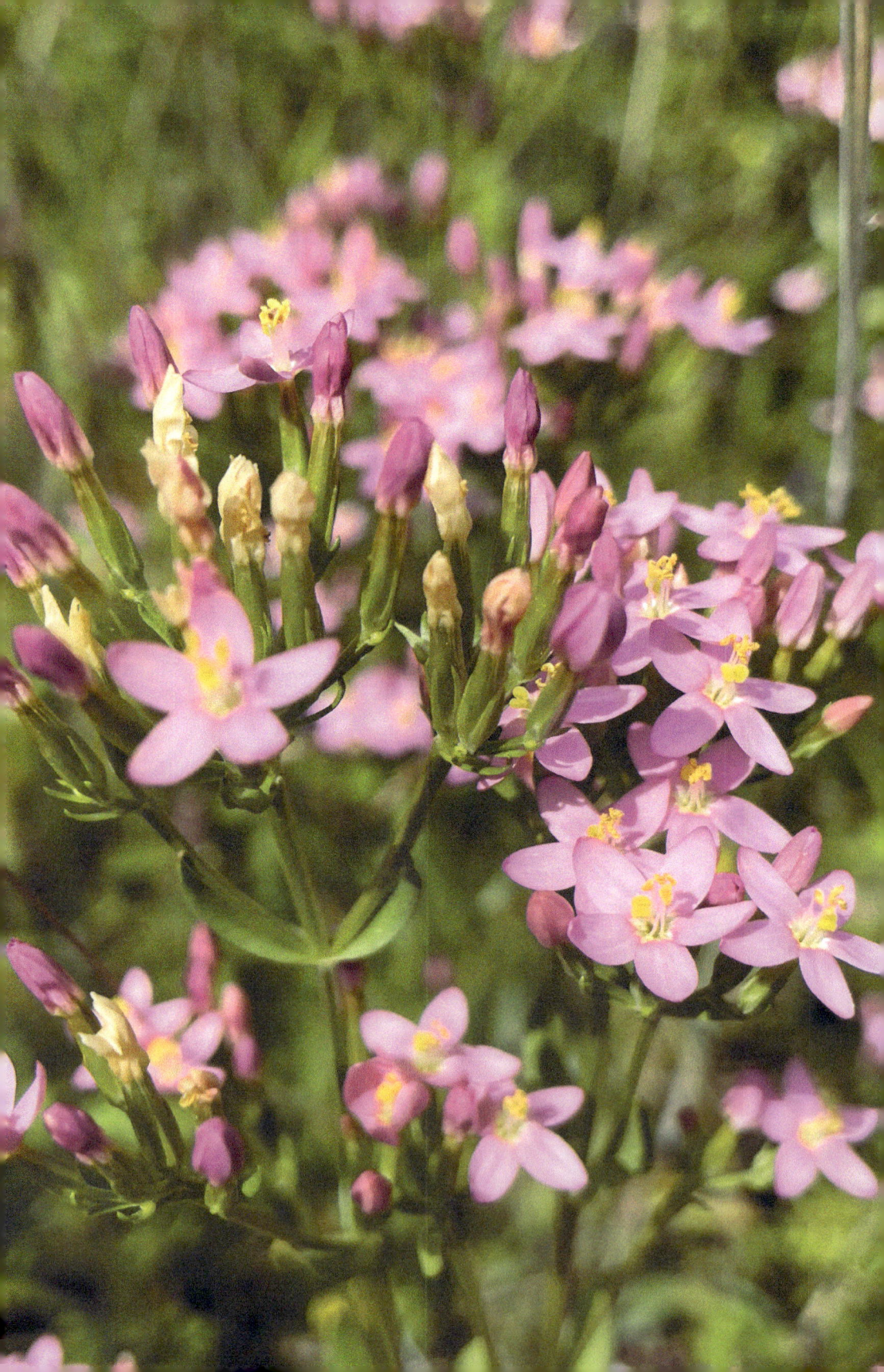

CENTAURY
Centaurium erythraea

Centaurium erythraea, commonly known as Centaury, is a plant in the Gentian family, *Gentianaceae*. It thrives in a variety of habitats, including grasslands, meadows and woodland clearings, and has a long history of use in traditional herbal medicine for its bitter principles, which stimulate digestion and promote appetite.

HISTORICAL USES

The herb was celebrated by the Anglo-Saxons for the cure of fevers, hence its alternative name of Feverwort, and was also used to kill worms, treat dropsy, as a sedative and to treat snakebites and other wounds.

According to John Gerard, Dioscorides, and Galen, *'the decoction draweth down by siege choler and thick humors, and helpeth the sciatica.'* Hildegard of Bingen meanwhile, in her 12th-century *Physica*, had already recommended it for loss of appetite, stomach complaints and biliousness.

Nicholas Culpeper's *Herbal* described how *'it helps those that have the dropsy, or the green sickness, being much used by the Italians in powder for that purpose. It kills worms … as is found by experience … A dram of the powder taken in wine, is a wonderful, good help against the biting*

ETYMOLOGY OF COMMON NAME
From late Latin *centaurea*, based on Greek *kentauros*, 'centaur' (because its medicinal properties were said to have been discovered by the centaur Chiron).

PLANT LORE
In European folklore, Centaury was sometimes used as a protective herb against evil spirits and negative energies. It was believed to ward off curses and bring good luck.

USE
All parts.

EDIBILITY
Only as a condiment. It is traditionally used as a flavouring in bitter herbal liqueurs and is an ingredient of vermouth.

HARVEST
In July, when just breaking into flower.

MEDICINAL PROPERTIES
Digestive, stomachic, tonic, antidiabetic and anticancerogenic.

ACTIVE CONSTITUENTS
Gentianin, xanthones, flavonoids, phenolic acids, triterpenes, alkaloids.

and poison of an adder. *The juice of the herb with a little honey put to it, is good to clear the eyes from dimness, mists and clouds that offend or hinder sight. It is singularly good both for green and fresh wounds, as also for old ulcers and sores, to close up the one and cleanse the other, and perfectly to cure them both. The decoction thereof dropped into the ears, cleanses them from worms ... and takes away all freckles, spots, and marks in the skin, being washed with it.'*

In his *Family Herbal* (1814), Robert Thornton described Centaury as '*justly esteemed as one of the most efficacious bitters indigenous to this island ... It was formerly much used as a stomachic bitter both in substance and infusion, and for the cure of intermittent fevers. It is recommended for worms, and, like chamomile, is made into tea for assisting the operation of emetics. It answers the purpose of any of the bitters and is often taken to create an appetite; but the long-continued use of any bitter impairs the coats of the stomach and produces an incurable debility of that organ.'*

Fray's Golden Recipes for the Use of All Ages (1897) considered Centaury '*an excellent general tonic, used extensively in jaundice, chronic liver complaint, and combined with agrimony and Colombo root* [Cocculus palmatus] *invaluable for indigestion.*'

MODERN RESEARCH

As the opposite allude to, Centaury is a strong bitter that helps with heartburn, gas pains in the intestines and stomach, bloating, constipation and colic. These and other properties are covered further as follows:

Digestive

A 2021 study confirmed this historical use when it showed that the active substances of Centaury, such as gentianine and apigenin, can affect the secretion of glands of the digestive tract, increase bile, enhance the contraction of uterine muscles, and have an anti-inflammatory, analgesic, weak laxative effect and antioxidant activity.

Antidiabetic

Centaury has been a traditional treatment for diabetes in the Mediterranean, and this use is supported by numerous studies. A 2011 study on rats clearly indicated that Centaury decreased oxidative stress and pancreatic damage, attributed to its antioxidant nature. The effect on the regulation of blood glucose was found to be similar to glibenclamide, an anti-diabetic drug (Stefkov et al., 2014). This hypoglycaemic effect is thought to arise from the stimulation of glycogen synthesis in the liver and gastrointestinal tract, as well as increased secretion of insulin from the pancreas.

Anticancerogenic

In a study on colorectal cancer cells Centaury has also shown anticancer activity. The xanthone it contains demonstrated the most significant inhibition effects of cell growth. Since xanthones are increasingly being used for their pharmacological properties, Centaury could be used as a useful source of plant material to produce drugs.

TOPICAL USE

Application of the crushed parts of the fresh herb is also said to be effective in healing lesions and pain. It can also be used as an antiseptic and as a treatment for dandruff.

DOSAGES

Tisane – ½tsp/2.5g. Drink half a cup, 3 times per day.
Tincture – 1:20, 50%, 200ml.

PRECAUTIONS

Centaury is contra-indicated for individuals with peptic ulcers. Not suitable for children or those who are pregnant or lactating.

Centaury recipes

Medicinal recipes

Centaury tisane

Pour 250ml boiling water over ½tsp/2.5g of the dried leaf and allow to steep for 10-15 minutes. Use as a digestive, to stimulate the appetite and for heartburn, gas pains, bloating and constipation.

Centaury infused tincture – 1:20 50%

If you are using 40% alcohol, ie vodka, make a simple tincture by covering 1 part herb to 20 parts fluid.

If you are using Everclear or other 100% proof, use the following method for a specific tincture:

- 100g dried herb
- 2lml alcohol
- 2l water

Take 100g of dried herb and split into two parts of 50g each. Place 50g in the alcohol and 50g in the water. Steep/infuse in the water for 10 minutes. Strain thoroughly and top up if the water is less than 2l. Add the infusion to the alcohol mix and leave for 14 days before straining. Use to aid digestion, as a liver tonic and to treat the gallbladder.

Centaury oxymel

An oxymel makes hard-to-take herbs much easier to stomach. Fill your jar a quarter full of herbs and then use the ratio of 1 part honey to 3 parts apple cider vinegar. Stir, seal and leave to steep/infuse for two weeks. Strain out the liquid into another jar and then take two spoonfuls diluted with water for each dose to aid digestion.

Centaury dandruff rinse

Add 2tbsp/30g Centaury to 250ml boiling water. Steep for half an hour. Cool and apply to the scalp for 1–2 hours and rinse.

Centaury cocktail bitters

Start by making a Centaury tincture but also add some dried Hogweed seeds, Avens root, Rose petals and the zest of 3 oranges. Let the mix sit for two weeks, then strain, but reserve the marc (tea), and decoct it for 10 minutes in 1 cup of water. Mix the 'tea' with the tincture and add 2tbsp honey. Try it as is or add a teaspoon in your next Manhattan or Old Fashioned!

CHICKWEED
Stellaria media

Stellaria media, commonly known as Chickweed, is a flowering plant in the Carnation family, *Caryophyllaceae*, together with its relatives, the Stitchworts. It thrives in a variety of habitats, including lawns, gardens, fields, meadows and disturbed areas such as roadsides and waste ground and has a long history of use in traditional herbal medicine for its soothing properties.

HISTORICAL USES

Hildegard of Bingen (1098–1179) recommended Chickweed in her *Physica* for occasions where a person has fallen or been struck so that his skin is bruised. She advised that the herb should be cooked in water, then squeezed out and the herb tied to the wound.

Nicholas Culpeper's *Herbal* said '*the bruised herb, or the juice applied, with cloths or sponges dipped therein, to the region of the liver, and as they dry to have fresh applied, doth wonderfully temper the heat of the liver and is effectual for all impostumes and swellings whatsoever; for all redness in the face, wheals, pushes, itch or scabs.*'

R.L. Hool, author of *Common Plants and Their Uses in Medicine* (1922), wrote '*Chickweed is a most wonderful remedy,*

ETYMOLOGY OF COMMON NAME
From the late 14th-century *chekwede*, so-called because it is enjoyed by chickens.

PLANT LORE
It is said that when chickweed expands its leaves fully, no rain will fall; its arrival in spring signalled the beginning of the planting season.

USE
All parts.

EDIBILITY
Edible and nutritious, and is used as a leaf vegetable, often raw in salads.

HARVEST
Between May and July.

MEDICINAL PROPERTIES
Demulcent, refrigerant, antimicrobial, anti-inflammatory, antidiabetic, anti-obesity, anxiolytic and antipruritic.

ACTIVE CONSTITUENTS
Saponins, flavonoids, triterpenes, polysaccharides, coumarins, mucilage.

for it is both strengthening and healing. Its properties are emollient, demulcent, resolvent, diuretic, and pectoral. It may be used in powder, infusion, decoction, fluid extract, solid extract, in pills, tincture, fomentations, ointment, and poultices, and may be used in all cases of weakness, inflammation of the stomach, lungs, bowels, or bronchial tubes, for bleeding of the lungs and bowels, bronchitis, asthma, consumption, etc. For peritonitis, or all or any form of internal inflammation it has a wonderful soothing and healing action on all the parts it comes in contact with, and in addition possesses as much nutriment as is contained in many articles used as food. While in all cases of weak constitutions, especially the asthmatic and consumptive, it will be found both strengthening and healing. As an outward application for all kinds of wounds, inflamed surfaces, boils, scalds, burns, skin diseases, piles, fistulas, old wounds, bad legs, inflamed or sore eyes, tumours, erysipelas, deafness, swelled testes, ulcerated throat or mouth, there is not its equal as a remedial agent in the Botanic practice.'

MODERN RESEARCH

A 2020 review of the chemical constituents and pharmacological activities of Chickweed found important secondary metabolites, which displayed the following diverse activities:

Antimicrobial

Extracts of Chickweed have been shown to significantly inhibit the microbial growth of pathogenic bacterias such as *Staphylococcus aureus*, *Escherichia coli*, *Salmonella typhi*, *Klebsiella pneumoniae* and *Bacillus cereus*. In 2015, a novel peptide isolated from leaves of Chickweed was reported to have potent inhibitory activity against plant pathogenic fungi.

Anti-inflammatory and antipruritic

The historical writers were right about treating itches, swellings, bruises/wheals and impostumes (abscesses), with Chickweed as it contains saponins that alleviate inflamed mucous membranes and is therefore excellent at relieving the irritation of eczema and psoriasis while promoting a drying effect. In 2012 the inflammatory effect of a methanolic leaf extract was investigated on paw oedema in rats and showed pronounced reduction in inflammation.

Anti-obesity

Chickweed's other traditional use is as an old wives' remedy for obesity. In a 2012 study of it on mice fed a high-fat diet for six weeks, Chickweed significantly suppressed the body weight of the mice. The inhibition in body weight did not depend upon the decreased food or energy intake but was caused by the delaying of fat and carbohydrate absorption through inhibition of digestive enzymes.

Anxiolytic

The anti-anxiety activity of various extracts of Chickweed was compared with the standard drug diazepam.

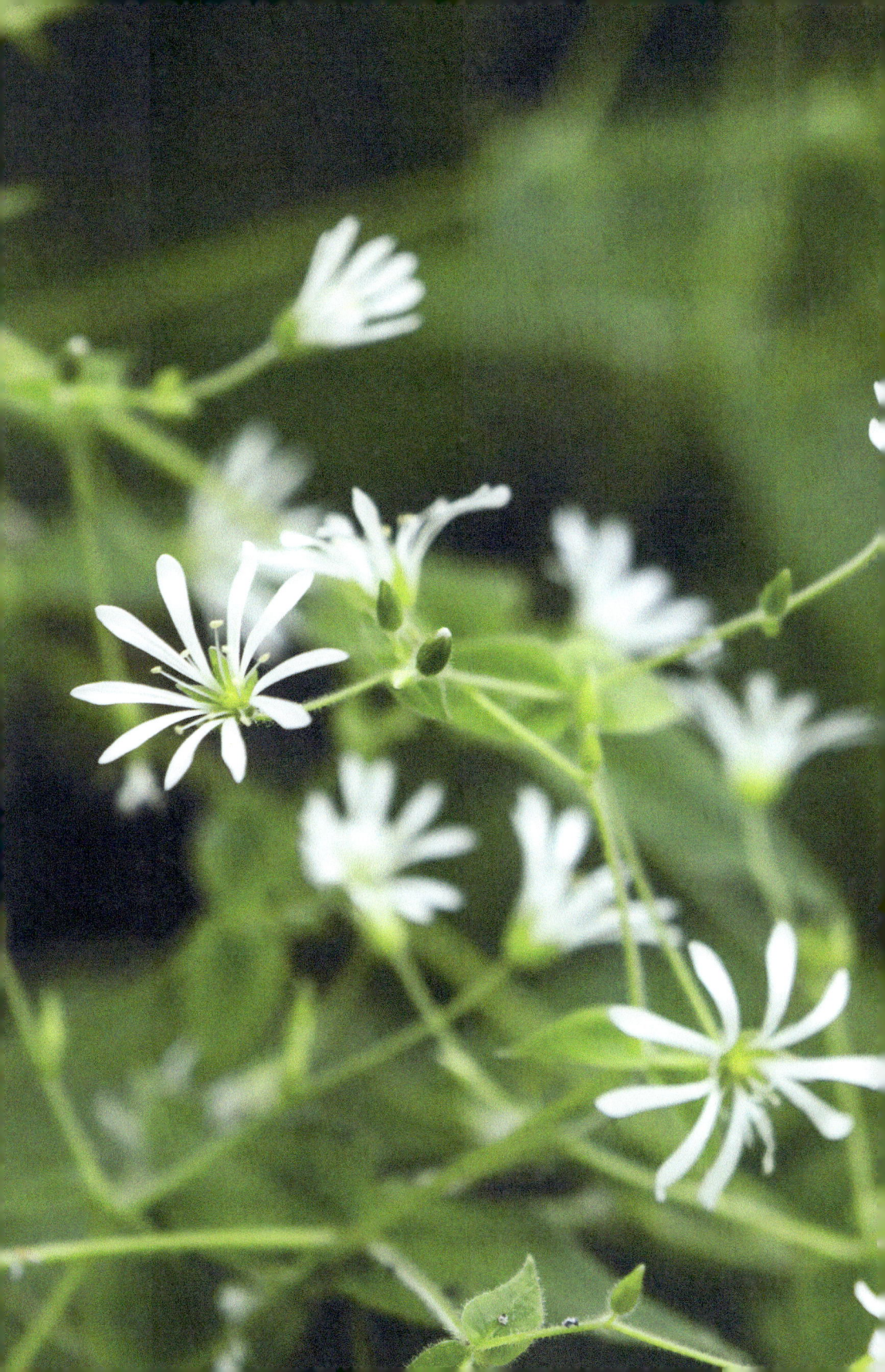

Among various extracts, activity was shown to be best in the methanol extract, and the activity could possibly be related to fats, flavonoids, steroids and/or triterpenoids that are known to interact with the GABAergic system, a common mechanism of action for many anxiolytic agents.

Antidiabetic

A 2021 animal study found that Chickweed tisane may be beneficial in cardiac dysfunction induced by diabetes since it ameliorates the cardiac output. This may prove useful against diabetic cardiomyopathy, one of the major consequences of diabetes.

TOPICAL USES

With anti-inflammatory, antiseptic and antifungal properties, infusions of Chickweed can be used to treat several skin complaints, including boils, sores, rashes, wounds, eczema and psoriasis. It will also relieve the itching and inflammation that accompanies many of these conditions.

A 2021 study showed that Chickweed extract applied on the wounds recorded the strongest and fastest wound closure and proliferation of skin cells compared with the control.

DOSAGE

Tisane – 2tsp, 3 times per day.
Tincture – 1:5 45% 2–10ml, 3 times per day – 20 drops = 1ml/1tsp = 5ml.

PRECAUTIONS

Overdose may cause diarrhoea and vomiting. Not suitable for children or those who are pregnant or lactating.

Chickweed recipes

Medicinal recipes

Chickweed tisane
Pour 250ml boiling water over 2tsp/10g of dried leaf and allow to steep for 10–15 minutes. Use to relieve inflammation and to soothe tension. Can also be used externally as an acne wash and to relieve the itching of eczema and psoriasis.

Chickweed infused tincture – 1:5 45%
If you are using 40% alcohol, ie vodka, make a simple tincture by covering 1 part herb to 5 parts fluid.

If you are using Everclear or other 100% proof, then use the following method for a specific tincture:
- 100g dried herb
- 225ml alcohol
- 275ml water

Take 100g of dried herb and split into two parts of 50g each. Place 50g in 225ml alcohol and 50g in 275ml of boiled water. Steep/infuse in the water for 10 minutes. Strain thoroughly and top up if the water is less than 275ml. Add the infusion to the alcohol mix and leave for 14 days before straining. Use for inflammation of the digestive, renal and respiratory tracts.

Chickweed oil
- 100g dried and powdered Chickweed plant
- 2 tbsp Everclear
- 1l grapeseed oil

Place the herbs in a jar with the alcohol and allow to steep for 10 minutes before adding the oil. Leave for 4 weeks and then strain. Use to soothe eczema and other skin irritations.

Eczema bath
- 20g Mallow root
- 20g Viola
- 20g Oats
- 20g Chamomile
- 20g Chickweed

Steep the herbs in 1l water for 15 minutes, then strain and add to the bathwater to soothe and ease irritated skin.

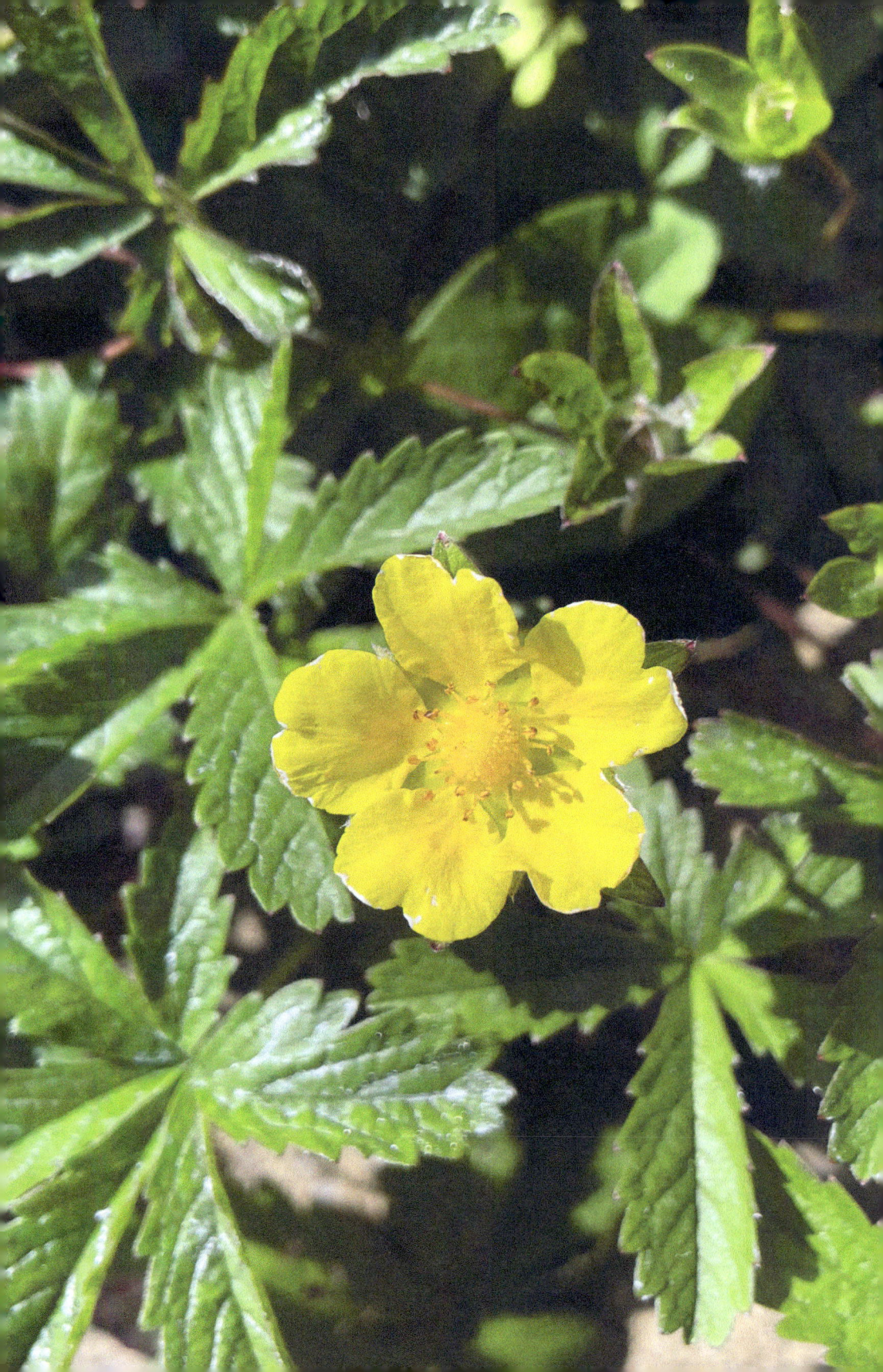

CINQUEFOILS
Potentilla spp.

In the UK, several species of *Potentilla* (commonly known as Cinquefoils) are found, including *Potentilla reptans*, commonly known as Creeping cinquefoil, Tormentil (*Potentilla erecta*) and Silverweed (*Potentilla anserina*). All are members of the Rose family and thrive in a variety of habitats, including meadows, pastures, heaths and open woodlands.

HISTORICAL USES

The roots of Tormentil were used in Ancient Greece by both Hippocrates and Dioscorides to cure the intermittent fevers that prevailed in marshy, ill-drained lands. Dioscorides stated in *De Materia Medica* that one leaf of Cinquefoil cured a quotidian (one-day) ague, three a tertian (three-day) and four a quarten (four-day) ague, while a decoction of the underground parts was used to bathe a purulent facial eczema and to rinse oral cavity ulceration.

Hildegard of Bingen (1098–1179) agreed with the above but recommended in her *Physica* that it '*be mixed with flour and water as a paste, then spread on a cloth and tied around the belly of the person with the fever.*'

John Gerard (1545–1612) related in his *Herball* that '*Ortolpho Morolto a learned physician, commended the leaves of Cinquefoil be boiled with water, and

ETYMOLOGY OF COMMON NAME
From the Latin *quinquefolium*, from *quinque*, 'five' + *folium*, 'leaf'.

PLANT LORE
Cinquefoil was often included in charms for its protective qualities. Its five leaves were thought to represent the five senses, and possessing it was believed to sharpen these senses.

USE
The root.

EDIBILITY
An emergency food, only eaten when all else fails.

HARVEST
In early autumn.

MEDICINAL PROPERTIES
Astringent, antimicrobial, anti-inflammatory, cardioprotective, antiulcerogenic and antitussive.

ACTIVE CONSTITUENTS
Tannins, flavonoids, phenolic acids, polysaccharides, essential oils, alkaloids.

LEFT: CREEPING CINQUEFOIL

some *Lignum vitæ* added, against the falling sickness [epilepsy], *if the patient be caused to sweat upon the taking thereof. He likewise commendeth the extraction of the roots against the bloody flux.*'

Nicholas Culpeper's *Herbal* said of Silverweed that it '*is a plant that deserves to be much more known in medicine than it is ... The leaves given in powder, will frequently effect a cure in agues and intermitments; while a strong infusion stops the immoderate bleeding of the piles; and, sweetened with a little honey, it is an excellent gargle for sore throats.*'

Culpeper described Tormentil as '*most excellent to stay all kind of fluxes of blood or humours, whether at nose, mouth, or belly, while the juice or powder of the root put in ointments, plaisters, and such things that are to be applied to wounds or sores, is very effectual and the juice of the leaves and the root bruised and applied to the throat or jaws, heals the king's evil, and eases the pain of the sciatica.*' He called Cinquefoil '*an especial herb used in all inflammations and fevers, whether infectious or pestilential, or to cool and temper the blood and humours in the body; as also for all lotions, gargles and infections; for sore mouths, ulcers, cancers, fistulas and other foul or running sores.*'

Robert Thornton's *Family Herbal* of 1814 maintained that that the root of Tormentil '*has a strong bitter taste but imparts no peculiar sapid flavour. As a proof of its powerful astringency, it has been substituted for oak bark in the tanning of skins for leather. This root has been long held in great estimation by physicians as a very useful astringent; and as the resin it contains is very inconsiderable, it seems more particularly adapted to those cases where the heating and stimulating medicines of this class are less proper; as in phthisical diarrheic, diarrhoea cruenta, etc.*'

Harold Ward's *Herbal Manual* of 1936 stated that Tormentil root '*is regarded as one of the best and most powerful of all the herbal astringents ... used in diarrhoea and as a gargle for relaxed throats. It may also be used with benefit as a lotion for application to ulcers.*'

MODERN RESEARCH

The Cinquefoils all share many of the same properties, particularly astringency. Modern pharmacological studies have generally confirmed the long traditional use of the species and their extracts as a treatment for the following:

Astringent

The astringent use was confirmed in a 2003 clinical trial by Russian authors (Subbotina et al., 2003). The study showed that Tormentil had a high efficacy in child diarrhoea caused by Rotavirus infection. The duration of diarrhoea in the Tormentil treatment group was 3 days, compared with 5 days in the control group. In the treatment group, 40% of the children were diarrhoea-free 48 hours after admission to the hospital, compared with 5% in the placebo group. The authors concluded that the treatment with Tormentil extract appeared to be an effective therapy.

The use of Silverweed's astringency meanwhile, has been confirmed in its approval by Commission E in Germany for:
- diarrhoea
- inflammation of the mouth and pharynx
- premenstrual syndrome (PMS)

The use of Silverweed for PMS is based on pharmacological studies showing that the herb increases the tone of the uterus in various animal species (Schulz et al., 1998).

Antimicrobial

Most of the biological effects of *Potentilla* species can be explained by the high number of tannins in the aerial and the underground parts. In 1978, moderate antiviral effects were demonstrated by Tormentil against *Herpes* virus types I and II, as well as against influenza and cowpox. Then, in 1985, animal tests demonstrated the antiviral effects of a Tormentil rhizome extract against viruses used in vaccines.

A 2017 study investigated the antimicrobial properties of the aerial parts of Cinquefoil against some important pathogenic microorganisms, which may have been the cause of pains in the bowels referred to by Culpeper. Results showed the highest effect on *Listeria*, *Candida albicans* and *Rhizopus* species of fungi with moderate inhibitory effect on *Bacillus cereus*, *Proteus vulgaris* and *Pseudomonas aeruginosa*.

A study in June 2019 evaluated the use of Cinquefoils in the treatment of mastitis using a decoction of the aerial parts (Kozuharova et al., 2012). The tests showed that Cinquefoil has moderate bacteriostatic activity against *Staphylococcus* but that preliminary tests also demonstrated agonistic activity to the oxytocin and vasopressin receptors that play an important role in the opening of milk ducts (Mincheva et al., unpubl. results).

Antiulcerogenic

Tannins are known to be of particular therapeutic importance as gastroprotective agents, and further verification of Culpeper's writings came in 2007, when Cinquefoils were used in the treatment of colitis in 16 patients. During treatment, colitis significantly declined, and although there was mild discomfort in six patients, the authors (Huber et al., 2007) suggest that the addition of the extract to conventional therapy may help to reduce some of the symptoms. This suggestion was substantiated in 2015 when further studies concluded that the extract, with the additional property of a free-radical scavenger, could be successfully used in the prevention of inflammatory colon disorders.

Anti-inflammatory

Culpeper's findings that the root of Cinquefoil heals inflammations, painful sores and shingles as well as joint pain and gout is also borne out. Silverweed meanwhile, is used as a cataplasm in the alleviation of rheumatic and arthritic pains and neuralgia (Youngken et al., 1949), and Tormentil root has been found to have very strong cyclooxygenase (an enzyme that creates inflammation) inhibiting properties, which confirms its anti-inflammatory activity (Tunón et al., 1995).

In 2005 and 2007, animal studies further significantly confirmed anti-inflammatory effects of Cinquefoils when applied to mouse ear oedema (Pilipović et al., 2005; Pilipović et al., 2007).

In 2021 these earlier findings were demonstrated again in rats and proved that Silverweed extracts have potential as a drug to treat and prevent high-altitude pulmonary oedema, a condition that usually requires treatment with steroids.

Cardioprotective

In 2021, six new triterpenoids were isolated from Cinquefoil root and evaluated for their cardioprotective effects. Triterpenoids can protect heart muscle cells (cardiomyocytes) from damage, particularly during events such as ischaemia-reperfusion injury, which occurs when blood supply returns to the heart after a period of ischaemia or lack of oxygen. Two of the compounds, tormentic acid and ursolic acid, exhibited significant inhibitory effects and could therefore be suitable natural candidates to prevent heart muscle injury.

Antitussive

In 2016, the antitussive and expectorant activities of Silverweed were evaluated. The results showed that the plant significantly inhibited the frequency of coughs and increased their latent period. Similarly, the extract also showed substantial expectorant activity. The result of the study shows that Silverweed can be used as an antitussive and expectorant herbal medicine and that polysaccharides may be the main active ingredients responsible for its bioactivities.

TOPICAL USES

Externally, the *Potentilla* species are also used for bathing skin conditions, such as eczema, psoriasis rosacea, etc. as well as fungal infections and in compresses for burns, frostbite and skin injuries.

A 2023 clinical trial involved individuals wearing masks for over 6 hours a day, while using a moisturiser containing Silverweed extract. Results demonstrated a notable reduction in skin redness and transepidermal water loss after 2 and 4 weeks, respectively, meaning that the moisturiser significantly enhanced skin hydration compared to the control group.

DOSAGE

Tisane – 1tsp/5g, 2–3 times per day.
Decoction – 1tbsp/15g root, leaf or stem decocted and taken throughout the day.
Tincture – 1:5 parts of plant and ethyl alcohol 70%, 2–4ml, 3 times per day.

PRECAUTIONS

There have been complaints of gastro-intestinal upset reported in the literature. Not suitable for children or those who are pregnant or lactating.

Cinquefoil recipes

Medicinal recipes

Tormentil tisane

Pour 250ml boiling water over 1tsp/5g of dried Tormentil root and allow to steep for 30 minutes. Use to treat diarrhoea, sore throats, IBS, ulcerative colitis and colitis. Can also be used externally in the form of a compress applied to inflamed areas and as a wash for mouth ulcers, infected gums and inflamed eyes.

Tormentil root decocted tincture – 1:5 70%

If you are using 40% alcohol, ie vodka, make a simple tincture by covering 1 part herb to 5 parts fluid.

If you are using Everclear or other 100% proof, use the following method for a specific tincture:

- 100g dried Tormentil root
- 350ml alcohol
- 150ml water

Split the dried herb into to equal 50g parts. Cover 50g dried herb with the alcohol. Place the other 50g in the water. Bring the water to a gentle boil, reduce heat and simmer for 20–40 minutes. Remove from heat and allow to cool a bit. Strain thoroughly and top up if the water is less than 150ml. Add the infusion to the alcohol mix and leave for 14 days before straining. Use to treat, diarrhoea, sore throats, irritable bowel syndrome and colitis.

Cinquefoil decoction

- 1tbsp/15g Cinquefoil root, leaves and stems
- 250ml water

Boil the plant content for 30 minutes to reduce and drink throughout the day to help with diarrhoea, gout, pain and mastitis. Use as a gargle, mouthwash or rinse and for toothache. Use also as a topical solution for inflammation of the body and joints.

Cinquefoil cough honey

In a medium pot, combine 500ml of Cinquefoil decoction with 128g honey. Use as needed.

Silverweed balm

- 100g dried Silverweed leaves
- 2tbsp alcohol, such as Everclear
- 1l grapeseed oil

Place the leaves in a jar with the alcohol and allow to steep for 10 minutes before adding the oil. Leave for 4 weeks and then strain. Make into a balm by using a 1:3 ratio of melted beeswax to your oil mix, ie 1 part wax to 3 parts liquid. Melt the wax pellets in the oil in a double boiler or bain-marie. Remove from the heat and allow to cool and set completely before using for the topical anti-inflammatory treatment of rashes and redness.

CLEAVERS
Galium aparine

Galium aparine, commonly known as Cleavers, Stickyweed or Goosegrass, is a member of the Bedstraw family and native to the UK. It is found in a variety of habitats, including woodlands, hedgerows, grasslands, meadows and disturbed areas such as gardens and waste grounds. Cleavers has a long history of use in traditional herbal medicine where it is valued for its diuretic and tonic properties.

HISTORICAL USES

We learn from Dioscorides in *De Materia Medica* that an ointment of great efficacy is made from the expressed juice of this plant mixed with hog's lard, for tumours in the breast.

Nicholas Culpeper's *Herbal* advised that:

> *The distilled water drunk twice a day helpeth the yellow jaundice; and stayeth laxes and bloody fluxes. The juice of the leaves, or they a little bruised and applied to any bleeding wound, stayeth the bleeding. The juice also is very good to close up the lips of green wounds, and the powder of the dried herb strewn thereupon doth the same, and likewise helpeth old ulcers. Being boiled in hog's grease, it helpeth all sorts of hard swellings or kernels in the throat, being anointed therewith. The juice*

ETYMOLOGY OF COMMON NAME
Possibly a derivative of Old English *clēofan*, 'to split', reflecting the tendency of the small seed to cleave (stick) to anything that passes.

PLANT LORE
Cleavers were traditionally used in springtime cleansing rituals to detoxify and purify the body after winter.

USE
All parts.

EDIBILITY
The whole plant is edible, but beware of the hooked hairs, which are like Velcro, so eat the young parts of the plant or use as a pot herb. The seeds can be dry-roasted to make a coffee substitute.

HARVEST
In May and June (autumn for the seeds).

MEDICINAL PROPERTIES
Antimicrobial, tonic, anticancerogenic.

ACTIVE CONSTITUENTS
Triterpenoids, coumarins, flavonoids, phenolic acids, polysaccharides, essential oils, mucilage and alkaloids.

dropped into the ears taketh away the pain of them. It is a good remedy in the spring, eaten (being first chopped small and boiled well) in water gruel, to cleanse the blood and strengthen the liver, thereby to keep the body in health, and fitting it for that change of season that is coming.

William Fernie in his 1897 *Herbal Simples* recorded that:

This herb has a special curative reputation with reference to cancerous growths and tumours. For open cancers an ointment is made from the leaves and stems wherewith to dress the ulcerated parts, and at the same time the expressed juice of the plant is given internally. Dr Tuthill Massy avers that it often produces a cure in from six to twelve months, and advises that the decoction shall be drank regularly afterwards in the Springtime.

MODERN RESEARCH

Related to the other bedstraws, this plant was used in medieval kitchens because it could be picked in frost or snow. Research has shown that it has the following medicinal properties:

Lymphatic tonic

Culpeper's recommendation of Cleavers as a spring remedy is accurate as we now know that Cleavers can play a crucial role in removing toxins and metabolic waste from the body while supporting the movement and drainage of lymph fluid, thereby enhancing the body's natural detoxification processes. This, as Culpeper says, effectively aids conditions such as jaundice, swollen glands, tonsillitis and adenoid trouble as well as cystitis and other urinary tract conditions.

Antimicrobial

With regard to its ability to heal open and ulcerous wounds, a June 1883 article in the *British Medical Journal* by Dr F.J.B. Qninlan, at St Vincent's Hospital, Dublin, described how he used poultices made with the fresh juice of Cleavers, and applied three times per day, to heal chronic ulcers on the legs. Its effects, he says, *in the most unlikely cases, were decisive and plain to all.*

The results of a 2016 study revealed that *Staphylococcus aureus*, *Pseudomonas aeruginosa* and *Candida albicans* were highly sensitive to Cleavers while *Bacillus subtilis* showed moderate sensitivity. *Staphylococcus* of course can lead to sepsis and death, while *Pseudomonas* will infect open wounds and pressure sores. Both could be the cause of the 'running sores' described by Culpeper and Fernie.

Anticancerogenic

Cleaver's activity in the fight against cancer was recorded as far back as Dioscorides and has been confirmed in numerous studies. For example, it has been reported that extracts were effective against colon and breast cancer cells (Vlase et al., 2014; Atmaca et al., 2016).

A 2017 study again confirmed

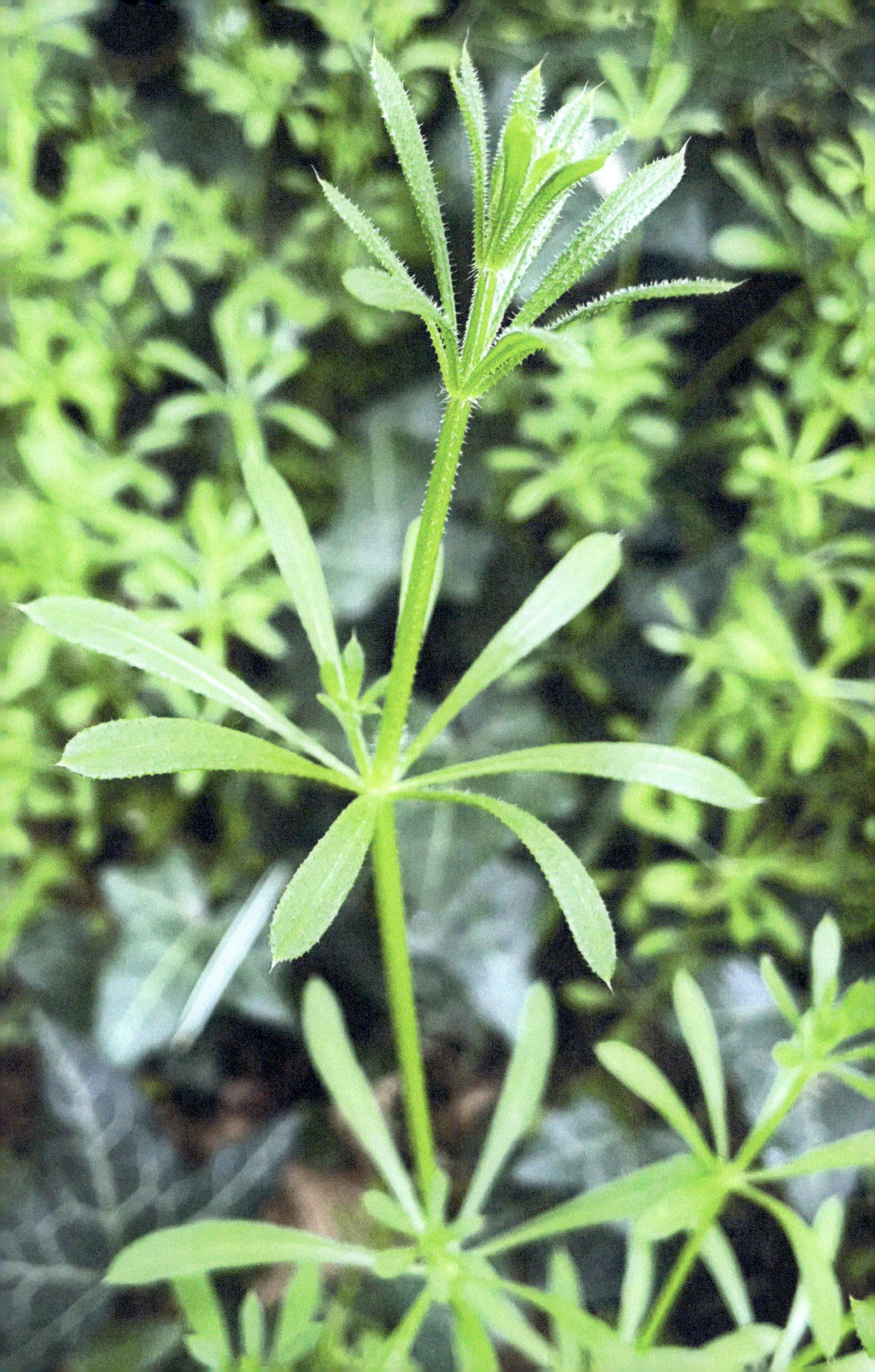

anticancer effects against colon and breast cancer cells and showed that Cleavers inhibits cancer cell growth through apoptosis (programmed cell death), but also acts as an immunomodulator by promoting the proliferation of lymphocytes (a type of white blood cell). This effect suggests the potential for immune system benefits and cancer cell reduction.

In a 2021 study, it was determined that extracts of Cleavers also exhibited strong cytotoxic effects on lung cancer cell lines. The same study confirmed that it has an important antioxidant potential and, together with the antimicrobial and high antifungal activity, means that Cleavers has a high biological activity and can be used as a natural agent in pharmacological studies.

TOPICAL USES

Cleavers can be used in a compress also on burn injuries, ulcers, grazes as well as various skin inflammations, and as a cream that may be applied topically to treat psoriasis.

DOSAGE

Tisane – 1tsp/5g. Drink half a cup, 3 times per day.

Tincture – 1:5 in 25%, 4–10ml, 3 times per day – 20 drops = 1ml/1tsp = 5ml.

PRECAUTIONS

This herb may be used freely. But it should be taken for only 2 weeks at a time and then skip 1–2 weeks. Not suitable for children or those who are pregnant or lactating.

Cleavers recipes

Medicinal recipes

Cleavers tisane

Pour 250ml boiling water over 1tsp/5g of dried leaf and allow to steep for 10-15 minutes. Take in mouthful doses throughout the day to support the lymphatic system and for general detoxification.

Cleavers cold infusion

Steep 3tbsp/90g dried herb in 1 litre of cold water overnight and drink at intervals of 3-4 hours a day as a lymphatic tonic. Use for tonsillitis and glandular fever, cystitis and urethritis. The cold infusion can also be used externally as a skin wash to improve the complexion and as a hair tonic to fight dandruff.

Cleavers infused tincture 1:5 25%

If you are using 40% alcohol, ie vodka, you will need to dilute this at the ratio of 60ml water to every 100ml vodka to make a 25% medium and then cover 1 part herb to 5 parts fluid.

If you are using Everclear or other 100% proof, use the following method for a specific tincture:

- 100g dried Cleavers herb
- 125ml alcohol
- 375ml water

Take 100g of dried herb and split into two parts of 50g each. Place 50g in 125ml alcohol and 50g in 375ml of boiled water. Steep/infuse in the water for 10 minutes. Strain thoroughly and top up if the water is less than 375ml. Add the infusion to the alcohol mix and leave for 14 days before straining. Use to support the lymphatic system and for general detoxification as well as for conditions such as water retention, cystic acne and fibrous breast tissue.

Cleavers seed coffee dessert

Harvest 100g seeds of Cleavers in autumn and then place your dessert glasses in the fridge to cool while you roast the seeds at 175°C for 45 minutes. Using a coffee grinder or pestle and mortar, grind the seeds to powder and set aside. Take your glasses from the fridge and place your choice of ice cream in the cold glasses. Make your Cleavers coffee on the stove using a cup of water and a tablespoon of Cleavers and then slowly pour over the ice cream. Serve immediately.

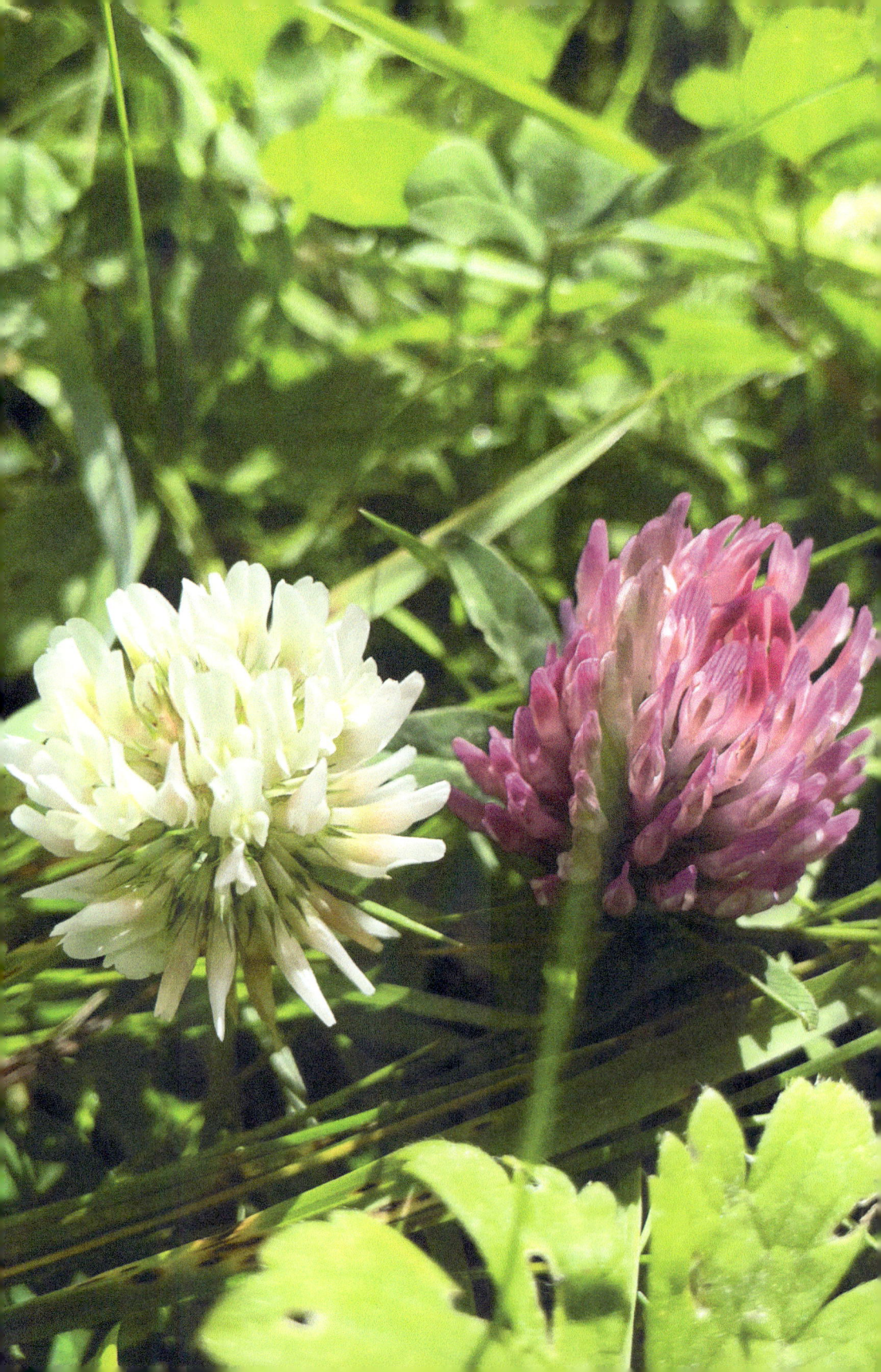

CLOVER
Trifolium spp.

Trifolium is a genus of plants commonly known as Clovers, and several species of *Trifolium* are found in the UK, including the well-known Red clover (*Trifolium pratense*) and White clover (*Trifolium repens*). Both are found in a wide range of habitats, including grasslands, meadows, lawns, roadsides and disturbed areas, and both have a long history of use in traditional herbal medicine.

HISTORICAL USES

In folk tradition, Red clover was first used by the Druids to signify the branches of learning, ie Bard, Ovate and Druid, then associated with the Christian doctrine of the Trinity because of its threefold leaves. It was worn as a magic charm to protect against evil.

John Gerard referred to Clover as Meadow Trefoil and says that the '*floures grow at the tops of the stalks in a tuft or small Fox-taile eare, of a purple colour, and sweet of taste*' while Culpeper does not refer to Clover but describes Trefoil with flowers that '*are small and white, numerous, in a round thick head, each cell containing four small seeds*'. If this is Clover, Culpeper goes on to say '*The leaves and flowers are good to ease the pains of the gout, if the*

ETYMOLOGY OF COMMON NAME
From the Old English word *clāfre*, which came from the Latin *trifolium*, 'trefoil, clover'; this refers to the cloven form of the leaf.

PLANT LORE
Well-known for good luck, particularly the four-leaf clover. Finding a four-leaf clover is considered a sign of good fortune and is believed to bring luck to the finder.

USE
The blossoms.

EDIBILITY
The leaves of both Red and White clover are consumed raw or as a potherb. The dried-out leaves of White clover pass on a vanilla flavour to cakes and other foods.

HARVEST
When in flower.

MEDICINAL PROPERTIES
Anti-inflammatory, hepatoprotective, oestrogenic and anticancerogenic.

ACTIVE CONSTITUENTS
Isoflavones, coumarins, flavonoids, phenolic acids, essential oils, polysaccharides.

herb be boiled and used as a clyster (enema). If the herb be made into a poultice, and applied to inflammations, it will ease them.'

Fray's Golden Recipes for the Use of All Ages (dated 1897) described Red clover as: *'A recipe worth a fortune – In ten cases of cancer this simple remedy has failed in none. Red clover tops are to be used in the manner of tea. This unpretentious plant cannot be urged on the public too strongly for its wonderful power and direct action over a cancer or for any cutaneous affection.'*

In the 1930s Red clover was still used as a cancer treatment; the blossoms, combined with other herbs, became commercially popular in the USA and numerous so-called Trifolium Compounds were marketed as blood purifiers, or alteratives, to help clear the body of metabolic toxins. The herb was listed in the National Formulary of the United States until 1946.

MODERN RESEARCH

Generally, Red clover is the preferred herb for medicinal use, but a 2012 study showed extracts obtained from several clovers and not just Red, have been shown to possess various properties as follows:

Anti-inflammatory

As Culpeper correctly said, Clover is anti-inflammatory and has traditionally been considered an alterative herb and mild lymphatic to clear the body of toxins. The anti-inflammatory effect of both Red and White clovers is related to the high content of isoflavones, which can help reduce inflammation and have been traditionally used to manage conditions like psoriasis, eczema and other inflammatory skin problems.

Hepatoprotective

It's quite easy to overlook White clover, but a 2019 study of the extract of its leaves was analysed and administered to mice to counter hepatoxicity (liver injury). The extract was found to be rich in phenolic compounds and shown to normalise liver functions. This may explain why, in Iran, the aerial parts of White clover are still used to treat neonatal jaundice (Tahvilian et al., 2014).

Oestrogenic

Red clover is also valued in the alleviation of menopausal symptoms, again owing to its isoflavones, including genistein and daidzein, which are a type of phytoestrogen that can mimic oestrogen in the body. A 2012 clinical trial was conducted on 72 menopausal women and demonstrated that these isoflavones reduced menopausal symptoms. A further 2015 clinical trial then studied the supplementation of 50mg of Rimostil (a Red clover commercial product) for two years in 189 menopausal women. Results showed significant improvement in premenstrual syndrome symptoms such as fatigue and swelling.

This was followed in 2017 by multiple studies on the use of 80mg a day of Red clover isoflavones to treat menopause, which showed a safe and clinically significant benefit to reducing hot flushes.

Anticancerogenic
Verifying the statements by Fray and the use back in the 1930s, a 2020 study to investigate the effects of Red clover and doxorubicin medication on breast cancer tumour-bearing mice showed that after 35 days the combination inhibited the proliferation of tumour cells. The interaction between Clover extracts and conventional anticancer agents therefore holds promise as a potential anticancer and antimetastatic supplement.

There is a lack of literature on the anticancer activities in White clover, but in 2020 its potential cytotoxicity was studied in lung cancer lines and chronic myeloid leukaemia cells by Sarno et al. The results reported that it blocked the proliferation of cancer cells and that the strong cytotoxic effects did not occur in normal cells, which suggests that the compounds in White clover might lead to the identification of new therapeutic agents active against cancers such as chronic myelogenous leukaemia.

TOPICAL USES
A 2006 study determined that Red clover isoflavones are effective in reducing skin ageing, while in a 2021 paper a combined extract made of *Ocimum basilicum* (Basil) and Red clover was used to demonstrate healing effect on skin pathologies. Results demonstrated the complete recovery of the skin layer when treated with the blend and improved wound contraction time and complete healing after 13 days of treatment. A clinical case of psoriasis was also treated with the same blend, and in one week of treatment there was significant improvement of the patient's health, leading to a conclusion that the topical use of the novel gel formulation containing Basil and Red clover is a successful therapeutic alternative in the treatment of dermal diseases.

DOSAGE
Tisane – 1tbsp/15g, 3 times per day.
Tincture – 5–10ml, 1:5 60% can be taken 3 times daily – 20 drops = 1ml/1tsp = 5ml.

PRECAUTIONS
No health hazards or side effects are known in conjunction with the proper administration of designated therapeutic dosages of clover. Not suitable for children or those who are pregnant or lactating.

Clover recipes

Medicinal recipes

Red clover tisane

Pour 250ml boiling water over 1tbsp/15g of the dried flowers and allow to steep for 10–15 minutes. Use for menopausal symptoms such as fatigue, hot flushes and inflammation.

Clover infused tincture 1:5 60%

If you are using 40% alcohol, ie. vodka, make a simple tincture by covering 1 part herb to 5 parts fluid.

If you are using Everclear or other 100% proof, use the following method for a specific tincture:

- 100g dried herb
- 300ml alcohol
- 200ml water

Take 100g of dried herb and split into two parts of 50g each. Place 50g in the alcohol and the other 50g in boiled water. Steep/infuse in the water for 10 minutes, strain and top up if the water is less than 200ml. Add the infusion to the alcohol mix and leave for 14 days before straining. Use for menopausal symptoms as above.

White clover iced tea

- 100g clover blossoms
- 1l water

Bring the water to the boil and then remove from the heat. Steep/infuse the blossoms in the water overnight, strain and serve over ice. Drink as an anti-inflammatory, as a boost for the immune system and a detoxifier.

Red clover blossom syrup

- 500ml tisane
- 500g sugar

Warm your tisane over a low heat and bring to a simmer. Then cover partially and reduce the liquid down to half its original volume, ie. 250ml. Add the sugar and stir constantly, but do not let the mix boil. Remove the syrup from the heat and allow to cool. If you are looking to preserve the syrup, add Red clover tincture at a ratio of 5%, otherwise syrups keep for up to two years unopened. If not adding tincture, after opening, store in the refrigerator and use within 1 month. A general dosage is a dessertspoon taken 1 to 3 times a day with increased frequency during an acute phase of symptoms.

COLTSFOOT
Tussilago farfara

Tussilago farfara, commonly known as Coltsfoot, is a native of the UK and is found in a variety of habitats, including damp woodlands, hedgerows, stream banks and waste areas. It is known for its distinctive yellow flowers, which emerge before the leaves, and has a long history of use in traditional herbal medicine, particularly for respiratory conditions.

HISTORICAL USES

The flower buds of Coltsfoot have been used for more than 2,000 years in China, for the treatment of coughs, phlegm, bronchial and asthmatic conditions. Coltsfoot is listed as a 'Middle grade' drug in the *Divine Farmer's Materia Medica* (Han Dynasty, 25–220AD), the oldest book on Chinese medicine. It was also recorded in books such as the *Compendium of Materia Medica* (Ming Dynasty), written by Li Shi Zhen, which extensively described the function of coltsfoot as a remedy for chronic cough and phlegm syndromes with blood.

In Europe the leaves of the plant were preferred, and John Gerard (1545–1612) recommended in his *Herball* that *'the fume of the dried leaves taken through a funnel, burned upon coals, effectually helpeth those that are troubled with the shortness of breath, and fetch*

ETYMOLOGY OF COMMON NAME
Named for the resemblance of the leaf to a colt's foot.

PLANT LORE
Coltsfoot's early blooming made it significant in springtime festivals and celebrations. It was sometimes included in rituals or offerings to welcome the arrival of spring and ensure good health.

USE
The leaves, flowers and root.

EDIBILITY
The flowers, stems and young leaves can be eaten raw or cooked. Coltsfoot flowers have a delicate aniseed flavour.

HARVEST
Flowers in spring and the leaves in summer.

MEDICINAL PROPERTIES
Antitussive.

ACTIVE CONSTITUENTS
Mucilage, tannins, flavonoids, polysaccharides, phenolic acids, pyrrolizidine alkaloids.

their wind thick and often, and breaketh without peril the impoſtumes [abscesses] *of the breaſt. Being taken in manner as they take Tobacco, it mightily prevaileth againſt the diseases aforesaid.'*

Nicholas Culpeper's *Herbal* stated that '*the fresh leaves, or juice, or syrup thereof, is good for a bad dry cough, or wheezing and shortness of breath. The dry leaves are beſt for those who have their rheums and diſtillations upon their lungs causing a cough: for which also the dried leaves taken as tobacco, or the root is very good.'*

British herbalist R.L. Hool, author of *Common Plants and Their Uses in Medicine* (1922), wrote of Coltsfoot:

> In all affeƈtions of the lungs and other organs conneƈted with them, its sanative and cleansing influence will be found highly beneficial. The Coltsfoot, being mucilaginous, soothes all the mucous surfaces that it comes in contaƈt with, through the blood and absorbent vessels, and by that means allays the inflammation of the lungs and bronchial tubes.

MODERN RESEARCH INTO THE ANTI-TUSSIVE EFFECTS

All of the above historical uses have been confirmed in modern research, with a 2013 study of the compounds verifying that both the leaves and flower buds contain caffeoylquinic acids, flavonoids and mucilage, which are thought to be responsible for its antitussive effects. These compounds exert their action by inhibiting airway inflammation, reducing sputum or directly relieving coughs.

Unfortunately, this plant has recently been implicated in safety issues owing to the presence of pyrrolizidine alkaloids. A report to the National Institute of Medical Herbalists (NIMH) in September 2018, however, found little human evidence of harm with the arguments in the literature extrapolated from two sources: evidence from human exposure to other plant species (not Coltsfoot) that contain pyrrolizidine alkaloids or evidence from animal studies, often utilising pyrrolizidine alkaloids that are not found in Coltsfoot.

A further NIMH review in 2020 concluded that: '*Based on these case reports, the evidence of harm caused by these plants is weak. These cases are up to thirty years old and insufficient detail and inconsiſtent information make it difficult for clear assessments of causality; nor is it possible to make such judgements with insufficient information about concomitant medication and without full relevant medical hiſtory.*' As with Comfrey, a risk/benefit analysis should be made before use and the potential benefits weighed against the risks and the weakness of the evidence, including dietary and supplementary recommendations to support protective liver function during treatment.

A 2020 study to investigate the mechanism of Coltsfoot flower bud

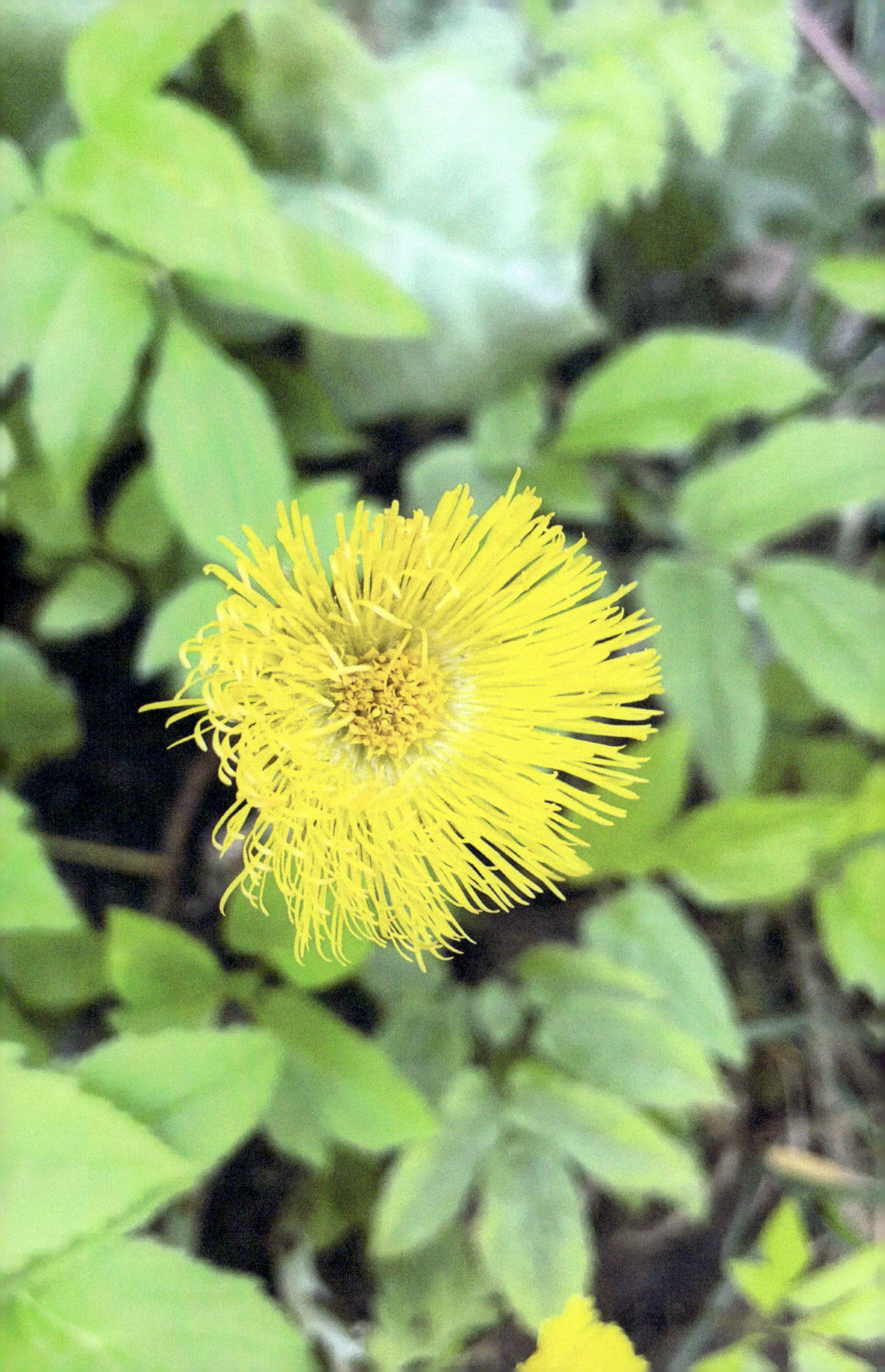

decoction against coronavirus disease (COVID-19) found that the compounds in the flowers can bind with SARS CoV-2 3CL hydrolase and ACE2, and exert a therapeutic effect on COVID-19.

TOPICAL USES

Coltsfoot flowers are also used in making a poultice or balm, which is applied for relief from skin complaints, such as eczema, sores, inflammations and even ulcers, while the fresh leaves of Coltsfoot are reported to be used in the Balkans region for the treatment of wound-healing (Jarić et al., 2018).

DOSAGE

Tisane – ½ tsp/2.5g, 3 times per day.
Tincture – 1:5 45%. 2–8ml – 20 drops = 1ml/1tsp = 5ml.

The total daily dose is 4.5–6gm of drug.

PRECAUTIONS

These plants should be avoided in individuals with liver conditions. Not suitable for children or those who are pregnant or lactating.

Coltsfoot recipes

Medicinal recipes

Coltsfoot tisane

Pour 250ml boiling water over ½tsp/5g of the dried leaf and allow to steep for 10-15 minutes. Drink this three times a day, as hot as possible for respiratory conditions, gout, flu, colds and fever. NB please note precautions regarding pyrrolizidine alkaloids.

Coltsfoot infused tincture: 1:5 45%

If you are using 40% alcohol, ie. vodka, make a simple tincture by covering 1 part herb to 5 parts fluid.

If you are using Everclear or other 100% proof, use the following method for a specific tincture:

- 100g dried herb
- 225ml alcohol
- 275ml water

Take 100g of the dried herb and split into two parts of 50g each. Place 50g in 225ml alcohol. Take the other 50g part and place in 275ml of boiled water. Steep/infuse in the water for 10 minutes. Strain thoroughly and top up if the water is less than 275ml. Add the infusion to the alcohol mix and leave for 14 days before straining. Useful for people with chronic coughs, such as those arising in emphysema or silicosis.

Coltsfoot steam

- 1tbsp/15g dried leaves and flowers
- 500ml boiling water

Add the flowers to a bowl and cover with the water. Cover the head with a towel and inhale the vapour.

Herbal cough syrup

- 1 part Coltsfoot leaves
- 1 part Lungwort
- 1 part Ribwort plantain
- 500g sugar

Bring the water to the boil and place the herbs in it for 10 minutes. Remove the herbs and place them in the jar that you intend to keep the syrup in. Now bring the remaining liquid back to a boil and dissolve the sugar in the water until it becomes syrupy. Pour the syrup over the herbs and then leave in the fridge for a few days before straining. Pour into air-tight jars and store in a cool place. Use for coughs in doses of 1-2tsp at a time.

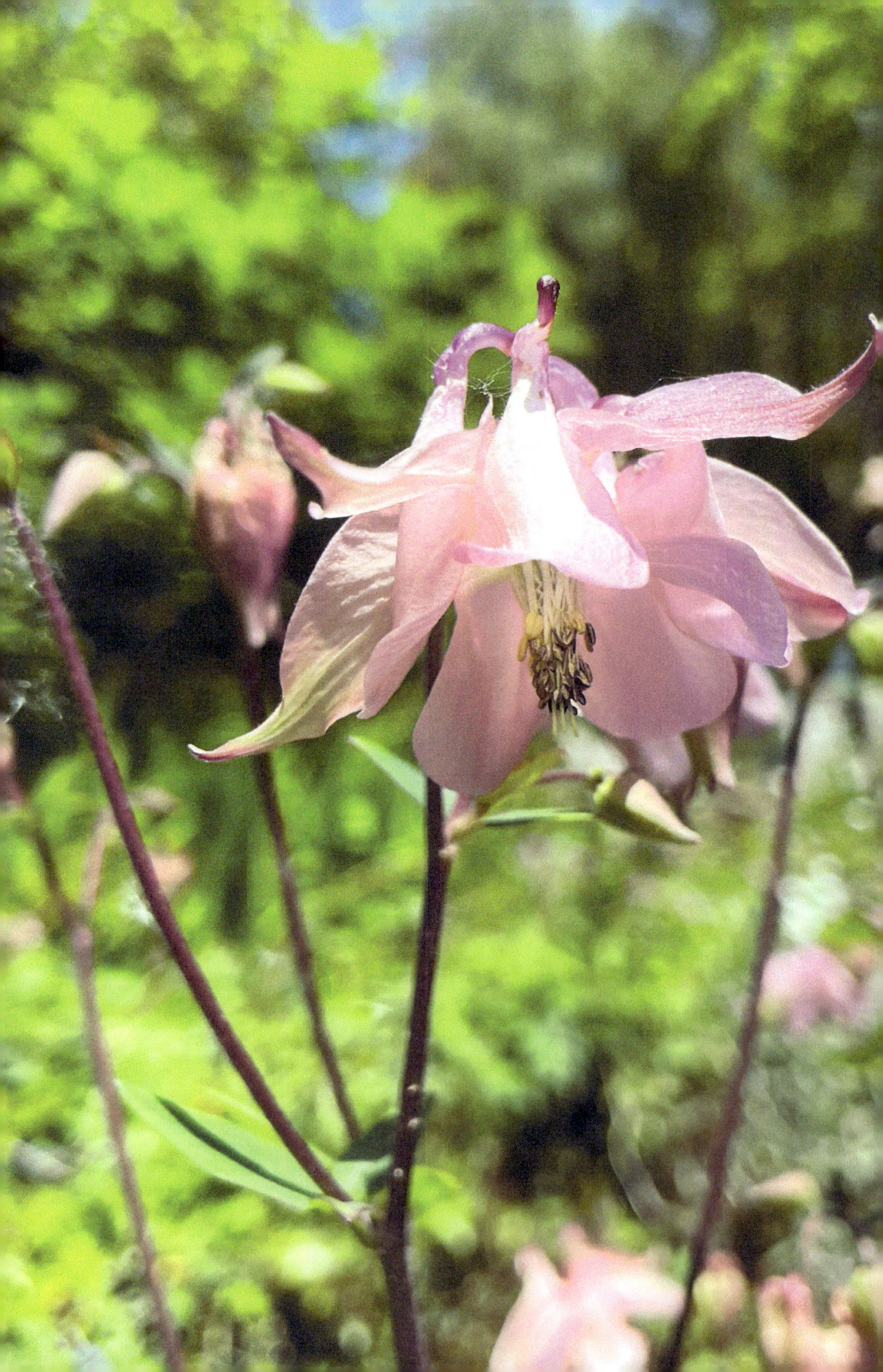

COLUMBINE
Aquilegia vulgaris

Aquilegia vulgaris, commonly known as Columbine, is native to the UK and can be found growing in woodlands, meadows, hedgerows and rocky areas. All parts of the Columbine plant contain toxic compounds, including alkaloids and glycosides, which can cause mild to moderate toxicity if ingested. Despite this toxicity, Columbine has been employed in traditional herbal medicine.

HISTORICAL USES

The crushed seeds of Columbine have been used for centuries by the indigenous populations of North America to treat skin conditions.

John Gerard (1545–1612) related in his *Herball* that the herbalist Clusius '*saith, that Dr Francis Rapard a physician of Bruges in Flanders, told him that the seed of common Columbine very finely beaten to powder, and given in wine, was a singular medicine to be given to women to hasten and facilitate their labour, and if the first taking were not sufficiently effectual, that then they should repeat it again.*'

Nicholas Culpeper wrote in his *Herbal* that '*the leaves are successfully used in lotions for sore mouths and throats … a dram of the seed taken in wine with a little saffron, opens obstructions of the liver, and is good for the yellow jaundice,*

ETYMOLOGY OF COMMON NAME
From medieval Latin *colombina*, for the supposed resemblance of the flower to a cluster of five doves.

PLANT LORE
Columbine was associated with Freya in Norse mythology and was also a symbol for Aphrodite, the goddess of love, in ancient Greece.

USE
The leaves, root and seeds.

EDIBILITY
The plant is often thought of as poisonous, but many leaves must be consumed for there to be ill effects. Drying the plant also eliminates any danger.

HARVEST
In May and June.

MEDICINAL PROPERTIES
Astringent, antimicrobial, anticonvulsant, anti-inflammatory and hepatoprotective.

ACTIVE CONSTITUENTS
Flavonoids, tannins, coumarins, phenolic acids, terpenoids, alkaloids, polysaccharides and essential oils.

LEFT: COLUMBINE

if the party after the taking thereof be laid to sweat well in bed.'

Culpeper also repeats the previous recommendation that *'The seed also taken in wine causes a speedy delivery of women in childbirth: if one draught suffice not, let her drink the second, and it will be effectual.'*

MODERN RESEARCH

As Culpeper stated, Columbine has long been used been used in folk medicine against liver and bile duct disorders, owing to the following properties:

Hepatoprotective

In 2009, a study was undertaken to evaluate the protective effects of Columbine on liver damage. Results demonstrated that the extract reduced the effects of liver damage by restoring the activity of some antioxidant enzymes and by inhibiting microsomal lipid peroxidation. A 2010 study then confirmed these protective effects, and again concluded that an increase in the antioxidant capacity and inhibition of lipid peroxidation was responsible.

Astringent

While I have not been able to verify Gerard and Culpeper's recommendation for inducement of labour, herbs with astringent properties have traditionally been used for stimulating uterine contractions during labour, and the properties of Columbine as a coagulant and astringent can also help to reduce bleeding after delivery.

Also, Columbine is still used by herbal practitioners to lessen menstrual bleeding and reduce some of the discomfort and symptoms associated with menstruation.

Antimicrobial

The antimicrobial activity of Columbine has shown to be particularly high towards *Staphylococcus aureus*, *Staphylococcus epidermidis* and *Aspergillus niger*, fully justifying the use of Columbine in folk medicine for treatment of skin rashes and infections.

Anticonvulsant

In addition to the above, a decoction of the leaves and stems harvested when flowering has been used in folk medicine to treat agitation, which led to its use in cases of epilepsy. Studies found that the plant had anticonvulsant effects, and a further study identified the responsible compounds as myo-inositol and oleamide, which, when administered orally in high concentrations, can reach the central nervous system and exert their effects.

TOPICAL USE

A decoction made from the seeds has been used as hair shampoo to get rid of head lice and scabs.

DOSAGE

Tisane – 1tsp/5g, 3 times per day.

PRECAUTIONS

The leaves contain hydrocyanic acid, but toxicity is destroyed when the leaves are dried. Not suitable for children or those who are pregnant or lactating.

Columbine recipes

Medicinal recipes

Columbine tisane
Pour 250ml boiling water over 1tsp/5g of the dried herb and allow to steep for 10–15 minutes. It can be used as an astringent and antidiarrhoeal 3–6 times a day.

Columbine compress
Soak a cloth in a tisane of the dried herb and use to soothe wounds and sore skin.

Columbine seed lice treatment
Seeds harvested in the autumn can be dried and powdered for use as a hair lice treatment paste when mixed with a small amount of water.

Columbine poultice
- 1tsp fresh leaves (if using dried, moisten with hot water)
- 2tsp coconut oil
- cheesecloth or cotton bandage

Finely chop the herb and add the coconut oil to make a paste. Spread the mix onto a clean cloth or piece of gauze. Fold the cloth or gauze over the herbs to form a small packet and place the poultice directly onto the affected skin area. Ensure that the herb paste is in contact with the skin and secure the poultice in place with a bandage, wrap or medical tape to keep it from moving. Use for sores, wounds and insect bites. Note: Discontinue use if skin irritation occurs.

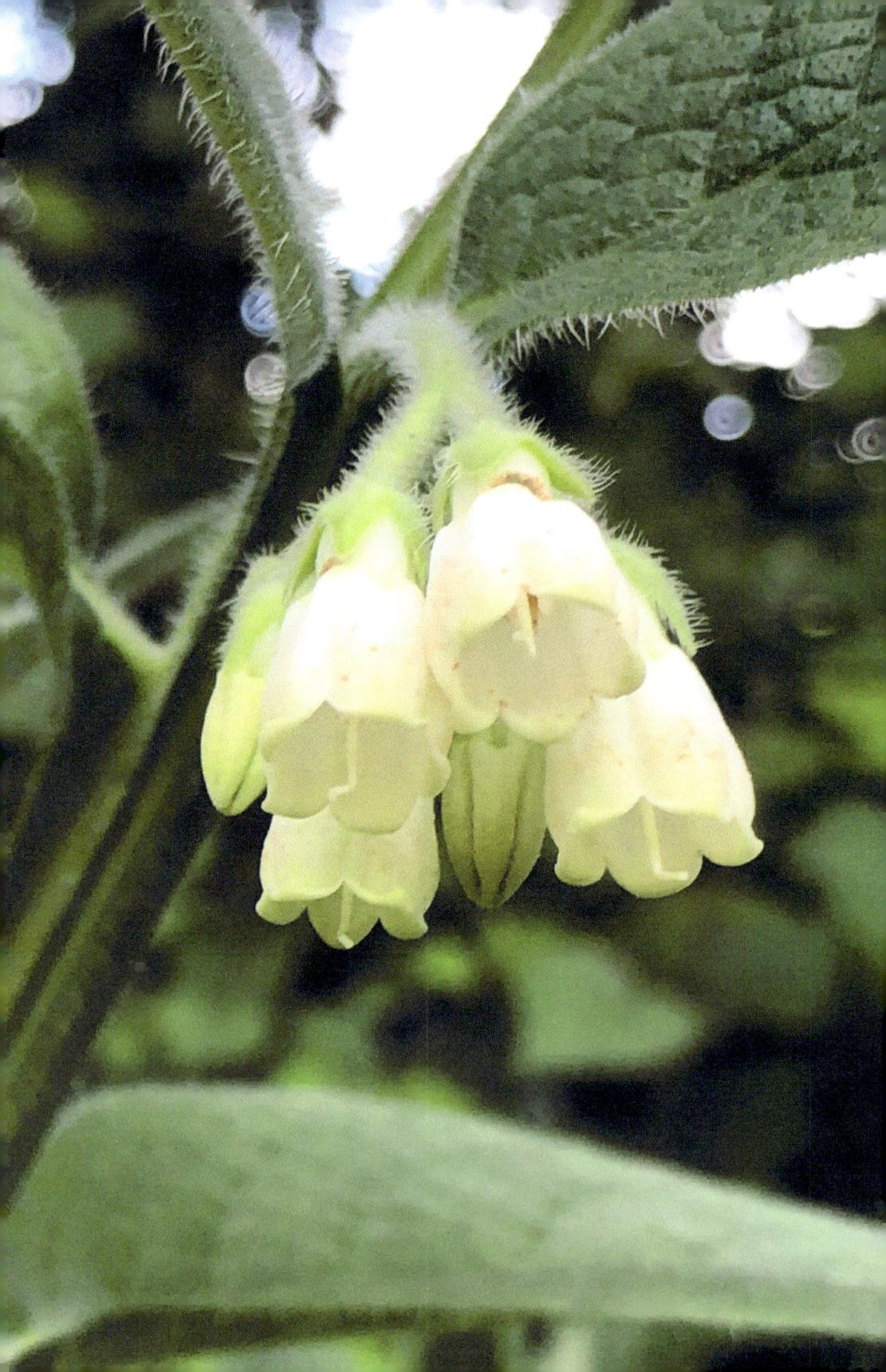

COMFREY
Symphytum officinale

Symphytum officinale, commonly known as Comfrey, is a perennial herb native to the UK. It belongs to the *Boraginaceae* family and has a long history of use in traditional herbal medicine. It is also valued in permaculture and organic gardening practices for its deep roots, which help break up compacted soil and leaves; these can be chopped up and used as a nutrient-rich mulch or added to compost piles to acceleratede composition.

HISTORICAL USES

In his *Naturalis Historia*, Pliny, the 1st-century Roman author, naturalist and natural philosopher, recommended, '*a syrup of the herb or a decoction of its Root for the treatment of bruises and sprains.*'

Another 1st-century author, Dioscorides, mentioned Comfrey in his *De Materia Medica*, with the words '*The roots below are black on the outside and white and slimy on the inside ... Finely ground and then drunk they are beneficial for those spitting blood and those suffering from internal abscesses. Used as a compress they also seal fresh wounds. They have a joining together effect when cooked with pieces of flesh.*'

John Gerard (1545–1612) confirmed this in his *Herball* '*A salve concocted from the fresh herb will certainly tend to*

ETYMOLOGY OF COMMON NAME
From the Latin *confirmare*, meaning to join together, after its traditional folk use to speed the healing of fractures, broken bones, bruises and burns.

PLANT LORE
Comfrey was believed to be a traveller's aide. Many nomadic peoples put it their shoes to avoid blisters.

USE
The root and leaves.

EDIBILITY
Not recommended for eating.

HARVEST
In summer.

MEDICINAL PROPERTIES
Anti-inflammatory, vulnerary, analgesic.

ACTIVE CONSTITUENTS
Aallantoin, mucilage, tannins, rosmarinic acid, phenolic acids, alkaloids, polysaccharides, essential oils.

LEFT: COMFREY

promote the healing of bruised and broken parts.'

Nicholas Culpeper, meanwhile wrote in his *Herbal* '*It is said to be so powerful to knit together; that if they be boyled with dissevered pieces of flesh in a pot, it will join them together again, and a Syrup made thereof is very effectual for all those inward Griefs and Hurts ... and for outward Wounds and Sores in the Fleshy or Sinewy part of the Body whatsoever ... A Decoction of the Leaves hereof is available to all the purposes, though not so effectual as the Roots.*'

In 1855, American herbalist Albert Isaiah Coffin wrote that the root of the plant is also '*a good tonic medicine and acts friendly on the Stomach; very useful in cases where, from maltreatment, the mouth, the throat and stomach have become sore.*'

MODERN RESEARCH

As you would expect from a plant that has been extensively used throughout history, there has been much research on this herb and it has found the following properties attributed to Comfrey:

Vulnerary, anti-inflammatory and analgesic

Comfrey, as can be seen from the historical writers, is mainly celebrated for its wound-healing effects, and a number of studies and clinical trials have shown that it works significantly better than a placebo, with five times the pain reduction and four times improvement in quality of life. (Talhouk et al., 2007 [1]; Neagu et al., 2011 [2]; Gokadze et al., 2013 [3]). Comfrey has also proven effective for the treatment of acute upper and lower back pain, osteoarthritis and blunt injuries (Koll et al., 2004; Predel et al., 2005; Grube et al., 2007; Giannetti et al., 2010).

However, like Coltsfoot, Comfrey has received bad press in recent years since it is said to contain pyrrolizidine alkaloids, particularly echimidine, though a report to the National Institute of Medical Herbalists (NIMH) in September 2018 found little evidence of human harm in *Symphytum officinale*, which rarely contains echimidine. The report concluded that when consideration is given to the use of these plants, a risk/benefit analysis should be made before use and the potential benefits weighed against the potential risks. If you are to use Comfrey internally, it should be the *officinale* species only along with with time limits and dietary and supplementary support for the liver during treatment.

A further NIMH review in 2020 concluded that: '*Based on these case reports, the evidence of harm caused by these plants is weak. These cases are up to thirty years old. Insufficient detail and inconsistent information make it difficult for clear assessments of causality; nor is it possible to make such judgements with insufficient information about concomitant medication and without full relevant medical history.*'

A 2019 study investigated the anti-inflammatory properties of a hydroalcoholic Comfrey root extract in an *in vitro* model of inflammation, and results confirmed that the extract does exert anti-inflammatory properties *in vitro*, substantiating the beneficial effects observed in animal and clinical studies.

It is important when using Comfrey to look for Common comfrey, *Symphytum officinale*, rather than the more poisonous Prickly comfrey (*Symphytum asperum*) or Russian comfrey (*Symphytum* x *uplandicum*) species. The Common comfrey tends to have cream or pale pink flowers whereas the other two are a darker blue or violet.

TOPICAL USES

Multiple randomised controlled trials have demonstrated the efficacy and safety of Comfrey preparations for the topical treatment of pain, inflammation and swelling of muscles and joints in degenerative arthritis, acute myalgia in the back, sprains, contusions and strains after sports injuries and accidents, also in children aged 3 or 4 and over.

DOSAGE

Tisane – 1tsp/5g, 3 times per day for no more than 8 weeks a year.
Tincture (leaf) – 1:5 50% – dose 2.5–5ml. Maximum weekly dosage – 100ml for no more than 8 weeks.
Tincture (root) – 1:5 50% – Maximum weekly dosage – 80ml, for 8 weeks.

PRECAUTIONS

Comfrey is such an excellent and speedy wound-healing remedy that it should not be used on deep wounds or lacerations. It could potentially heal the top layer of skin before the bottom layer, resulting in an abscess. If using internally, see above dosages and time limits.

Comfrey recipes

Medicinal recipes

Comfrey root decoction

- 1tsp/5g root
- 250ml water

Use the dried root and break it up or grind it down to powder. Bring the water to a gentle boil, add the root, reduce the heat and simmer for 20–40 minutes. Remove from the heat and allow to cool before straining. Serve cold or reheat when ready, adding additional water and sweetener to taste.

Comfrey leaf infused tincture – 1:5 50%

If you are using 40% alcohol, ie. vodka, make a simple tincture by covering 1 part herb to 5 parts fluid.

If you are using Everclear or other 100% proof, use the following method for a specific tincture:

- 100g Comfrey leaf
- 250ml alcohol
- 25ml water

Take 100g of dried herb and split into two parts of 50g each. Place the first 50g in the alcohol and the other 50g in the boiled water. Steep/infuse in the water for 10 minutes. Strain thoroughly and top up if the water is less than 250ml. Add the infusion to the alcohol mix and leave for 14 days before straining.

Comfrey root decocted tincture – 1:5 50%

- 100g Comfrey root
- 250ml alcohol
- 25ml water

Take 100g of dried herb and split into two parts of 50g each. Place the first 50g in the alcohol. Take the other 50g part and place in the boiled water. Simmer the water and root for 20 minutes. Strain thoroughly and top up if the water is less than 250ml. Add the infusion to the alcohol mix and leave for 14 days before straining.

All of the above can be used for ulceration anywhere along the gastrointestinal tract, colitis, hiatus hernia, bleeding from stomach, throat, bowel, bladder and lungs. They can also be used to promote formation of a callus in fractures and for varicose ulcers and wounds that refuse to heal. However, if using Comfrey internally, please undertake a risk/benefit analysis as described in the preceding chapter, use supplements to support protective liver function during treatment and observe the dosages and time limits provided.

Comfrey salve

- 100g mixed powdered Comfrey root and leaf
- 2tbsp alcohol, such as Everclear
- 1l grapeseed oil

Roughly chop the root and leaf and place in the bottom of a jar with the Everclear. Allow to steep for 10 minutes and then add the oil. Infuse in a warm oven (75–100°) for 3–4 hours. Once infused, strain and make into a tincture infused salve as follows:

Use 80ml oil and 20ml tincture, then apply a 1:4 ratio of melted beeswax to your tincture/oil mix, ie. 1 part wax to 4 parts liquid. Weigh or measure out the wax pellets and place them with the herbal infused oil in a double boiler or bain-marie. Heat over a low heat until the wax is fully melted and then stir well. This is the time to slowly add your tincture to the mix, whisking it lightly as you do. Remove from the heat and allow to cool and set completely before using for healing burns, skin ulcerations, abrasions, lacerations, insect bites and any skin irritation plus fractures. Few other medicinal plants replenish wasted bone cells with the speed of Comfrey. See precautions.

Comfrey poultice

- 1tsp fresh Comfrey leaves (if using dried, moisten with hot water)
- 2tsp coconut oil
- cheesecloth or cotton bandage

Finely chop the herb and add the coconut oil to make a paste. Spread the mix onto a clean cloth or piece of gauze. Fold the cloth or gauze over the herbs to form a small packet and place the poultice directly onto the affected skin area. Ensure that the herb paste is in contact with the skin and secure the poultice in place with a bandage, wrap or medical tape to keep it from moving. Use to speed the healing of wounds, bruises, sprains and fractures. Note: Discontinue use if skin irritation occurs.

COW PARSLEY
Anthriscus sylvestris

Anthriscus forms a genus of plants in the *Apiaceae* family, commonly known as the umbellifers or Carrot family. In the UK, the most well-known species of *Anthriscus* is *Anthriscus sylvestris*, Cow parsley or Wild chervil. This is not to be confused with *Anthriscus cerefolium* or French Parsley which is also known as Chervil. It is found in a variety of habitats, including woodlands, hedgerows, grasslands, meadows and roadside verges.

HISTORICAL USES

Hildegard of Bingen (1098–1179) advised in *Physica* that Chervil, '*heals broken wounds of the bowels*' but also that a person should eat Chervil if evil humours of foods '*rise to the spleen, causing pain there.*' It is possible that Hildegard is not referring to Wild chervil here but rather *Anthriscus cerefolium*, particularly as it was a herb commonly grown in monastery and abbey gardens.

Nevertheless the aerial parts of Cow parsley were traditionally used in Ireland and Tunisia to treat headaches and in Serbia as a diuretic and tonic. In Asia, the roots have traditionally been used for fever-reducing and pain-relieving, as a diuretic and a cough remedy. In India, the plant is still used by the indigenous communities to treat

ETYMOLOGY OF COMMON NAME
Cow parsley, a rather dismissive name, is an inferior version of Garden parsley; the name wild chervil is sometimes used, with its origin in Ancient Greek *chairephyllon*, meaning 'leaves of joy'.

PLANT LORE
Folklore has it that Cow parsley makes one merry, sharpens the wit, bestows youth upon the aged and symbolises sincerity.

USE
All parts.

EDIBILITY
Leaves can be eaten raw or used as a pot herb.

HARVEST
Spring and summer.

MEDICINAL PROPERTIES
Digestive, tonic, antibacterial, anti-inflammatory, analgesic and anticancerogenic.

ACTIVE CONSTITUENTS
Coumarins, flavonoids, phenolic acids, triterpenes, carotenoids, essential oils, polysaccharides.

LEFT: COW PARSLEY

rheumatism and other inflammatory ailments.

Nicholas Culpeper's *Herbal* wrote, '*The wild chervil bruised and applied, dissolveth swellings in any part, or the marks of congealed blood by bruises or blows in a little space.*'

MODERN RESEARCH

Research has found the following properties attributed to Cow parsley:

Digestive and tonic

Cow parsley contains terpenoid compounds that have carminative properties, such as limonene, α-pinene and myristicin. An infusion of fresh leaves can settle the stomach and may be why it eases the pricking in the sides, or a stitch as we would call it, described by Culpeper as 'pricking' and the evil humours described by Hildegard. It is also used as a spring tonic that lifts the spirits. as it is rich in vitamins and minerals, including vitamin C, vitamin A, vitamin K, potassium and iron.

Diuretic

Cow parsley, when taken as an herbal tisane, reduces cellulitis and fluid retention. This can be beneficial for conditions such as hypertension (high blood pressure) and oedema (swelling caused by fluid retention).

Anti-inflammatory and analgesic

The analgesic and anti-inflammatory activity of Cow parsley has been shown to be because of deoxypodophyllotoxin, a potent anti-inflammatory lignan contained largely in the root. A 2015 study showed that the activity of deoxypodophyllotoxin was stronger than that of the drugs prednisolone and indomethacin, suggesting that it may be beneficial in regulating allergic reactions.

The effects of Cow parsley on respiratory diseases were investigated further in 2021 and were found, when combined with a mixture of Mulberry tree twigs and Mexican sage, to improve asthma and cough symptoms by reducing inflammation.

A 2022 investigation into the efficacy of Cow parsley in paw oedema confirmed that the leaves were effective in alleviating inflammation and improving joints.

Anticancerogenic

It has also been shown that deoxypodophyllotoxin might be used to synthesise epipodophyllotoxin, the starting material for anticancer drugs such as etoposide and teniposide. Its ability to grow rapidly and in almost any type of soil makes Cow parsley a highly valuable source of both lignan and flavonoid compounds.

TOPICAL USES

Cow parsley leaves are also beneficial for suppurative and inflammatory skin conditions such as eczema, psoriasis, systemic lupus erythematosus and acne. In respect of its effectiveness in skin treatments, this herb is also used in creams for haemorrhoids and varicose veins.

DOSAGE

Tisane – ½ tsp/2.5g, 3 times per day.

PRECAUTIONS

Cow parsley has been known to cause skin irritations in some people. Not suitable for children or those who are pregnant or lactating.

Caution – this plant can be confused with the highly poisonous Hemlock, *Conium maculatum*.

Cow parsley recipes

Medicinal recipes

Cow parsley tisane

Pour 250ml boiling water over ½tsp/2.5g of the dried leaf and allow to steep for 15 minutes. Use to aid digestion and relieve gas and bloating, but also to improve blood circulation and reduce cellulitis and fluid retention.

Cow parsley infused oil

- 100g dried and powdered plant
- 2tbsp Everclear
- 1l grapeseed oil

Place the herbs in a jar with the alcohol and allow to steep for 10 minutes before adding the oil. Leave for 4 weeks and then strain. Make into a salve by using a 1:3 ratio of melted beeswax to oil. Apply externally for the treatment of skin irritations, eczema, wounds and abscesses.

Cow parsley poultice

- 1tsp fresh leaves (if using dried, moisten with hot water)
- 2tsp coconut oil
- cheesecloth or cotton bandage

Finely chop the herb and add the coconut oil to make a paste. Spread the mix onto a clean cloth or piece of gauze. Fold the cloth or gauze over the herbs to form a small packet and place the poultice directly onto the affected skin area. Ensure that the herb paste is in contact with the skin and secure the poultice in place with a bandage, wrap or medical tape to keep it from moving. Use to help soothe skin irritations, insect bites and minor wounds. Note: Discontinue use if skin irritation occurs.

Cow parsley compress

Use to help relieve joint pain and inflammation. Soak a cloth in a tisane of the dried leaves and apply it to the affected areas 2–3 times a day.

COWSLIP
Primula veris

Primula veris, commonly known as Cowslip, is native to the UK and a member of the Primrose family, *Primulaceae*. It is related to the Primrose and can be found growing in various habitats, including meadows, grasslands, woodland edges and hedgerows.

HISTORICAL USES

John Gerard described in his *Herball* of an unguent made with the juice of Cowslips and oil of linseed, which *'cureth all scaldings or burnings with fire, water, or otherwise.'*

Nicholas Culpeper's *Herbal* also recommended an ointment made with the flowers, which *'taketh away spots and wrinkles of the skin, sunburn, and freckles, and remedy all infirmities of the head coming of heat and wind, as vertigo, ephialtes* [nightmares]*, false apparitions, phrenzies, falling-sickness, palsies, convulsions, cramps, and pain in the nerves.'* He also says that the roots ease pains in the back and bladder and open the passage of urine.

MODERN RESEARCH

Cowslips are in decline in the wild, and this should be borne in mind if using this plant. Modern research of Cowslip has confirmed the following uses:

ETYMOLOGY OF COMMON NAME
A distorted pronunciation of 'cow slop', so named because the flowers were believed to grow near cow pats in meadows and fields.

PLANT LORE
Cowslips have been called 'keys of heaven' because the flowers look like a set of keys.

USE
Leaves and flowers.

EDIBILITY
Young Cowslip leaves were at one time eaten in country salads and mixed with other herbs to stuff meat and flavour soups, while the flowers were made into a delicate conserve.

HARVEST
In spring.

MEDICINAL PROPERTIES
Sedative, antispasmodic, antimicrobial, anti-inflammatory, analgesic, cardioprotective and expectorant.

ACTIVE CONSTITUENTS
Flavonoids, saponins, phenolic glycosides, triterpenes, polysaccharides, carotenoids, mucilage, essential oils.

Sedative and anxiolytic

Cowslip has been traditionally used for its sedative properties, and recent scientific studies support this. In 2013, Zielińska-Pisklak et al. highlighted the sedative effects, which were believed to arise from bioactive compounds such as flavonoids and saponins. These are known to have calming effects, and may be why Culpeper recommended the plant for 'infirmities of the head' such as vertigo, ephialtes (anxiety), phrenzies (hysteria), falling-sickness (epilepsy), palsies, convulsions, etc.

Expectorant

According to the European Medicines Agency (EMA), Cowslip flowers and roots are used against coughs, bronchitis and catarrhs of the respiratory tract. In 2022, studies provided conclusive evidence that Cowslips can be used as an expectorant medicine and that triterpene saponins are the main active ingredients responsible for these bioactivities.

Antimicrobial

These triterpene saponins also have antibacterial activity, and in a 2014 study the extracts showed inhibitory effect against both gram-positive and gram-negative microorganisms at varying degrees and also contain constituents that can stop mitosis (cell division) in any part of the cell cycle.

In 2021, these inhibitory effects were also shown against human pathogenic yeasts (*Candida albicans*, *Candida parapsilosis*, *Candida glabrata*) and bacteria such as *Pseudomonas aeruginosa*, *Enterococcus faecalis* and *Staphylococcus aureus* (Erzsébet et al., 2021). This would make sense of Culpeper's remedy for the skin.

Returning to the EMA comments on Cowslip's respiratory illness, the leaves and flower extracts have shown to be active against *Mycobacterium tuberculosis*; extracts caused a 41% inhibition of the bacteria (Tosun et al., 2005).

A 2022 investigation into anti-influenza activity showed Cowslip to have virucidal properties, which confer prophylactic and therapeutic effects against the flu virus *in vitro*. The authors asserted that combining Cowslip with extracts of medicinal plants with proven anti-influenza activity such as Echinacea and Cretan rockrose could achieve an impressive protective effect against infection by the influenza virus.

Anti-inflammatory and analgesic

In 2017, the anti-inflammatory effects of Cowslip leaves and roots were investigated and proven in rat paw oedema. The most desirable action of both types of extracts was at the dose level 200mg/kg, and extract of the leaves possessed the most effect, owing to the phenolic content. This may be why it was suggested for headaches and other pains by the historical writers.

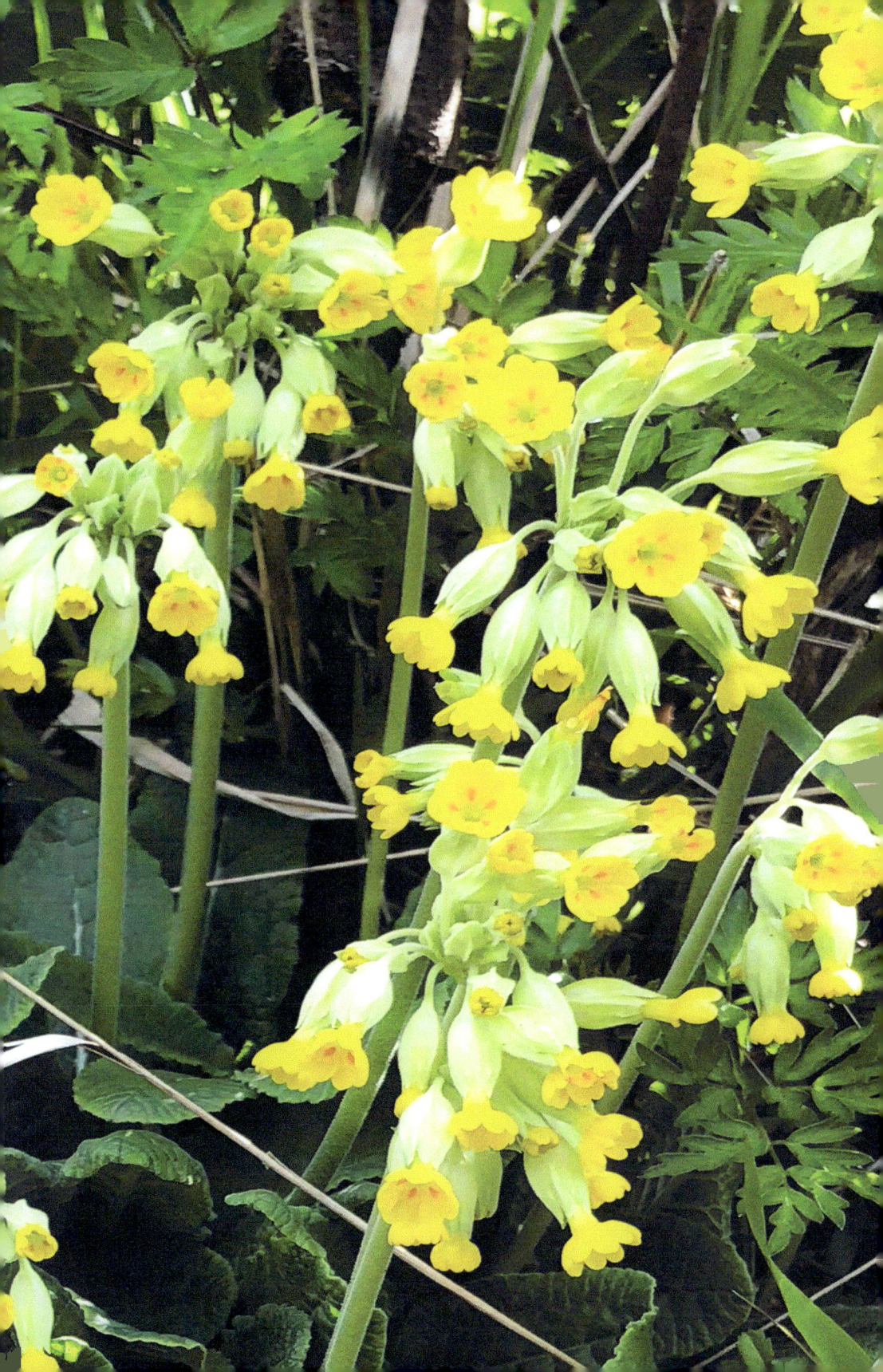

Cardioprotective

A 2019 study investigated the composition of Cowslip herbal extract and its effects on the myocardial contractile function in animals with chronic heart failure. The extract was found to contain flavonoid aglycons, flavonoid glycosides and polyethoxylated flavonoids, which demonstrated a cardioprotective effect by increasing the contractions of the heart.

TOPICAL USE

Since Culpeper's time, herbalists have been recommending Cowslip flower water as a lotion for treating skin complaints. The petals of the flower have astringent properties and the essential oil is applied externally to the skin to prevent wounds and infection and to treat bruises.

DOSAGE

Tisane – 2tsp/10g, 3 times per day.

PRECAUTIONS

Cowslip should never be given to patients who are taking anti-coagulant medications like warfarin or who are sensitive to aspirin. Has hypertensive effects. Not suitable for children or those who are pregnant or lactating.

Cowslip recipes

Medicinal recipes

Cowslip tisane
Pour 250ml boiling water over 1tsp/5g of the dried flowers and allow to steep for 10–15 minutes. Use as an expectorant, mild sedative and anti-inflammatory.

Cowslip root decoction
Add 2tsp to 250ml of water and bring to a gentle boil, reduce heat and simmer for 20–40 minutes. Remove from the heat and allow to cool before straining. Use as an anti-inflammatory for sciatica and rheumatism.

Cowslip cough syrup
- 1 cup fresh Cowslip flowers (or ½ cup dried Cowslip flowers)
- 1 cup raw honey
- 1 cup water

If using fresh Cowslip flowers, ensure they are clean and free from any dirt or insects.

Bring the water to a boil in a saucepan and add the Cowslip flowers. Reduce the heat and let it simmer for 10–15 minutes. Remove the saucepan from the heat and strain the mixture to remove the flowers, then return the liquid to the pan and add the honey. Heat the mixture gently, stirring until the honey is dissolved. Do not let the mixture boil. Remove from the heat and allow to cool before transferring to sterilised bottles or jars. The syrup will keep in the fridge for up to two months. Take 1–2tsp up to 3 times per day to help with coughs and alleviate respiratory symptoms.

Cowslip compress
Use to help relieve joint pain and inflammation. Soak a cloth in a tisane of the dried flowers and apply it to the affected areas 2–3 times a day.

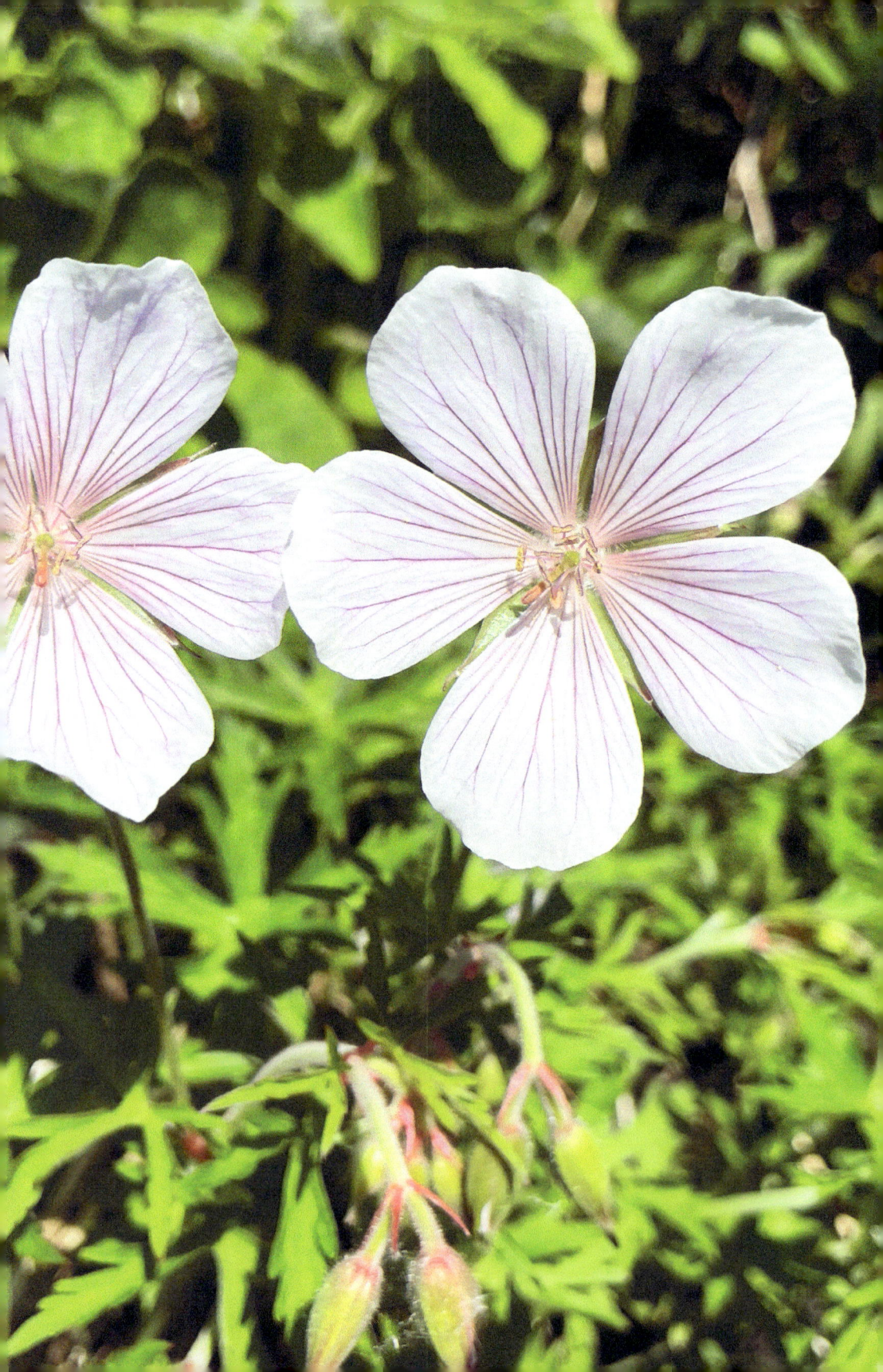

CRANESBILL
Geranium spp.

The UK is home to several native species of Wild geraniums, also known as Cranesbills, including the Wood cranesbill (*Geranium sylvaticum*), Meadow cranesbill (Geranium *pratense*), Dove's-foot cranesbill (*Geranium molle*) and Herb Robert, which has its own chapter in this book.

HISTORICAL USES

Early Native Americans recognised the value of Wild geranium. It was used by the Cherokee, Choctaw, Haudenosaunee, Menominee, Meskwaki and Ojibwa for medicinal purposes, including for relief from a sore mouth, as a laxative, an antiseptic and an emetic.

Nicholas Culpeper wrote in his *Herbal*, 'crane's-bill or dove's foot, is reckoned among the number of vulnerary plants, being useful in inward wounds bruises, and haemorrhages, and all fluxes in general. It is mightily commended for the cure of ruptures in children, given in powder. It likewise helps the stone and provokes urine.'

Fray's Golden Recipes for the Use of All Ages in 1897 suggested '*A bruised geranium leaf applied to a cut quickly heals it.*'

ETYMOLOGY OF COMMON NAME
The English name 'cranesbill' derives from the resemblance of the fruit capsule of some of the species to a crane's head and bill.

PLANT LORE
Cranesbill has been used in various magical and spiritual practices. It was believed to get rid of ghosts and demons in spells and by superstition.

USE
The root and leaves.

EDIBILITY
Edible raw or cooked, and less tough when young. Has a flavour like Parsley.

HARVEST
In spring and summer before the seeds appear.

MEDICINAL PROPERTIES
Haemostatic/styptic, anticancerogenic, anti-inflammatory, antibacterial and antihypertensive.

ACTIVE CONSTITUENTS
Tannins, flavonoids, phenolic acids, triterpenoids, polysaccharides, alkaloids and essential oils.

MODERN RESEARCH

Cranesbill, as mentioned above, is valued as a useful astringent and haemostatic owing to its tannin content. Tannins also act as a diuretic by stimulating regional blood flow and initial vasodilation, which makes Cranesbill a good remedy, as Culpeper says, for flushing out kidney stones. Modern research also supports the historical use of the plant for the following:

Astringent and vulnerary

The roots and leaves contain large amounts of tannin, and various Geranium species are used internally for the treatment of diarrhoea. Their astringent effects were also studied in 1999 as a treatment for herpes, when they were found to block virus replication *in vitro* and delay vesiculation (swellings) when administered orally to guinea pigs after primary infection.

Anticancerogenic

In 2008, geraniin, a form of tannin from Cranesbill, was found to cause cell death through induction of apoptosis (programmed cell death), which may provide a pivotal mechanism for cancer-preventive action. In 2009, Mazzio et al. found that an extract of Cranesbill also exhibited cytotoxicity against a neuro 2-a murine neuroblastoma (brain cancer) cell line.

A 2016 study by Graca et al. of the effects of Dove's-foot cranesbill against several cancer cell lines (breast, non-small cell lung, cervical and hepatocellular) found that all extracts possessed cytotoxic activity, with the acetone extract being the most effective.

Antihypertensive

In 2013, Ivanov et al. found that a 70% aqueous extract of Meadow cranesbill possessed remarkable *in vitro* inhibitory activity against angiotensin-converting enzyme (ACE), an enzyme that plays a central role in the regulation of blood pressure.

Anti-inflammatory

Cranesbill has also demonstrated significant anti-inflammatory properties owing to its high content of tannins and flavonoids. These compounds work by inhibiting inflammatory pathways and reducing the production of inflammatory mediators. Further, in 2014, Piwowarski et al. demonstrated the anti-inflammatory action of Meadow cranesbill on macrophages (white blood cells) when it was shown that the extract was a source of urolithin metabolites, which had an inhibitory effect on pro-inflammatory cytokines.

Antibacterial

Cranesbill exhibits significant antibacterial activity, again owing to its high content of tannins, flavonoids and phenolic acids, which work by disrupting bacterial cell walls, inhibiting bacterial enzymes and preventing bacterial proliferation. In 2022, the extracts of about twenty Geranium species were tested against a large panel of gram-positive and gram-negative bacteria among which some important human pathogens, including methicillin-resistant *Staphylococcu aureus* (MRSA) were included. The extracts were found to possess a broad spectrum of inhibitory activities, and, in most cases, minimum inhibitory concentrations (MICs) against the bacterias were determined.

TOPICAL USES

A poultice from the base or pounded roots of the plant was used to treat wounds, burns and haemorrhoids.

DOSAGE

Tisane – 1–2tsp/5–10g, 3 times per day.
Decoction – 1tsp/5g, 3 times per day.
Tincture – 1:5 45% – approximately ½ teaspoon or 3ml, 3 times per day – 20 drops = 1ml/1tsp = 5ml.

PRECAUTIONS

You should not take this medication for over three weeks at a stretch unless a qualified practitioner of herbal medicine has recommended otherwise. Not suitable for children or those who are pregnant or lactating.

Cranesbill recipes

Medicinal recipes

Cranesbill tisane

Pour 250ml boiling water over 1-2tsp/ 5-10g of the dried herb and allow to steep for 10-15 minutes. Use to soothe gastrointestinal issues, for incontinence and blood in the urine. Also as a gargle for ulceration of the mouth and throat.

Cranesbill root decoction

Boil 1tsp/5g of the root for 10-15 minutes in 2 cups (500ml) of water. Use for diarrhoea, inflammation in the bladder and symptoms related to Crohn's disease.

Cranesbill decocted tincture – 1:5 45%

If you are using 40% alcohol, ie. vodka, make a simple tincture by covering 1 part herb to 5 parts fluid.

If you are using Everclear or other 100% proof, use the following method for a specific tincture:

- 100g Cranesbill root
- 300ml alcohol
- 200ml water

Take 100g powdered root and split into two parts of 50g each. Place 50g in 125ml alcohol. Take the other 50g part and place in 375ml of water. Bring the water to a gentle boil, reduce heat and simmer for 20-40 minutes. Remove from heat and allow to cool a bit. Strain thoroughly and top up if the water is less than 375ml. Add the decoction to the dried root and alcohol mix, and leave for 14 days before straining. Use for duodenal ulcers, diarrhoea, metrorrhagia, heavy menstruation and dysmenorrhea.

Cranesbill poultice

- 1tsp fresh Cranesbill leaves and roots (if using dried, moisten with hot water)
- 2tsp coconut oil
- cheesecloth or cotton bandage

Finely chop the herb and add the coconut oil to make a paste. Spread the mix onto a clean cloth or piece of gauze. Fold the cloth or gauze over the herbs to form a small packet, then place the poultice directly onto the affected skin area. Ensure that the herb paste is in contact with the skin and secure the poultice in place with a bandage, wrap or medical tape to keep it from moving. Use to help to help heal wounds, reduce inflammation and soothe skin conditions. Note: Discontinue use if skin irritation occurs.

DAISY
Bellis perennis

Bellis perennis, the Common or English daisy, is a well-known and widespread plant native to the UK. It is a member of the huge *Asteraceae* family and has a long history of use in traditional herbal medicine for a wide-ranging variety of ailments.

HISTORICAL USES

John Gerard wrote in his *Herball*, '*Daisies do mitigate all kinde of paines, but especially in the joints, and gout, if they be stamped with new butter unsalted, and applied upon the pained place but they worke more effectually if Mallowes be added thereto. The juice of the leaves and roots snift up into the nostrils, purgeth the head mightily, and helpeth the megrim* [migraine]. *The leaves stamped take away bruises and swellings proceeding of some stroke, if they be stamped and laid thereon; whereupon it was called in old time Bruisewort. The juice put into the eies cleareth them, and taketh away the watering of them. The decoction of the field Daisie made in water and drunke, is good against agues.*'

Nicholas Culpeper's *Herbal* stated that '*the leaves and sometimes the roots ... are used in wound drinks and are accounted good to dissolve congealed and coagulated blood.*'

In his *Herbal Simples*, William

ETYMOLOGY OF COMMON NAME
The word comes from Old English *dægesege*, meaning 'day's eye', because the petals open at dawn and close at dusk.

PLANT LORE
Wearing a daisy chain was said to protect a child from being kidnapped by fairies.

USE
The root, leaves and flowers.

EDIBILITY
The young buds and leaves can be added to salads, soups or sandwiches.

HARVEST
In spring and summer.

MEDICINAL PROPERTIES
Anti-inflammatory, antioxidant, antibacterial, anticancerogenic and anxiolytic.

ACTIVE CONSTITUENTS
Saponins, tannins, flavonoids, triterpenes, polyphenols, inulin, mucilage.

Fernie (second edition, 1897) quoted Gerard but went on to say '*The root was named* consolida minima *by older physicians. Fabricius speaks of its efficacy in curing wounds and contusions. A decoction of the leaves and flowers was given internally, and the bruised herb blended with lard was applied outside. The leaves stamped take away bruises, whereupon it was called in old time Bruisewort.*'

Interestingly, Fernie also mentioned that '*the infusion of the plant in tablespoonful doses, or the diluted tincture, will answer admirably to renovate and re-establish the health and strength of the sufferer.*'

MODERN RESEARCH

This small but much overlooked plant, also known as Bruisewort, as Fernie says, should be regarded as of much higher worth than it is. The aerial parts have been used for the treatment of rheumatism (Morikawa et al., 2011), common cold (Cakılcıoglu et al., 2010) and headache (Uzun et al., 2004) as well as for their expectorant, sedative and anti-inflammatory activities (Siatka and Kasparova, 2010) in traditional medicine. Research appears to confirm the following of the historical writers' findings:

Anti-inflammatory and vulnerary

In a study published in 2012, 100% of the wounds on rats treated with an extract of Daisy healed perfectly without any scarring. The researchers concluded with the claim: '*Thus, the traditional usage of wound healing of [Daisy] was scientifically verified for the first time.*' It is thought that its mechanism was to act upon muscle fibres of blood vessels and promote collagen synthesis.

A 2015 paper by al-Snafi, 'The Pharmacological Importance of *Bellis perennis*', examined various of its actions, such as anti-inflammatory, fever-reducing, wound-healing, cytotoxicity and antioxidant effects, and concluded that: '*it is a promising medicinal plant with a wide range of pharmacological activities which could be utilised in several medical applications because of its effectiveness and safety.*'

In 2020, Lotan et al. published the results of their trial of 55 patients, who underwent mastectomy and immediate breast reconstruction. Patients were randomly assigned and treated with Arnica and Daisy or a placebo after surgery and up to the time of drain removal. Results showed that seroma (abnormal accumulation of fluid) formation and opioid intake was reduced in the group taking the Arnica/Daisy treatment. The authors concluded that as this treatment lacked side effects and was inexpensive, it should serve as a valuable treatment adjunct in patients undergoing mastectomy and reconstruction.

The above results will be why Gerard found this little plant useful for pains, headaches, bruises, swelling and agues, though I have found no

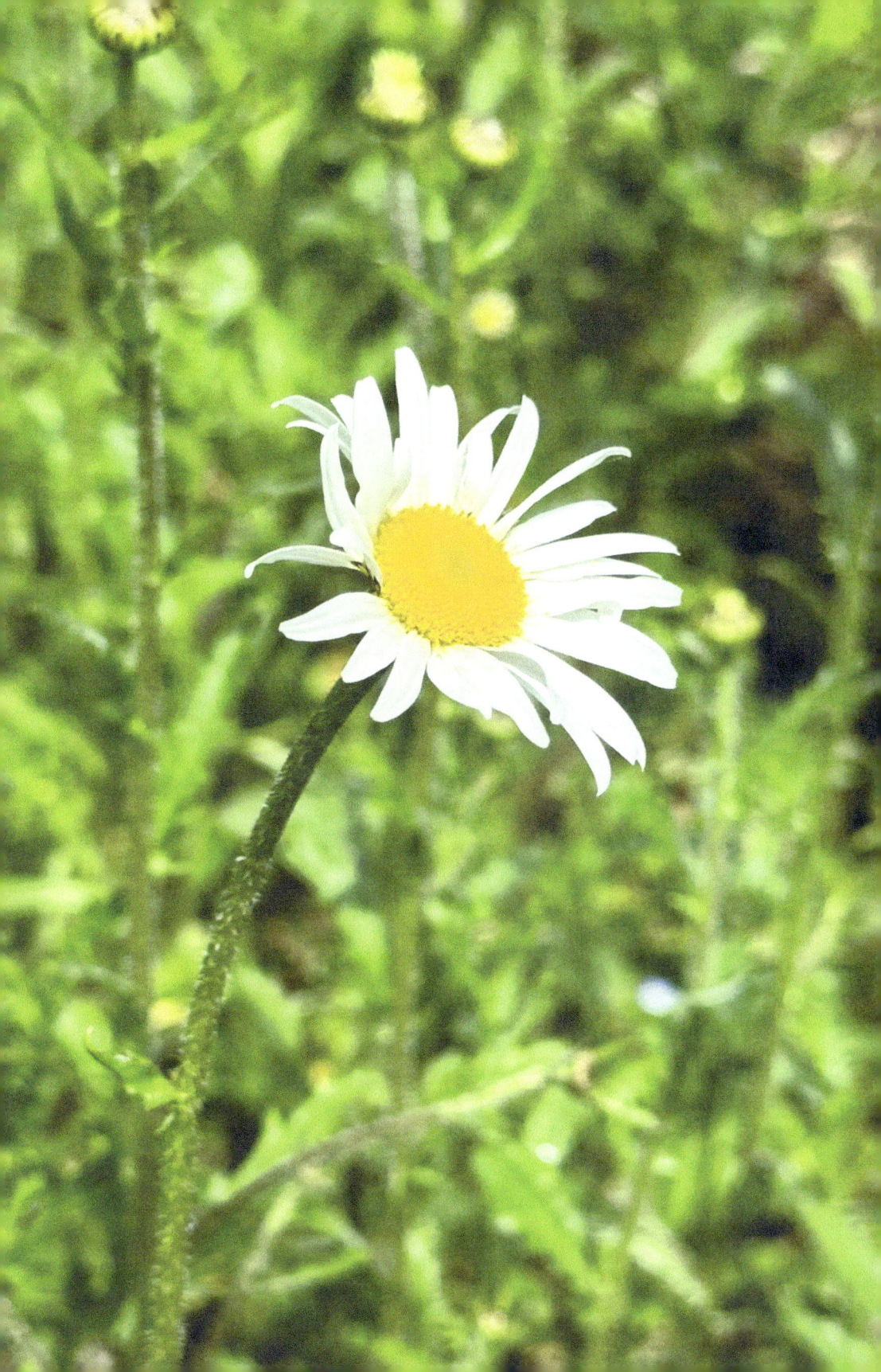

evidence that sniffing the juice up the nostrils is any more effective than drinking it as a tea!

Antibacterial

In addition to the above, results from *in vitro* studies also suggest that Daisies could be an alternative source in the fight against bacterial infections. The methanol and ethanol extracts of flowers have exhibited broad-spectrum antibacterial activity against *Streptococcus pyogenes*, *Staphylococcus aureus*, *Staphylococcus epidermidis* and *Enterobacter cloacae*, the causes of many wound and skin infections.

Anticancerogenic

Daisy flowers have also been utilised as herbal tea to treat breast and uterine cancer. Li et al. (2005) indicated the cytotoxic activities of six triterpenoid saponins from the roots of Daisy against human leukaemia cells, and Karakas et al. (2015) showed that Daisy had moderate antiproliferative activity on human breast cancer and human hepatocellular carcinoma cells. In one study, 19 extracts and two fractions were obtained from wild-grown flowers and foliage and evaluated for biological activity. The greatest cytotoxic activity against chosen cell lines was found in leaf extracts and the active constituent was a saponin that inhibits tumour growth and shows great promise for future research.

Anxiolytic

Somewhat confirming both the use of Daisy as a mild sedative and Fernie's description of Daisy for re-establishing health and strength, a 2011 study to investigate the effects of Daisy on anxiety and spatial memory performance of rats was shown to produce an anxiolytic and anaesthetic effect of high-dose extracts. It is thought that Daisy may act like 'benzodiazepines', which are widely used drugs in reducing anxiety-like behaviours.

In 2012, Marques et al. tested extract of Daisy in mice and noted an anxiolytic effect in the open field test and swimming test. They then tested combinations of antidepressant with Daisy extracts and found that a combination of imipramine (a tricyclic antidepressant) and Daisy extract showed a greater reduction of anxiety-related behaviours than imipramine or the Daisy extract alone, while other antidepressants such as paroxetine (an SSRI) and reserpine (an adrenergic) had no effect (reserpine blocked the effect of the Daisy extract). Based on these results, the authors suggested that Daisy may have an effect on the noradrenergic activity of the central nervous system, which may in turn stimulate alertness, arousal and readiness for action.

TOPICAL USES

As Gerard said, Daisy once had a great reputation as a cure for bruises, aches, pains and strains in the way that people now use Arnica. Extracts of Daisy can be found in many of cosmetic rejuvenating eye care treatments because it contains L-arbutin, which suppresses melanin activity and brightens skin.

DOSAGE

Tisane – ½ cup of Daisy flowers to 2 cups of water. 2tsp, 3 times per day.

PRECAUTIONS

No health hazards or side effects are known in conjunction with the proper administration of designated therapeutic dosages. Not suitable for those who are pregnant or breastfeeding.

Daisy recipes

Medicinal recipes

Daisy tisane

Pour 2 cups of boiling water over a half cup of flower heads and bring to a gentle simmer. Once reached, remove from the heat and allow to cool. Strain and take 2tsp, 3 times per day as a mild sedative and anti-inflammatory for headaches as well as bloating and indigestion. The tisane can also be applied externally to the skin for the treatment of skin diseases such as sores, wounds, acne, rash and pyoderma.

Daisy wound balm

- 100g dried Daisy flowers
- 2tbsp alcohol, such as Everclear
- 1l grapeseed oil

Place the flowers in a jar with the alcohol and allow to steep for 10 minutes before adding the oil. Leave for 4 weeks and then strain. Make into a balm by using a 1:3 ratio of melted beeswax to your oil mix, ie. 1 part wax to 3 parts liquid. Melt the wax pellets in the oil in a double boiler or bain-marie. Remove from the heat and allow to cool and set completely before using topically for healing bruises and skin irritation.

Daisy syrup

- 1 part Daisy tisane
- 1 part sugar

Simmer your strained tisane or decoction until it is reduced by half and then add the sugar. You will always end up using double the amount of sugar to tisane. Stir until the sugar has dissolved and then continue cooking till the mixture has thickened to a syrup. Leave to cool. Pour into sterilised bottles closed with a cork. This will keep for a maximum of 3 months. Use as a sedative, expectorant, antiseptic and anti-inflammatory. To fully preserve a syrup, it's wise to add 5% of your end volume with a tincture of the herb (or one of the herbs) in the syrup.

Daisy flower vinegar hair rinse

- fresh Daisy flowers (enough to fill a glass jar)
- apple cider vinegar

Fill a glass jar with fresh Daisy flowers and pour in apple cider vinegar until they are completely covered. Seal the jar tightly with a lid and leave in a cool, dark place to infuse for 2–4 weeks. Strain the vinegar through a fine mesh strainer or cheesecloth into a clean bottle and use as a hair rinse after shampooing to condition the hair and soothe the scalp.

DANDELION
Taraxacum officinale

While there are actually several species of Taraxacum in the UK, including several hybridised species, the best known is *Taraxacum officinale*, the common Dandelion, a widespread plant found in gardens, grass verges and waste grounds. It is a member of the Daisy and Sunflower family, the *Asteraceae*, and is native to the UK. It has a long history of use in traditional medicine and culinary applications.

HISTORICAL USES

Dandelion has been recorded in ancient writings, and Arabian physicians recommended the plant in medicine in the 10th and 11th centuries, while in China and India Dandelion was used to treat liver diseases and digestive problems.

Nicholas Culpeper's *Herbal* commented, '*It is of an opening and cleansing quality, and therefore very effectual for obstructions of the liver, gall and spleen, and the diseases that arise from them, as the jaundice, and hypochondriac. It openeth the passages of the urine both in young and old; powerfully cleanseth imposthumes [abscesses] and inward ulcers in the urinary passages, and by its drying and temperate quality doth afterwards heal them.*'

Fray's Golden Recipes for the Use of All

ETYMOLOGY OF COMMON NAME
From French *dent-de-lion*, or lion's tooth (because of the jagged shape of the leaves)

PLANT LORE
In folklore, blowing dandelion seeds while making a wish is a common practice. It is believed that the number of seeds left after blowing indicates the number of children a person will have or the fulfilment of wishes.

USE
All parts.

EDIBILITY
The young leaves are added to salads and are packed with many vitamins and minerals. The root when roasted makes a wonderful substitute for coffee.

HARVEST
Leaves in spring, flowers in spring and summer, roots in autumn (best in November).

MEDICINAL PROPERTIES
Diuretic, antidiabetic, anti-inflammatory and hepatoprotective.

ACTIVE CONSTITUENTS
Polysaccharides, sesquiterpenes, carotenoids, flavonoids, sterols, triterpenes, phenolic acids.

Ages (1897) said of Dandelion, '*no herb acts on a sluggish liver with better effect.*'

MODERN RESEARCH

The historical uses are accurate in that Dandelion is now a well-known diuretic and is chiefly used in kidney and liver disorders. Modern research has found or confirmed the following properties:

Diuretic

Dandelion leaves are a potent diuretic owing to their high potassium content and are far superior to over-the-counter diuretics (Râcz–Kotilla et al., 1974). A study by Clare et al. in 2009 showed that the leaves increase urinary frequency and fluid excretion in healthy individuals, while a further two studies demonstrated a positive effect on the treatment and prevention of kidney diseases, such as urolithiasis (Karakus et al., 2017; Ghale-Salimi et al., 2018).

Antidiabetic

Some 40% of the mature Dandelion root is composed of inulin, a mixture of complex carbohydrates that acts as energy storage and promotes beneficial intestinal microflora, improves bowel function, stabilises blood sugar and helps absorption of calcium and magnesium. In 2007, studies revealed that extracts of the root exhibited considerable inhibitory activities on the digestion of carbohydrates and slowed down the absorption, making the plant a good candidate for the management of diabetes.

Anti-inflammatory

A 2018 study showed that Dandelion root extract can exert therapeutic effects in ulcerative colitis (Ding and Wen, 2018), while another study found that it able to prevent colitis altogether. In this study, the extract was reported to have a stronger effect than a comparable anti-inflammatory drug in the prevention of colitis, seemingly through anti-oxidative, anti-inflammatory and regenerative activities (Han et al., 2017). A study by Chen et al. in 2019 showed that Dandelion extract is able to improve the symptoms of colitis, controlling fatty acid metabolism and dysbiosis (imbalance in microbiomes).

Hepatoprotective

In July 2020, a study confirmed the long use of Dandelion for the liver when it found that liver histology was remarkably improved after treatment. The total antioxidant study of dandelion extract revealed that it has notable antioxidant power and concluded that it prevents the progression of hepatic fibrosis (liver damage) owing to its ability to scavenge free radicals and reduce the force of inflammatory cells.

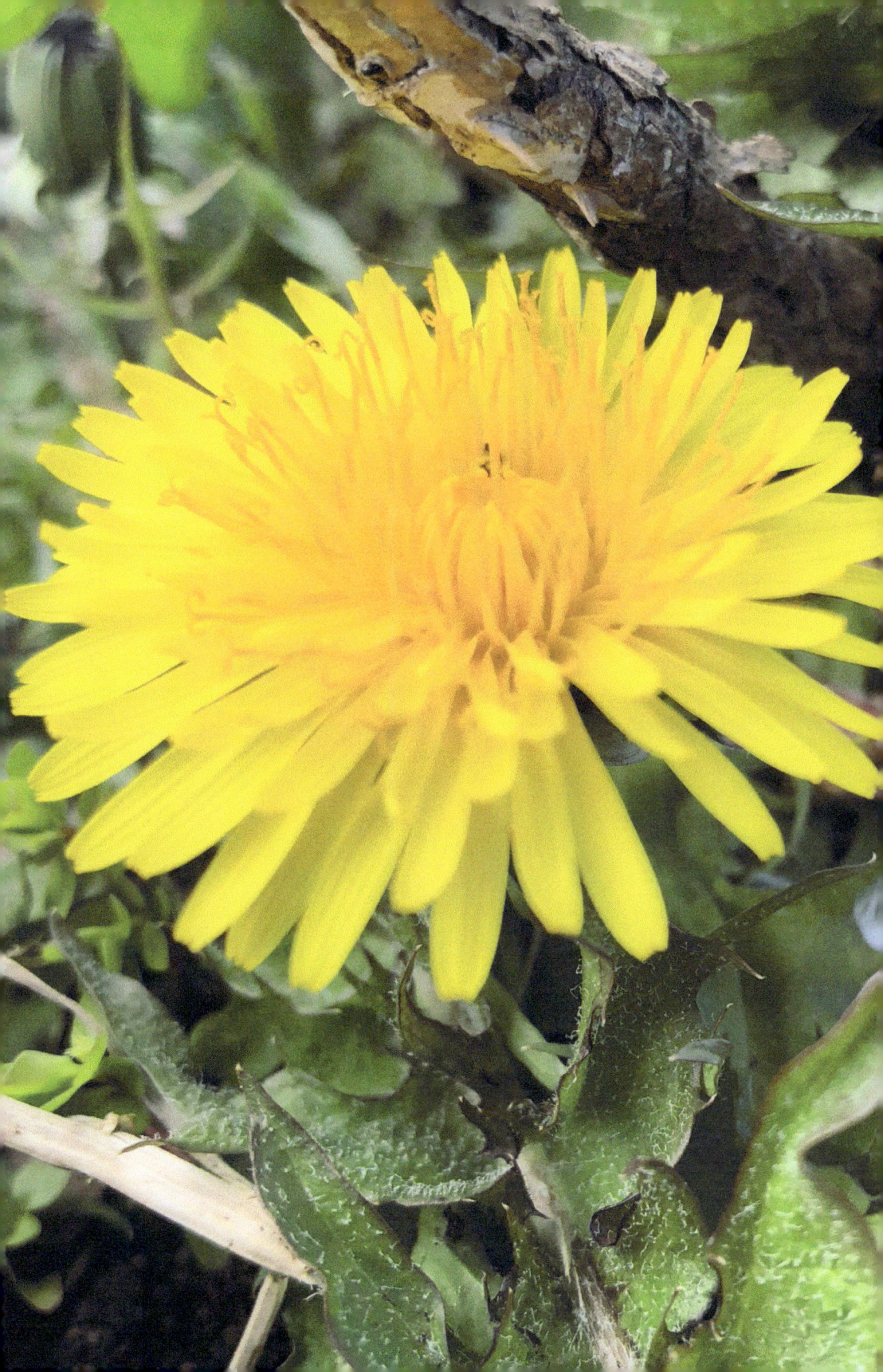

SARS spike protein blocker

A 2021 report on Dandelion leaf against SARS-CoV-2 variants showed that the leaf can block spike proteins from binding to surface receptors in human lung and kidney cells. The water-based extract has been shown to be effective against spike protein mutation and a host of other mutant strains. This could be a major advantage in prevention of SARS-CoV-2 infection.

TOPICAL USE

As a natural anti-inflammatory, Dandelion is perfect for sensitive skin or chronic conditions like rosacea and eczema. The root can be ground and mixed with water for skin disorders like acne, eczema, psoriasis, rashes and boils. A 2015 study from Canada reported that extracts can block harmful ultraviolet radiation, protecting the skin from sun damage and lowering the risk of skin cancer.

DOSAGE

Tisane – 3–4tsp/15–20g per 250ml boiling water. Half–1 cup freely.
Root decoction – 1tsp/5g per 250ml boiling water. Half–1 cup freely.
Tincture – 1:5 25% – 5–10ml, 3 times per day – 20 drops = 1ml/1tsp = 5ml.

PRECAUTIONS

Contact dermatitis has been reported, and Dandelion may potentiate diuretics. Avoid Dandelion use if you have diarrhoea, hyperacidity, acute irritable bowel syndrome or ulcerative colitis. Not suitable for children or those who are pregnant or lactating.

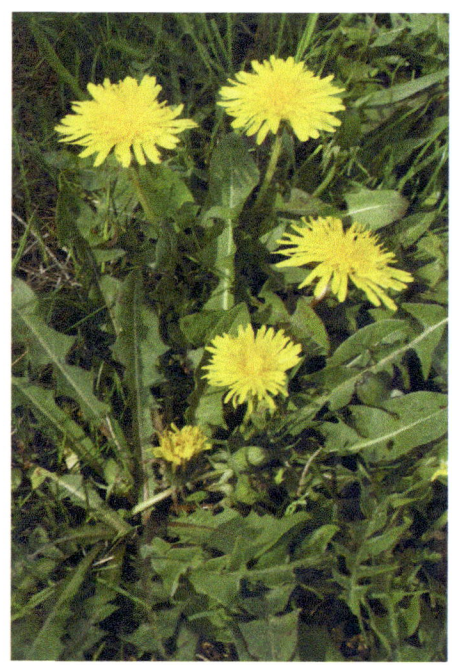

Dandelion recipes

Medicinal recipes

Dandelion leaf tisane

Pour 250ml boiling water over 3-4tsp/ 15-20g of the dried leaf and allow to steep for 10-15 minutes. Use as a diuretic and to support digestion and promote liver health, as well as an anti-inflammatory for joints. It may also prove to be therapeutic when dealing with COVID-19 infection.

Dandelion decocted tincture – 1:5 25%

If you are using 40% alcohol, ie. vodka, you will need to dilute this at the ratio of 60ml water to every 100ml of vodka to make a 25% medium and then cover 1 part herb to 5 parts fluid.

If you are using Everclear or other 100% proof, use the following method for a specific tincture:

- 100g Dandelion root
- 125ml alcohol
- 375ml water

Take 100g of powdered root and split into two parts of 50g each. Place 50g in the alcohol and the other 50g part in the water. Bring the water to a gentle boil, reduce heat and simmer for 20-40 minutes. Remove from heat and strain thoroughly. Top up if the water is less than 375ml. Add the decoction to the alcohol mix and leave for 14 days before straining. Use for the treatment of gallstones, constipation, dyspepsia, chronic arthritis and rheumatic diseases.

Dandelion honey

- 100-150 Dandelion blooms
- 1l water
- 3 cups (750g) sugar
- 1 lemon

Leave the blooms outside to allow bugs to escape, but do not wash them. Cut off the green stems and place the petals in a pan with half of the lemon. Cover with water and simmer for 30 minutes. Allow to cool, cover and leave to infuse overnight. Drain the water into a pan, add the sugar and remaining lemon, then stir and heat the liquid until the sugar is dissolved. Once dissolved, simmer for 30 to 60 minutes until the desired consistency is achieved

Dandelion coffee

- Dandelion root (washed)

Chop the root into small pieces, spread on a baking sheet and roast in a 180-200°C oven for 20-30 minutes. Ideally, run the roasted root through a coffee grinder to make a finer grind and then pop them in the cafetière with hot water for about 10 minutes to make a nice strong pot. Use as a tonic, diuretic, digestive, anti-inflammatory and antitussive.

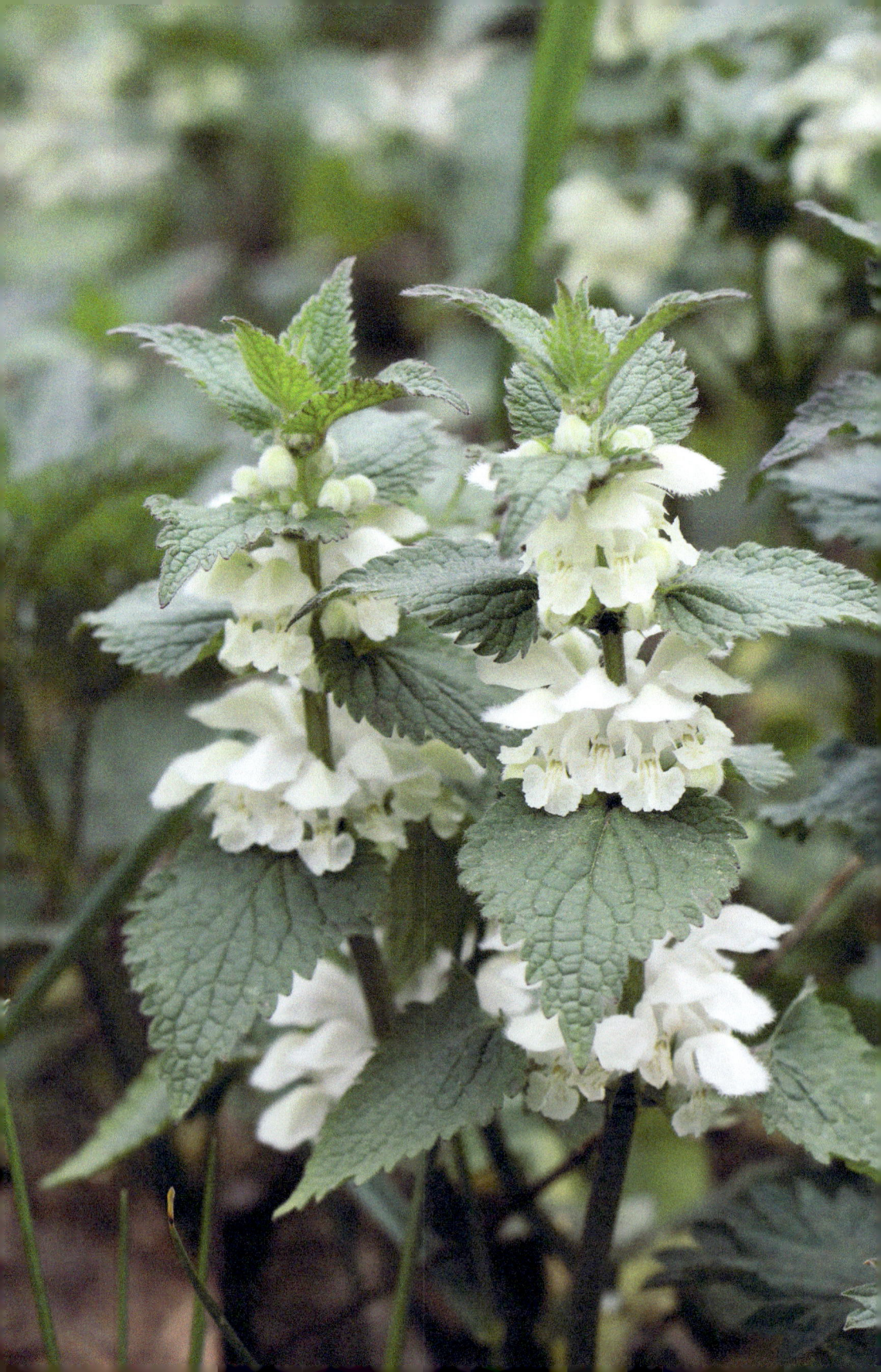

DEADNETTLES
Lamium spp.

In the UK, there are several native species of *Lamium*, all members of the Mint family, *Lamiaceae*, including White deadnettle (*Lamium album*), found in hedgerows, woodlands and disturbed habitats; Red deadnettle (*Lamium purpureum*), found in urban areas, along roadsides and in waste areas; and Yellow archangel (*Lamium galeobdolon*), found in woodland areas. All three of these species have been used in traditional herbal medicine.

HISTORICAL USES

In her *Physica*, Hildegard of Bingen (1098–1179) referred to these as 'Blindnettle' with the words, '*a person who eats it smiles with pleasure, since its heat touches his spleen and thence his heart is made happy.*' She went on to recommend it as a treatment for leucoma, saying '*place it in spring water for the night and having taken it from the water, heat it in a small dish and place, it warm, over the affected eye.*'

In his *Herball*, John Gerard (1545–1612) wrote of the Deadnettles, '*The floures* [flowers] *are baked with sugar, which is used to make the heart merry, to make a good colour in the face, and to refresh the vital spirits.*'

Nicholas Culpeper's *Herbal* described them as '*somewhat hot and drier than*

ETYMOLOGY OF COMMON NAME
Middle English origin, referring to the resemblance to stinging nettles, but without stinging hairs and therefore apparently 'dead'.

PLANT LORE
Also called archangel as it appears around the Feast of the Apparition (8 May), the day when the archangel Michael is said to have appeared on Mount Gargano, in the 6th century.

USE
All aerial parts.

EDIBILITY
Young leaves and shoots can be eaten raw

HARVEST
In spring.

MEDICINAL PROPERTIES
Antioxidant, vulnerary, anti-inflammatory, anticancerogenic, diuretic and haemostatic/styptic.

ACTIVE CONSTITUENTS
Flavonoids, iridoid glycosides, phenolic compounds, tannins, mucilage, saponins, essential oils.

LEFT: WHITE DEADNETTLE

the stinging nettles and used with better success for the stopping and hardness of the spleen ... It makes the head merry, drives away melancholy, quickens the spirits, is good against quartan agues [four-day fevers], stancheth bleeding at mouth and nose, if it be applied, doth much allay the pains, and give ease to the gout, sciatica, and other pains of the joints and sinews. It is also very effectual to heal green [fresh] wounds, and old ulcers; also, to stay their spreading. It draweth forth splinters and is very good against bruises and burnings.'

William Fernie (1897 second edition, *Herbal Simples*) wrote of White deadnettle, *'If the plant be macerated in alcohol for a week, the liquid is as efficacious for staying bleeding, when applied to the spot.'*

MODERN RESEARCH

The historical authors are united in referring to the ability of the Deadnettles to lift the spirits. While specific studies aimed at this characteristic are lacking, a study of the composition of essential oils in different *Lamium* species showed that in Red deadnettle the content of α- and β-pinene was as high as 75.3% in the flowers. Among other properties such as anti-inflammatory and pain-relieving, pinene is often also associated with energetic and euphoric experiences.

A 2003 analysis of populations of *Lamium* species, including the three native UK species, showed that significant amounts of squalene were found in all samples. Squalene is also a substance that possesses significant biological activity which may contribute to the following:

Antioxidant

In 2013 two of the species, Red deadnettle and White deadnettle, were evaluated for their antioxidant activity and while the former variety exhibited a higher scavenging activity, the latter showed stronger total antioxidant activity.

Vulnerary and bactericidal

The effects on wounds seen by Culpeper are no doubt also a consequence of squalene, which manages wound-healing by immunomodulation of macrophages (the main cells involved in wound-healing). It is useful in the last stages of healing owing to its anti-inflammatory properties and wound closure.

Chipeva et al. (2013) found that White deadnettle extracts possess a broad spectrum of antibacterial activity against bacteria strains such as *Bacillus subtilis Enterobacter aerogenes, Enterococcus faecalis, Escherichia coli, Klebsiella pneumoniae, Micrococcus luteus, Proteus hauseri, Pseudomonas aeruginosa, Salmonella enterica, Staphylococcus aureus* and *Staphylococcus epidermidis*, while a 2021 study reconfirmed the wound-healing effects of White deadnettle during an experiment on rats. Wound size was measured on days 3, 5, 7 and 12 of the experiment and showed that the wound-healing rate was significantly increased in the group treated with White deadnettle ointment.

Antiviral

A study by Zhang et al. (2009) reported that the aqueous extract of White deadnettle proved effective in the treatment of hepatitis C infections. Moreover, the antiviral activity of chloroform extracts has been shown to significantly inhibit *Herpes simplex* virus-1 and virus-2 cells (Todorov et al., 2013). When the chloroform extracts were applied at maximum concentrations, the virus replication was suppressed by over 90%.

There also may be some evidence here for the use by Hildegard for 'leucoma' as the causes of corneal leucoma can be diverse and may include bacterial or viral infections, including the *Herpes* virus.

Anticancerogenic

A 2019 study of Red deadnettle's chemical composition and potential for anticancer activity observed cell death and showed that the essential oil of Red deadnettle had compounds that showed cytotoxic activities. A 2022 study into the bioactive properties of Yellow archangel essential oil showed antiproliferative activity on the skin melanoma cell line.

TOPICAL USES

As we have seen, Deadnettles are antioxidant, antimicrobial and vulnerary. Because of their squalene content, they also make an excellent skin moisturiser. Squalene does not clog pores, making it suitable for all skin types, including oily and acne-prone skin. It helps strengthen the skin's barrier, protecting it from environmental damage and preventing trans epidermal water loss. For this reason, it also is excellent in an external compress for sores, bruises, burns and ulcers. White deadnettle dermatological products are already on the market featuring the squalene properties already mentioned.

DOSAGE

Tisane – 1–2tsp dried herb to 1 cup, 3 times per day.

Tincture – 1:5 45% – 5–10 drops, in a quantity of water especially against stomach ache.

PRECAUTIONS

Not suitable for children or those who are pregnant or lactating.

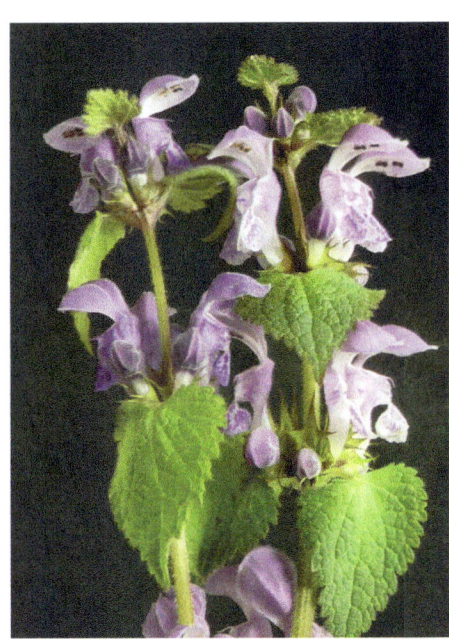

RIGHT: PURPLE DEADNETTLE

Deadnettle recipes

Medicinal recipes

Deadnettle tisane

Pour 250ml boiling water over 1tsp/5g of the dried herb and allow to steep for 10-15 minutes. Use as an antioxidant to prevent illness and as a mild diuretic.

Deadnettle infused tincture 1:5 45%

If you are using 40% alcohol, ie vodka, make a simple tincture by covering 1 part herb to 5 parts fluid.

If you are using Everclear or other 100% proof, use the following method for a specific tincture:

- 100g dried Deadnettle leaves and flowers
- 150ml alcohol
- 150ml water

Take 100g of dried herb and split into two parts of 50g each. Place 50g in 150ml alcohol. Take the other 50g part and place in 150ml of boiled water. Steep/infuse in the water for 10 minutes. Strain thoroughly and top up if the water is less than 150ml. Add the infusion to the alcohol mix and leave for 14 days before straining. Use to support healthy immune system function, fight free radicals, reduce pain and inflammation, and support healthy kidney function.

Deadnettle douche

- 50g dried herb (or a handful of fresh herb)
- 2 pints boiling water

Pour the water over the herb and allow to steep/infuse for 30 minutes. Use for vaginal discharge, wounds, bleeding after birth and prostatitis.

White deadnettle infused oil

- 100g dried herb
- 2tbsp alcohol, such as Everclear
- 1l grapeseed oil

Roughly chop the herb and place in the bottom of a jar with the Everclear. Allow to steep for 10 minutes and then add the oil. Allow the mix to steep/infuse for 4 weeks and use topically for wounds and skin care.

DOG'S MERCURY
Mercurialis perennis

Mercurialis perennis, commonly known as Dog's mercury, is a poisonous woodland plant, native to the UK and found in a wide range of woodlands and hedgerows, where it is frequently regarded as an indicator of ancient, semi-natural woodland.

HISTORICAL USES

Nicholas Culpeper's *Herbal* explained as follows, '*The decoction of the leaves of Mercury, or the juice thereof in broth, or drank with a little sugar put to it, purges choleric and waterish humours. Hippocrates commended it wonderfully for women's diseases, and applied to the secret parts, to ease the pains of the mother; and used the decoction of it, both to procure women's courses, and to expel the afterbirth; and gave the decoction thereof with myrrh or pepper or used to apply the leaves outwardly against the stranguary and diseases of the reins and bladder. He used it also for sore and watering eyes, and for the deafness and pains in the ears, by dropping the juice thereof into them, and bathing them afterwards in white wine. The juice or distilled water snuffed up into the nostrils, purges the head and eyes of catarrhs and rheums.*'

In his 1897, second edition of *Herbal Simples*, William Fernie described how '*A medicinal tincture is made from*

ETYMOLOGY OF COMMON NAME
A derisory name to distinguish it from 'true' mercuries such as Good-King-Henry, also known as Mercury goosefoot.

PLANT LORE
Another name is 'Boggart's posy' (a malevolent spirit), indicating the plant's toxicity. As a result, it has garnered negative associations in folklore and is often seen as an inauspicious or unlucky plant.

USE
The leaves.

EDIBILITY
Not edible – TOXIC!

HARVEST
When in flower

MEDICINAL PROPERTIES
Abortifacient, anti-inflammatory and antihyperglycaemic.

ACTIVE CONSTITUENTS
Methylamine, trimethylamine, saponins, glycosides, mercurialine, tannins, flavonoids, essential oils.

the whole plant freshly collected when in flower and fruit, with spirit of wine; and the dose of this in a diluted form is from five to ten drops of the third decimal strength, two or three times a day, with a spoonful of water. The condition which indicates its medicinal use, is that of a severe catarrh, with chilliness, a heavy head, sneezing, a dry mouth, and general aching, lassitude, with stupor, and heat of face.'

MODERN RESEARCH

Given its toxicity, Dog's mercury is rarely used in modern herbal medicine. The information about this plant is scant but what has been discovered is as follows:

Respiratory support

The historical writers refer to the use of Dog's mercury against ailments of the lungs, and this may be related to the presence of the sterol β-sitosterol, which has been demonstrated to affect the ability of *Streptococcus pneumoniae* to colonise the lungs.

Diuretic

Culpeper recommended the plant for the strangury (painful, frequent urination) and diseases of the reins (kidneys) and the bladder. The diuretic properties of Dog's mercury are attributed to its saponins, alkaloids, flavonoids and methylamine, which collectively stimulate urine production and promote the excretion of fluids. Methylamine in particular is thought to stimulate the renal tubules, enhancing the excretion of sodium and water.

Abortifacient

The exact mechanism by which Dog's mercury acts as an abortifacient is not well documented, but it is likely to be related to its toxic components, such as saponins, alkaloids and methylamine, which could be involved in triggering the uterine contractions needed, as Culpeper said, for expelling the afterbirth or indeed the termination of pregnancy.

Anti-inflammatory

The plant has been used traditionally to alleviate symptoms of gout and rheumatism, including pain and swelling. Compounds present in Dog's mercury that could contribute to its anti-inflammatory effect include kaempferol, which has proven efficacy in the treatment of arthrosis (which includes gout and rheumatism). This is the only anti-inflammatory use reported for Dog's mercury.

Antihyperglycaemic

Dog's mercury has been used to control blood sugar levels, which is an effect that can be attributed to the presence of rutin and ferulic acid. The antihyperglycaemic properties of rutin have been widely demonstrated, as has its potential to prevent and treat pathologies associated with diabetes, nephropathy, neuropathy, liver damage and cardiovascular disorders.

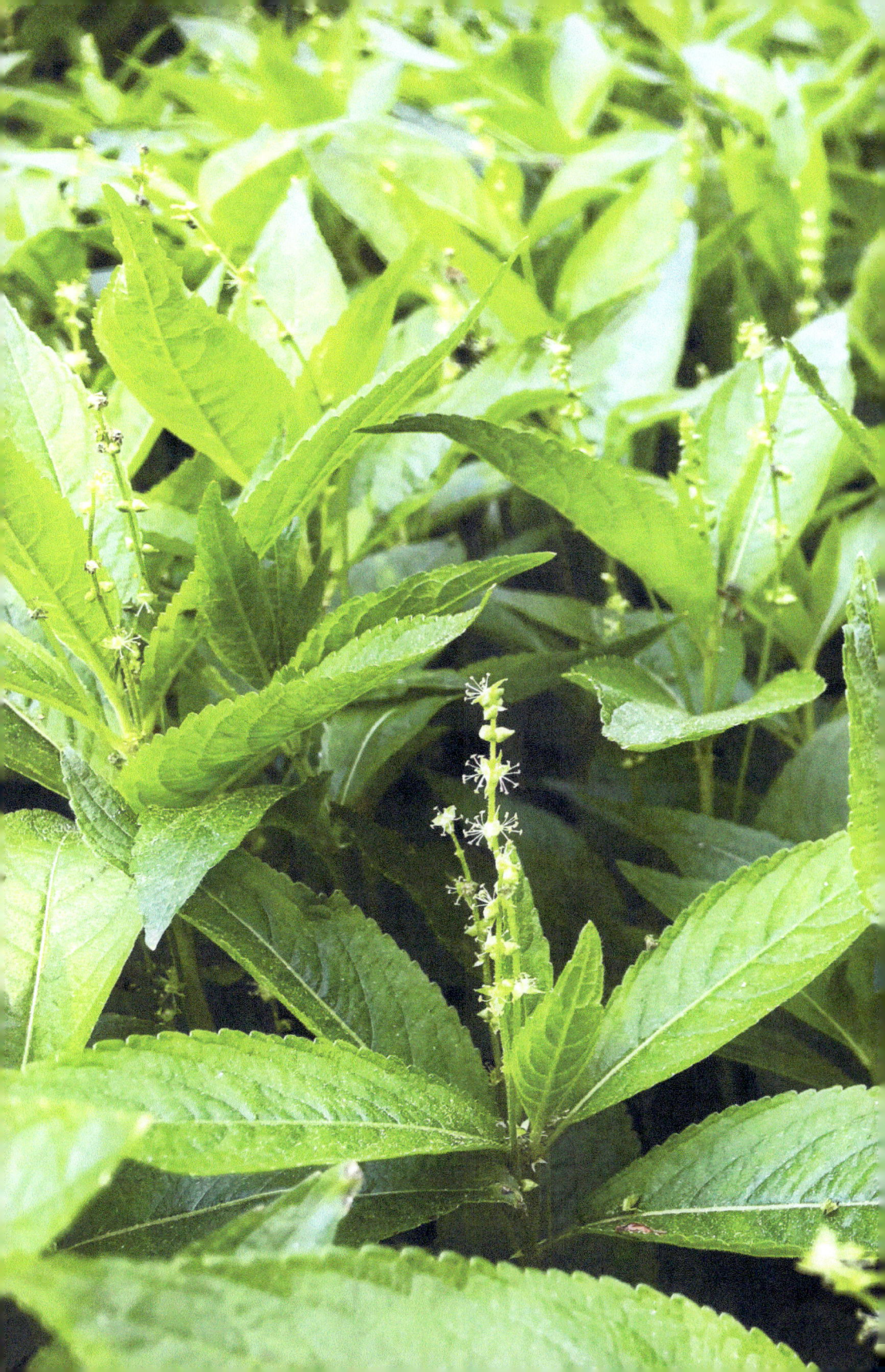

TOPICAL USE

The juice of the whole plant, collected when in flower, mixed with sugar or with vinegar, is a traditional external remedy for warts. When applied as a poultice, it is used to reduce swellings and to cleanse old sores.

The treatment of dark spots on the skin using *Dog's mercury* could be attributed to the presence of 4-methoxyphenol, which inhibits the formation of melanin precursors, the cause of darkening pigments. It is also used topically to treat depigmentation in patients with vitiligo when extensive body surface areas are unresponsive to regimentation therapies.

DOSAGE

External use only.

PRECAUTIONS

Dog's mercury is poisonous by itself but with a thorough drying/heating its poisonous quality can be destroyed. Poisoning in humans is generally caused by mistaken consumption of the herb and has been described in the literature (eg Rugman and Meecham, 1983) as causing nausea, vomiting, haemorrhagic inflammation of the gastrointestinal tract and of the kidneys as typical symptoms of an intoxication. Not suitable for children or those who are pregnant or lactating.

Dog's mercury recipes

Medicinal recipes
Dog's mercury infused oil

- 100g *dried* herb
- 2tbsp alcohol, such as Everclear
- 1l grapeseed oil

Roughly chop the herb and place in the bottom of a jar with the Everclear. Allow to steep for 10 minutes and then add the oil. Allow the mix to steep/infuse for 4 weeks.

Make into an infused salve by using a 1:3 ratio of melted beeswax to your oil mix, ie 1 part wax to 3 parts liquid as follows:

Weigh or measure out the wax pellets and place them with the herbal infused oil in a double boiler or bain-marie. Heat over a low heat until the wax is fully melted and then stir well. Remove from the heat and allow to cool and set completely before using topically for wounds and dark spots on the skin.

EYEBRIGHT
Euphrasia officinalis

Euphrasia officinalis, commonly known as Eyebright, is a small plant native to the UK, found in a variety of habitats, including grasslands, heathlands, meadows and open woodlands. It has a long history of use in traditional herbal medicine, particularly, as its name suggests, for eye conditions.

HISTORICAL USES

Hildegard of Bingen (1098–1179) is often credited with introducing the use of Eyebright as an eye remedy, though I was unable to find mention of it in the English translation of her work *Physica*.

John Gerard (1545–1612), however, said in his *Herball* that it was very much commended for the eyes, '*Being taken it selfe alone, or any way else, it preserves the sight, and being feeble and loſt it reſtores the same … Eye-bright ſtamped and laid upon the eyes, or the juice thereof mixed with white Wine, and dropped into the eyes, or the diſtilled water, taketh away the darknesse and dimnesse of the eyes, and cleareth the sight.*'

ETYMOLOGY OF COMMON NAME
Also called Eyewort. Named for its affinity with the eyes.

PLANT LORE
A herb sacred to the Druids that promotes clairvoyance. The knowledge of the plant was believed to have been passed to mankind by a linnet who used it to restore its eyesight.

USE
All parts.

EDIBILITY
The leaves can be used in salads but are slightly bitter.

HARVEST
When in full flower.

MEDICINAL PROPERTIES
Antibacterial, anti-inflammatory and astringent.

ACTIVE CONSTITUENTS
Iridoid glycosides, flavonoids, phenolic acids, tannins, volatile oils, lignans.

One of my favourite Nicholas Culpeper quotes is made about Eyebright and can be found in his *Herbal*:

If the herb was but as much used as it is neglected, it would half spoil the spectacle maker's trade and a man would think that reason should teach people to prefer the preservation of their natural before artificial spectacles ... It is then recommended that the juice or distilled water of the Eyebright taken inwardly in white wine, or broth, or dropped into the eyes for several days together helpeth all infirmities of the eye that cause dimness of sight. Some make conserve of the flowers to the same effect. Being used any of the ways, it strengthens the week brain or memory.

In his 1897, second edition book *Herbal Simples*, William Fernie commented, '*An attack of cold in the head, with copious running from the eyes and nose, may be aborted straightway by giving a dose of the* [Eyebright] *infusion (made with an ounce of the herb to a pint of boiling water) every two hours; as, likewise, for hay fever.*'

MODERN RESEARCH

As its name, and the above authors imply, Eyebright has an affinity to the eyes, and was and still is commonly used for eye problems. While I have not been able to find any proof that it improves eyesight, the plant has been confirmed to have the following properties:

Anti-inflammatory and antibacterial
Eyebright contains aucubin, an iridoid compound, which acts as an anti-inflammatory as well as an antibacterial. In a 2014 test-tube study, Eyebright extracts helped control inflammation in human cornea cells, and in a 2017 study, when combined with Chamomile, Eyebright was found to protect cornea cells from sun-related inflammation and damage.

Eyebright is also taken by mouth to treat inflamed nasal passages, allergies, hayfever, common cold, bronchial conditions and inflamed sinuses.

A 2022 study confirmed the use of Eyebright in the treatment of irritated eyes caused by allergic or non-infectious conjunctivitis and catarrhal inflammation accompanied by symptoms like redness, swelling, pain and increased tears. Results demonstrated inhibition of pain and inflammation plus inhibition of proteins involved in regulation of immune responses. Altogether, these mechanisms contribute to a general anti-inflammatory response and prevention of oxidative damage, which ultimately promotes the wound-healing process of the affected tissue in irritated eyes.

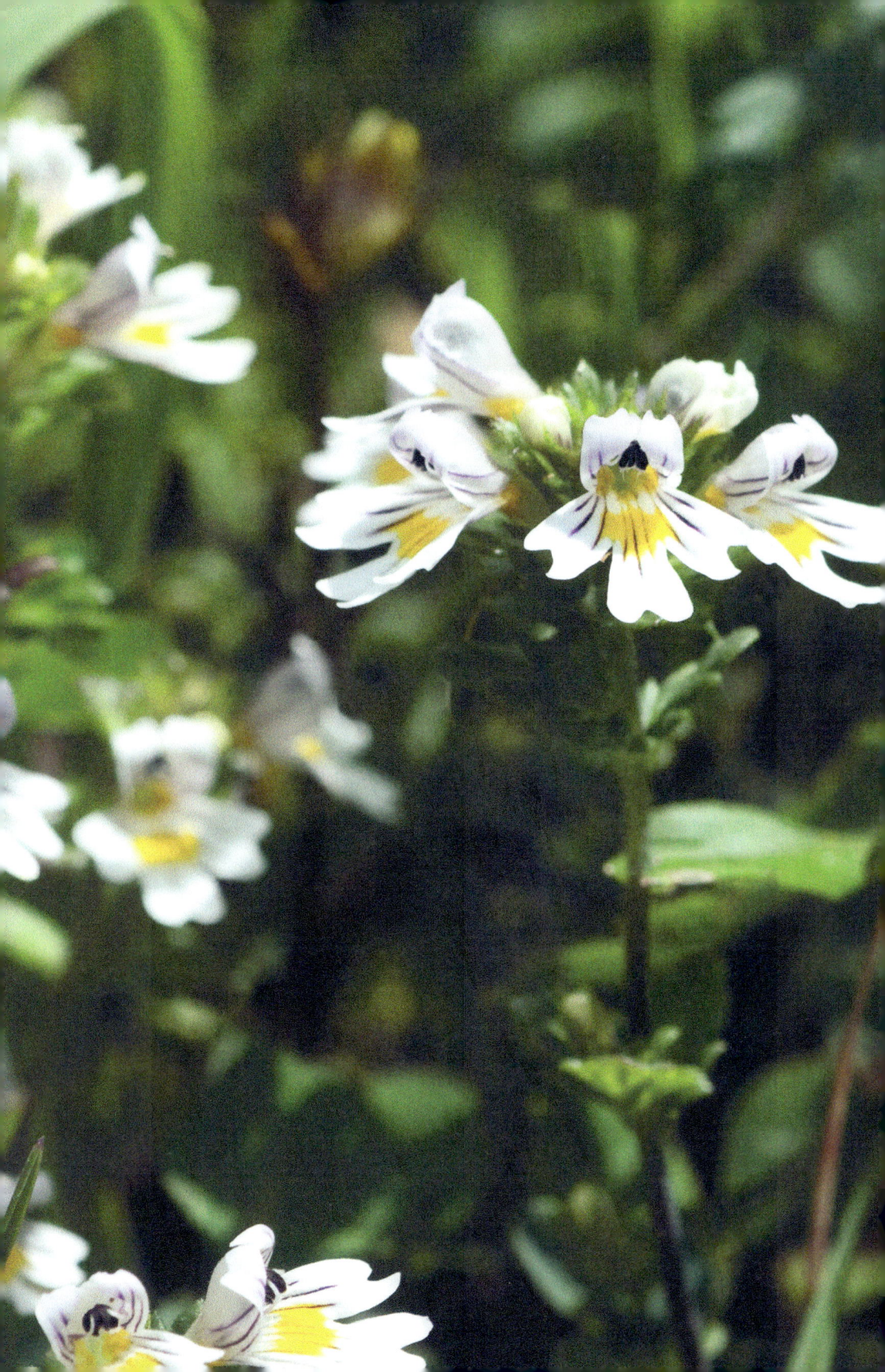

TOPICAL USES

The cooled herbal decoction can be used as an eye wash for infected eyes and enable rapid reduction in inflammation.

DOSAGE

Tisane – 1tsp/5g. Drink a half-cup, 3 times per day.
Tincture – fresh leaf, 1:5 45%, 2–6ml, 3 times per day – 20 drops = 1ml/1tsp = 5ml.

PRECAUTIONS

Not suitable for children or those who are pregnant or lactating.

Eyebright recipes

Medicinal recipes

Eyebright tisane
Pour 250ml boiling water over 1tsp/5g of the dried herb and allow to steep for 10 minutes. Use as a mucolytic, in the treatment of sinusitis and seasonal allergies.

Eyebright decoction
Boil 1tbsp/15g of the herb for 10–15 minutes in 250ml of water. Use as above and as an eye wash for infected eyes and to treat styes.

Eyebright infused tincture: 1:5 45%
If you are using 40% alcohol, ie. vodka, make a simple tincture by covering 1 part herb to 5 parts fluid.

If you are using Everclear or other 100% proof, use the following method for a specific tincture:
- 100g dried Eyebright herb
- 225ml alcohol
- 275ml water

Take 100g of the dried herb and split into two parts of 50g each. Place 50g in the alcohol and the other 50g in the boiled water. Steep/infuse in the water for 10 minutes. Strain thoroughly and top up if the water is less than 275ml. Add the infusion to the alcohol mix and leave for 14 days before straining. Use for anti-inflammatory effects and to treat conjunctivitis or blepharitis, allergies, colds, sinusitis and general respiratory discomfort.

Hayfever tea
- 1 part Eyebright
- 1 part Nettle
- 1 part Plantain

Mix the herbs and then pour 250ml boiling water over 1tsp/5g of the dried herb mix and allow to steep for 10 minutes.

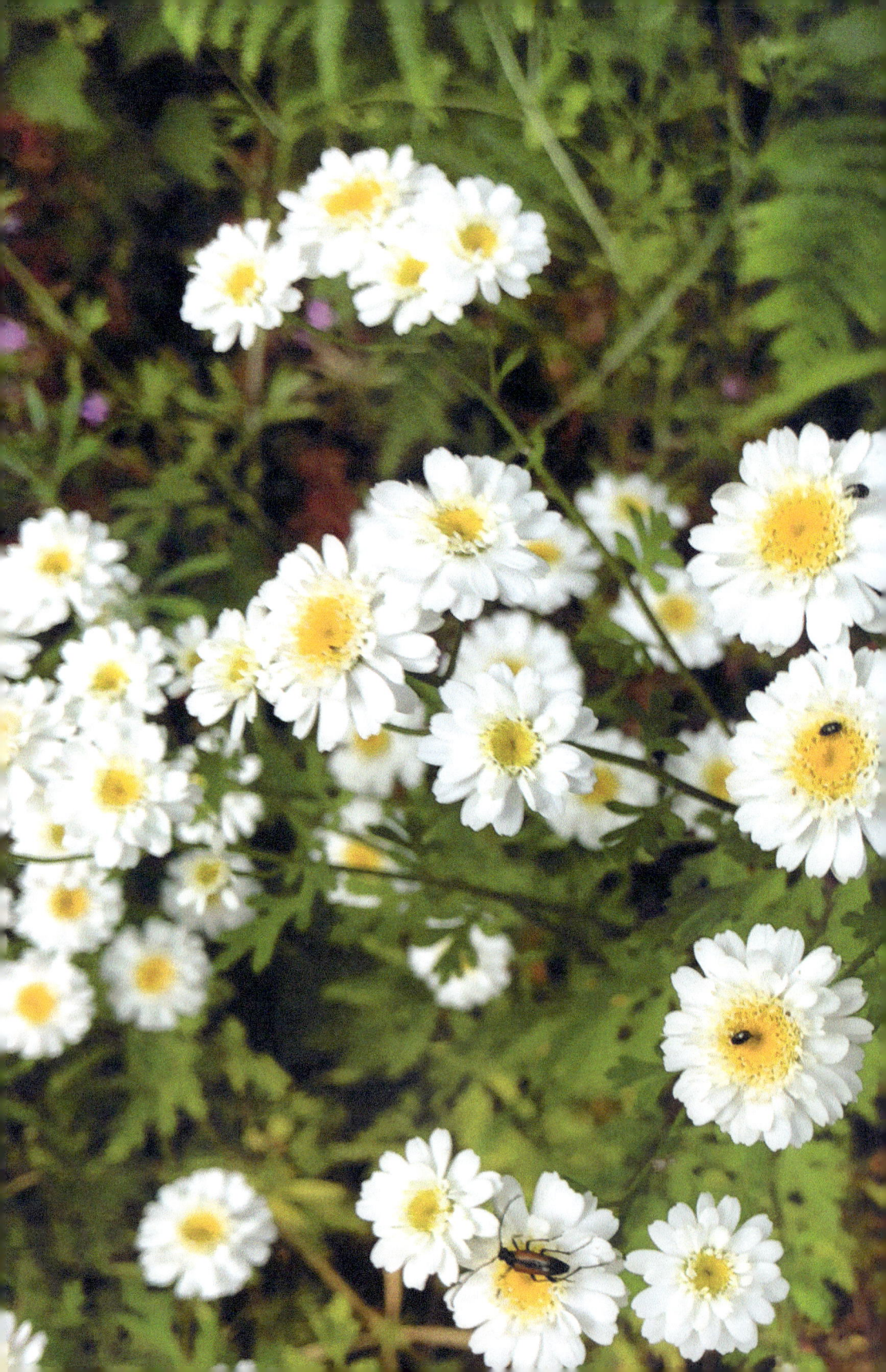

FEVERFEW
Tanacetum parthenium

Tanacetum parthenium, commonly known as Feverfew, is native to the Balkans, but has been widely cultivated and naturalised in the UK since around 1600. It is found in gardens, but also growing wild on roadsides, in waste areas and disturbed habitats. Feverfew has a long history of medicinal use and also as a natural insect repellent.

HISTORICAL USES

Hildegard of Bingen (1098–1179) strongly endorsed Feverfew, writing in *Physica*: *If a person eats it frequently, it will chase illness from him and keep him from getting sick.*

In his *Herball*, John Gerard (1545–1612) recommended Feverfew '*dried and made into powder, taken with honey or sweet wine, [it] purgeth by siege melancholy and flegme; wherefore it is very good for them that are giddie in the head, or which have the turning called Vertigo, that is, a swimming and turning in the head.*'

Nicholas Culpeper's *Herbal* advised that '*a decoction of the flowers in wine, with a little nutmeg and drank often is an approved remedy to bring down women's menstruation speedily and help expel the afterbirth. The decoction, made with some sugar or honey is used by many with good success to help the cough and stuffing of the chest, by colds as also to cleanse the reins*

ETYMOLOGY OF COMMON NAME
Etymology of common name
From the Latin *febrifugia*, from *febris*, 'fever' + *fugō*, 'I drive away'.

PLANT LORE
Planting Feverfew near the house, especially the door, was said to protect those inside from the plague.

USE
All aerial parts.

EDIBILITY
The dried flowers are used as a flavouring in cooking certain pastries. It imparts a deliciously aromatic bitter taste to certain foods

HARVEST
Just as it flowers.

MEDICINAL PROPERTIES
Analgesic, anticoagulant, uterine stimulant and sedative.

ACTIVE CONSTITUENTS
Flavonoids, essential oil, glycosides, sesquiterpenes, terpenoids, pinenes.

LEFT: FEVERFEW

[kidneys] *and bladder and help to expel the stone.'*

Dr John Hill, in *The British Herbal* (1756) stated, *'In the worst headaches this Herb exceeds whatever else is known.'*

MODERN RESEARCH

The plant's name means 'fever reducer', and there is evidence that Feverfew is indeed antipyretic, but that is not typically its main use. A 2011 review established that the most important active principles in the plant are the sesquiterpene lactones, particularly parthenolide, which has significant analgesic, anti-inflammatory and antipyretic activities. This confirms the folk uses of Feverfew for treatment of migraine headache, fever, common cold and arthritis. These and other findings from modern research are shown below:

Uterine stimulant

The uterine effect of the plant as described by Culpeper was confirmed in 2019, with a study finding the extract of the flower to be the most potent, followed by the leaf extract. This finding agreed with the folk uses of the plant as an abortifacient, emmenagogue and in certain labour difficulties. It also agreed with the warning of drug producers that Feverfew should not be used during pregnancy.

Analgesic

Feverfew has received mixed results in clinical trials in relation to migraine, but a 2019 study on children showed that it significantly reduced the frequency of tension-type headache during treatment, and the efficacy was maintained after 16 weeks of treatment withdrawal. The frequency of migraine attacks was also reduced in the migraine with aura (classic migraine with sensory disturbances) group during treatment and after withdrawal. Conversely, migraine without aura patients showed reduction in migraine's frequency during treatment but not at the end of the study.

Sedative

In some traditional medicinal books, Feverfew is described as having sedative or hypnotic effects (Khorasani, 1371). Studies showed that some components of this plant, namely α-pinene derivatives, may indeed have sedative and mild tranquillising properties (Pareek et al., 2011), and this was confirmed in a 2020 study in mice that showed significant sedative-hypnotic effects; this meant that future isolation of the active constituent could be trialled as a sedative agent.

Anticoagulant

Feverfew has been called the 'aspirin of the Middle Ages' because it was widely used to treat various inflammatory diseases, fevers and headaches. A 2022 study was carried out to see if it could be considered an herbal alternative to aspirin, particularly regarding the coagulation effects. Sixty individuals were randomly recruited into control and intervention groups. Participants consumed 1 capsule (250mg) of Feverfew or placebo every day for 2 weeks. Results showed that Feverfew produced no significant side effects in healthy individuals but demonstrated anticoagulant properties and a regulatory role in the immune system.

TOPICAL USES

The parthenolides in Feverfew can cause sensitivity to skin but are also believed to have insecticidal properties. Hanging dried Feverfew bouquets in indoor spaces was a traditional measure to help deter insects as the scent released from the dried flowers and leaves acted as a natural insect deterrent.

DOSAGE

The leaves are ingested fresh (2.5mg) or dried (50mg) leaves.

Tincture – 1:5 45%, 5–20 drops every 2 hours, 20 drops = 1ml/1tsp = 5ml.

PRECAUTIONS

Feverfew may inhibit the activity of platelets (which have a role in blood clotting), so individuals taking blood-thinning medications (such as aspirin and warfarin) should consult a healthcare provider before taking this herb. Children below 2 years of age must not be given Feverfew herb. Furthermore, the herbal remedy is not recommended for use during a term of pregnancy or by lactating women. Topical uses can cause contact dermatitis owing to the parthenolides. Dried Feverfew leaf or Feverfew extract are likely to be safe when taken for up to 4 months.

Feverfew recipes

Medicinal recipes

Feverfew cold infusion

This herb is said to be less effective when subjected to heat, hence the recipe for a cold infusion. The fresh leaf can also be chewed at a dose of 3 leaves per day. Steep 2tsp/10g dried herb in 1 litre of cold water overnight and drink at intervals of 3–4 hours to relieve headaches, migraines, arthritis, neuritis, neuralgia, indigestion, colds and muscle tension.

Feverfew oxymel

Feverfew is very bitter and so an oxymel makes it much easier to stomach. Put the herb in your jar to about a quarter depth and then fill with the liquid part in the ratio of 1 part honey to 3 parts apple cider vinegar. Stir, seal and leave to steep/infuse for 2 weeks. Strain out the liquid into another jar and then take 2 spoonfuls diluted with water at each dose.

Feverfew infused tincture: 1:5 45%

If you are using 40% alcohol, ie. vodka, make a simple tincture by covering 1 part herb to 5 parts fluid.

If you are using Everclear or other 100% proof, use the following method for a specific tincture:

- 100g dried Feverfew flowers
- 225ml alcohol
- 275ml water

Take 100g of the dried herb and split into two parts of 50g each. Place 50g in the alcohol and the other 50g in the boiled water. Steep/infuse in the water for 10 minutes. Strain thoroughly and top up if the water is less than 275ml. Add the infusion to the alcohol mix and leave for 14 days before straining. Use as a painkiller, anti-inflammatory, for anti-rheumatism and for hypertension.

FIGWORT
Scrophularia nodosa/auriculata

The *Scrophulariaceae* family is commonly known as the Figworts. In the UK, there are several species, including Common figwort (*Scrophularia nodosa*), the most widespread species, and Water figwort (*Scrophularia auriculata*), which prefers wet habitats such as marshes, riverbanks and damp woodland edges. Both of these Figworts have a history of use in traditional herbal medicine.

HISTORICAL USES

Nicholas Culpeper's *Herbal* stated that '*the decoction of the herb taken inwardly, and the bruised herb applied outwardly dissolved clotted and congealed blood coming from wounds, bruises and falls.*'

Dr John Hill wrote in *The British Herbal* (1756) that Figwort '*is famous as a remedy for the evil* [scrophula]; *the method is to take a strong decoction of the roots daily for a great length of time … A strong decoction of the root is good against all foulness of the skin, the itch not excepted: it should be taken inwardly, and the parts washed with some of it also warm. An ointment is made in some places of the leaves, boiled in lard, and used for the same purposes; but the decoction, or a poultice, made from the fresh root, boiled soft with bread and milk, will answer the purpose better.*'

ETYMOLOGY OF COMMON NAME
Figwort refers to an early use of these plants in treating haemorrhoids, an ailment then known as 'figs'.

PLANT LORE
The plant was once known as 'scrophula herb' because it was believed to cure this condition.

USE
All parts.

EDIBILITY
Only in times of famine!

HARVEST
In summer.

MEDICINAL PROPERTIES
Antispasmodic, vulnerary and anti-inflammatory.

ACTIVE CONSTITUENTS
Flavonoids, iridoid glycosides, phenolic acids, saponins, triterpenoids, sterols, phenylpropanoids, essential oils.

In his 1897, second edition book *Herbal Simples*, William Fernie advised that, *'when an ointment is made with it, using the whole plant bruised and treated with unsalted lard,* [it is] *a sovereign remedy against 'burnt holes' or gangrenous chickenpox.'*

MODERN RESEARCH

Figwort's scientific name derives from the folklore belief that the plant cured scrophula, an old term for lymphatic infections in the neck connected to tuberculosis. However, most people nowadays take Figwort as a diuretic, though it is still sometimes applied externally, as Culpeper and Fernie directed, for eczema, itching, psoriasis and rashes. Modern research has found the following properties for Figwort:

Anti-inflammatory

Water figwort in particular is used in traditional medicine against inflammatory skin diseases as above. It has shown a marked effect on both acute and chronic models of inflammation in studies (Cuéllar et al., 1998), while research in 2000 confirmed showed that iridoids in the plant were responsible for delayed reactions in contact dermatitis, which led to significantly reduced inflammatory lesions and suppression of cellular infiltration.

Vulnerary

A 2002 study confirmed the wound-healing properties of Woodland (ie common) figwort again via iridoids isolated from dried seed pods. These were shown, *in vitro*, to stimulate the growth of human dermal fibroblasts (connective tissues). Both this and the above anti-inflammatory properties would have been the reason for effects on wounds, etc. described by the historical authors.

Antispasmodic

A January 2012 study found that Figwort clearly demonstrated the presence of antispasmodic constituents and provided additional support to the other above activities.

Some people also use Figwort as a substitute for Devil's claw (*Hargophytum procumbens*), because the two herbs contain similar chemicals. The uses for Devil's claw are also stated as anti-inflammatory.

TOPICAL USES

As previously mentioned, Figwort is helpful in healing chronic skin conditions including psoriasis and eczema when it is applied topically to the affected areas as well as for hastening the healing wounds, burn injuries, ulcers and haemorrhoids. Water figwort is particularly useful in treating contact dermatitis.

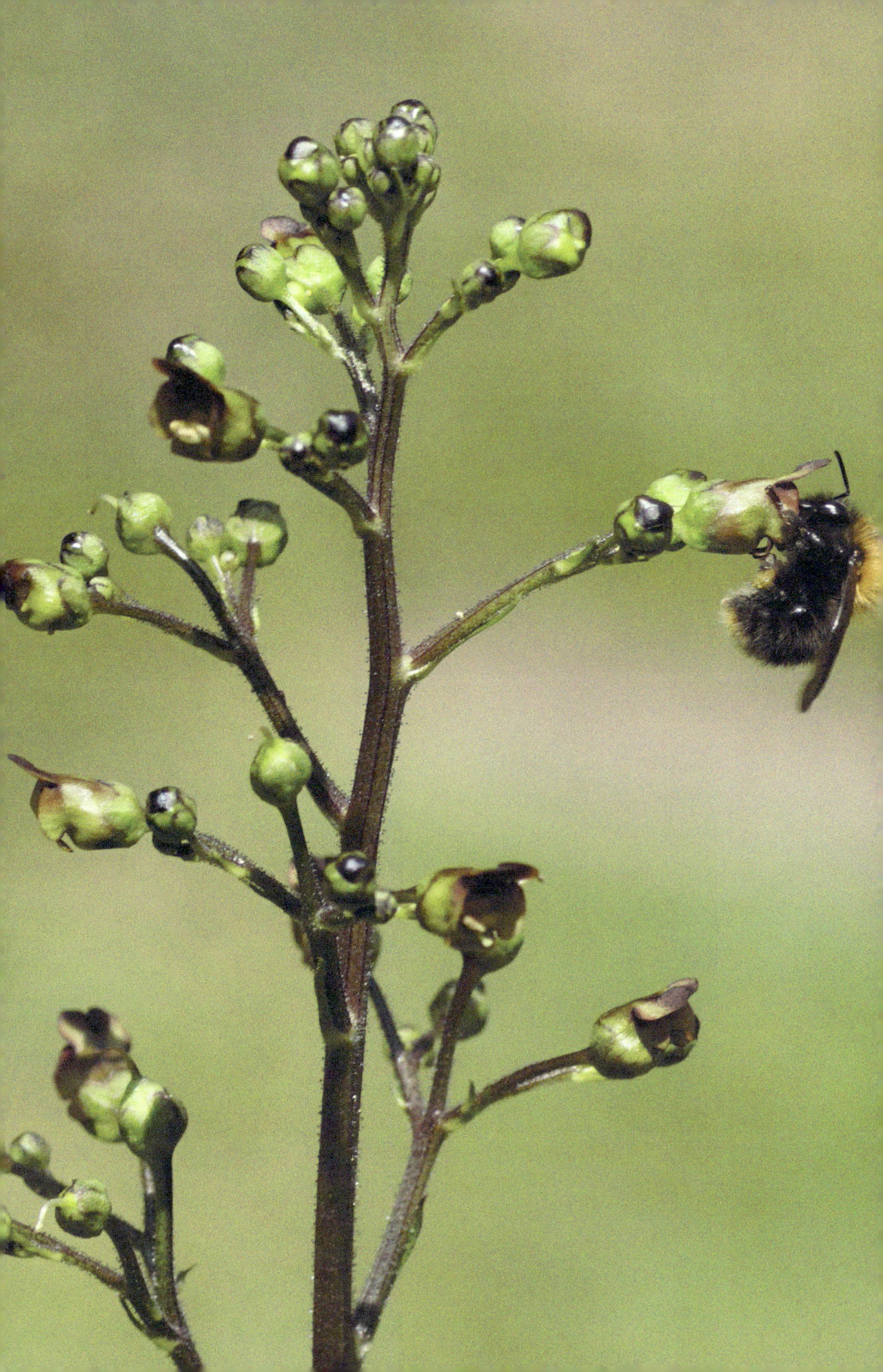

DOSAGE

Tisane – 1tsp/5g, 3 times per day.
Tincture – 1:10 45% – 2–4ml, 3 times daily – 20 drops = 1ml/1tsp = 5ml.

PRECAUTIONS

Like its close family member Foxglove (*Digitalis purpurea*), Figwort is cardioactive and therefore should not be used by those with heart conditions or arrhythmia. In addition, Figwort also possesses potent and potentially harmful laxative as well as emetic properties. Not suitable for children or those who are pregnant or lactating.

Figwort recipes

Medicinal recipes

Figwort tisane

Pour 250ml boiling water over 1tsp/5g of the dried herb and allow to steep for 10 minutes. Use for whole body detoxification and in lymphatic conditions, swellings and swollen lymph nodes.

Figwort compress

Soak a cloth in a tisane of the dried herb and use to soothe sprains, swellings, burns, inflammations etc.

Figwort infused tincture: 1:10 45%

If you are using 40% alcohol, ie vodka, cover one part herb to 10 parts fluid.

If you are using Everclear or other 100% proof, use the following method for a specific tincture:

- 100g dried Figwort herb
- 450ml alcohol
- 650ml water

Take 100g of dried herb and split into two parts of 50g each. Place 50g in the alcohol and the other 50g in the boiled water. Steep/infuse in the water for 10 minutes. Strain thoroughly and top up if the water is less than 650ml. Add the infusion to the alcohol mix and leave for 14 days before straining. Use topically for joints affected by arthritis or other inflammatory conditions. Dilute, if necessary, with water before applying. Also, a specific for skin conditions like eczema and/or psoriasis or any chronic skin condition (especially those accompanied by eruptions, itchiness and irritation).

Figwort salve for wounds

- 100g Figwort leaves and flowers
- 2tbsp alcohol, such as Everclear
- 1l grapeseed oil

Place the chopped herb in a jar with the alcohol and allow to steep for 10 minutes before adding the oil. Leave for 4 weeks and then strain. Make into a salve by using a 1:4 ratio of melted beeswax to your oil mix, ie 1 part wax to 4 parts liquid. Melt the wax pellets in the oil in a double boiler or bain-marie. Remove from the heat and allow to cool and set completely before using topically for healing wounds, burns and other and skin irritations/injuries.

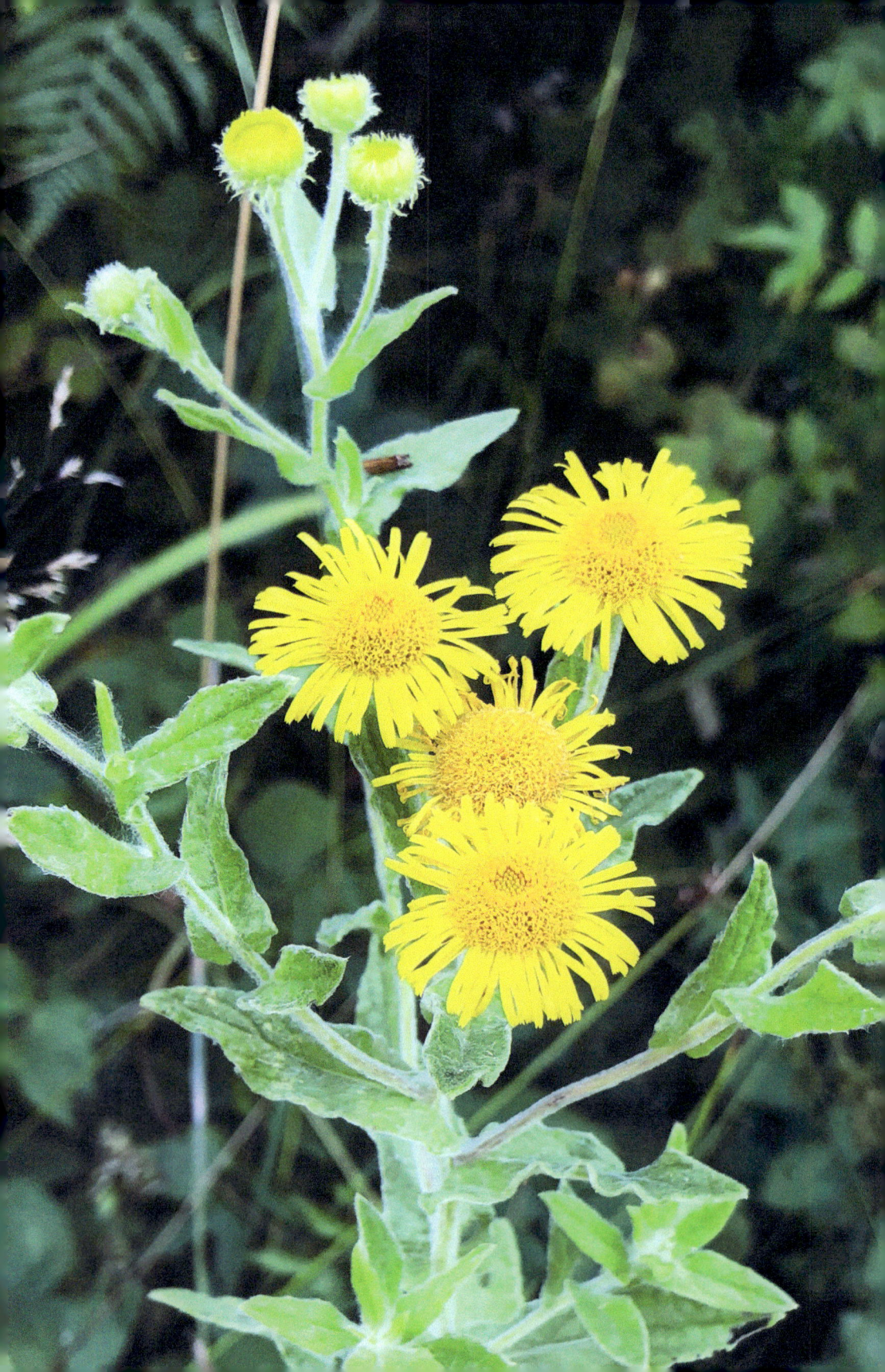

FLEABANE
Pulicaria dysenterica

Pulicaria dysenterica, Common fleabane, is a species in the Daisy and Sunflower family, the *Asteraceae*. It is native to the UK and commonly found in moist or wet areas, such as marshes, riverbanks and damp meadows. Common fleabane has a history of use in traditional herbal medicine for gastrointestinal issues, and to treat skin conditions such as wounds, ulcers and insect bites.

HISTORICAL USES

Maud Grieve's 1931 classic *A Modern Herbal* related that Fleabane *'was formerly used in dysentery, and on this account received its specific name from Linnaeus, who in his* Flora Svecica *says that he had been informed by General Keit, of the Russian Army, that his soldiers, in one of their expeditions against Persia, were cured of dysentery by means of this plant.'*

Old authors knew it as 'Middle fleabane', the Latin name being derived from the fact that, if burnt, the smoke drives away fleas and other insects.

Nicholas Culpeper's *Herbal* stated that *'The smell is supposed delightful to insects, and the juice destructive to them. The juice provokes urine and expels gravel in the reins or the kidneys ... It helps also the sciatica, griping of the belly, the colic, defects of the liver and provokes the women's courses.'*

ETYMOLOGY OF COMMON NAME
Derived from a belief that the dried plants repelled fleas or that the plants were poisonous to fleas.

PLANT LORE
'fleabane bound to the forehead is a great helpe to cure one of the frensie'.

USE
All parts.

EDIBILITY
The leaves of Fleabane are cooked (they can be eaten raw, but cooking will remove the small hairs on the leaves and stems) and served along with other greens.

HARVEST
In late summer.

MEDICINAL PROPERTIES
Antimicrobial, cytotoxic, anti-inflammatory, anxiolytic and antioxidant.

ACTIVE CONSTITUENTS
Flavonoids, essential oils, terpenoids, tannins, polyacetylenes, coumarins.

LEFT: FLEABANE

MODERN RESEARCH

Cadinol, nerolidol and caryophyllene were identified as components of Fleabane in a 2007 study, and their presence underlies the following properties:

Antimicrobial

The data from a study in 2002 indicates that extracts from Fleabane were found active against three tested bacteria (*Staphylococcus aureus*, *Bacillus cereus* and *Vibrio cholerae*) with *V. cholerae* the most sensitive. The extracts appeared to inhibit the growth of cholera, and this was further confirmed in a 2010 study. In 2023, further results showed that the essential oil of Fleabane inhibited the growth of *Pseudomonas aeruginosa* and *Escherichia coli* as well as the previous bacterial strains and was related to the presence of the three compounds mentioned. I have not found any evidence that Fleabane has been tested against shigella or entamoeba, the causes of dysentery, but this does not mean that it could not theoretically have the response described by Maud Grieve.

Antioxidant and cytotoxic

A 2022 study analysing the polyphenols in the plant and their cytotoxic activities on cervical cancer cells showed good antioxidant properties, with stronger activity recorded in extracts from underground compared to aerial parts of the plant. There was also a good cytotoxicity against the cancer cells reported, which could be further investigated.

Anti-inflammatory and gastroprotective

As we know from the historical writers, Fleabane was believed to have properties that could help alleviate abdominal pain, cramping and diarrhoea. We now know that cadinol, nerolidol and caryophyllene, in addition to their antimicrobial qualities, also possesses anti-inflammatory properties, which can specifically help reduce inflammation in the gastrointestinal tract. Then, the use of Fleabane in gastrointestinal issues was finally confirmed in a 2022 study, which found that the essential oil acts as a moderate acetylcholinesterase inhibitor and increased gastrointestinal motility. This together with its anti-inflammatory and antimicrobial activity means that Fleabane essential oil is further corroborated for treating digestive problems caused by some microorganisms.

Anxiolytic and sedative

While cadinol has been reported to have sedative effects, which could promote relaxation and aid in sleep, some studies suggest that caryophyllene may have anxiolytic effects, meaning it could help reduce anxiety. Caryophyllene is actually a cannabinoid, though it is one of the few that is not psychoactive, and the anxiolytic effects are thought to be mediated through interactions with the endocannabinoid system, specifically the CB2 cannabinoid receptors.

TOPICAL USES

A salve or poultice made from Fleabane root can be used to treat open sores, using the antimicrobial and anti-inflammatory properties.

DOSAGE

Tisane – 1tsp/5g. Drink half a cup, 3 times per day.
Tincture – 1:5 60%, 5–10ml, 3 times per day – 20 drops = 1ml/1tsp = 5ml.

PRECAUTIONS

Not suitable for children or those who are pregnant or lactating.

Fleabane recipes

Medicinal recipes

Fleabane tisane

Pour 250ml boiling water over 1tsp/5g of the herb and allow to steep for 10 minutes. Use as an anti-inflammatory in cases of digestive distress and diarrhoea, as well as for its sedative properties.

Fleabane infused tincture: 1:5 60%

If you are using 40% alcohol, ie. vodka, then cover 1 part herb to 10 parts fluid.

If you are using Everclear or other 100% proof, then use the following method for a specific tincture:

- 100g dried Fleabane herb
- 300ml alcohol
- 200ml water

Take 100g of fresh herb when in bloom and split into two parts of 50g each. Place 50g in the alcohol and the other 50g in the boiled water. Steep/infuse in the water for 10 minutes. Strain thoroughly and top up if the water is less than 200ml. Add the infusion to the alcohol mix and leave for 14 days before straining. Use in cases of diarrhoea and as above.

Fleabane poultice

- 1tsp fresh Fleabane root (if using dried you will need to moisten with water first)
- 2tsp coconut oil
- cheesecloth or cotton bandage

Finely chop or grate the root into a pulp and add the coconut oil to make a paste. Spread the paste evenly over the desired area and wrap with the cloth or bandage. Use for irritated skin and for scratches and insect bites.

FUMITORY, COMMON
Fumaria officinalis

Fumaria officinalis, commonly known as Fumitory, or earth smoke, is a species in the Poppy family, *Papaveraceae*. It is native to the UK and is typically found in disturbed habitats, such as arable fields, gardens, roadsides and waste areas. Fumitory has a history of use in traditional herbal medicine for its cooling and cleansing properties and for skin conditions such as eczema and acne.

HISTORICAL USES

Fumitory was widely used in the past as far back as Ancient Greece, while the Roman naturalist Pliny said in his *Natural History* that the juice of the plant brings on such a flow of tears that the sight becomes dim as with smoke (Delaveau, 1980), hence its reputed use in afflictions of the eye.

In his *Herball*, John Gerard noted its external use externally by stating that '*it helpeth in the summertime those that are troubled with scabs.*'

Nicholas Culpeper's *Herbal* agreed, '*it helps such as are itchy and scabbed, clears the skin, opens stoppings of the liver and spleen, helps rickets, hypochondriac melancholy, madness, frenzies.*'

Fumitory has been a part of many European herbal traditions, where it was used to prepare remedies for various ailments. In Portugal, it was used

ETYMOLOGY OF COMMON NAME
From late Middle English *fumyter*, 'smoke of the earth', from the fact that the colour of the flowers gives the appearance of smoke rising from the ground.

PLANT LORE
When gathered before a wedding and boiled in water, milk and whey, it was traditionally used as a wash for the complexion of rustic maids.

USE
The leaves.

EDIBILITY
Not edible

HARVEST
As flowering begins, summer.

MEDICINAL PROPERTIES
Hepatoprotective, stimulant and analgesic.

ACTIVE CONSTITUENTS
Alkaloids flavonoids, fumaric acid, phenolic compounds, glycosides, tannins.

in a tea against liver and gallbladder diseases. In Italy, the plant was used as bile stimulant, hypertensive, antispasmodic, respiratory stimulant and anti-arteriosclerosis. The plant was also used in hypertension, constipation, as liver detoxification, and spasmolytic in Cyprus and for the treatment of hypertension and cardiac disease in Morocco.

MODERN RESEARCH

I have been unable to confirm the use described by Pliny of an eye lotion, save for one reference in the *British Herbal Pharmacopoeia* (1976). Fumitory, however, is still widely used in traditional and folkloric systems of medicine and modern research has confirmed the following properties:

Bile stimulant

The historical writers are justified insofar as the plant has been used in impairments of the biliary duct and in cases of gallstones when surgery is not possible. In 1973, the bile-stimulating activity of Fumitory was demonstrated in animals and shown to decrease bile flow that had been artificially increased while increasing artificially reduced flow. Fumitory also inhibited the formation of gallbladder calculi in animal tests.

In 1979, a double-blind clinical trial was performed in a group of 30 patients with different biliary disorders (dyskinesia, cholecystitis, hepatopathy, cholelithiasis and post-operation cholecystectomy syndrome). Patients took 3 tablets of Fumaria-Nebulisat 250mg daily (two before meals and the third before sleep), for 28 days. The results were successful, especially against the symptoms of fullness and flatulence.

Fumitory was recognised by the European Medicines Agency in 2011 as a traditional herbal medicine used to increase bile flow and for the relief of symptoms of indigestion (such as sensation of fullness, flatulence and slow digestion).

Muscle relaxant

In 2015, the effect of an ethanolic extract of Fumitory on muscle relaxation and motor coordination was evaluated. The results indicated that the extract influences muscle coordination, which could be caused by an interaction of flavonoids with the GABA receptors in the brain. This muscle relaxation property has the potential to be used in the same way as centrally acting muscle relaxants like diazepam.

Hepatoprotective

Fumitory has also been shown to protect the liver by reducing elevated levels of bilirubin (higher than usual levels of bilirubin may indicate different types of liver injury), cholesterol and triglycerides in liver-injured rats.

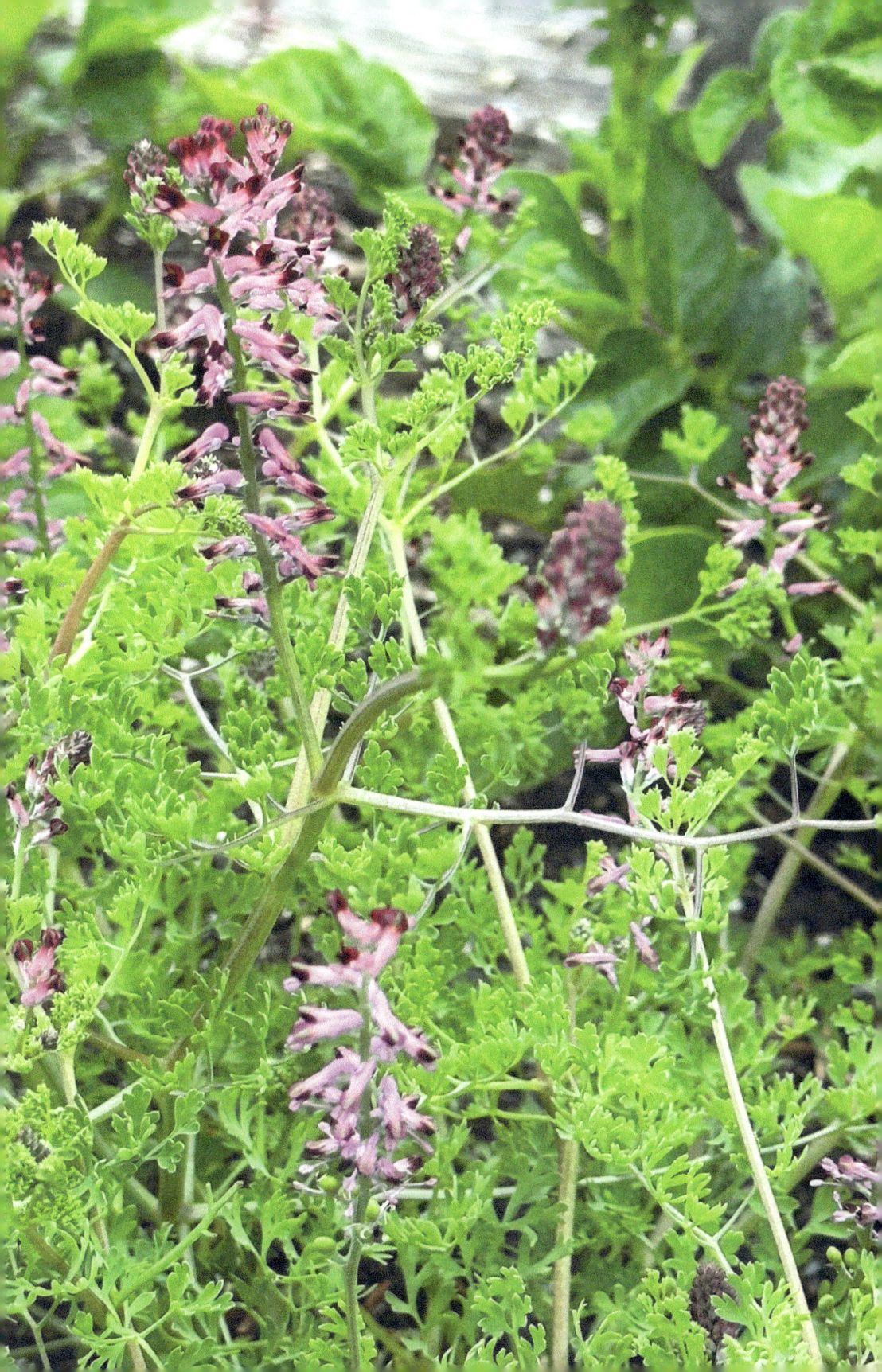

Analgesic

Studies have also shown that Fumitory has pain-relieving effects, particularly in an ethanol extract. At a dose of 500mg/kg Fumitory had better pain-relieving activity than the diclofenac-treated group.

TOPICAL USES

So far as the historical writers' assertions regarding the use of Fumitory for 'scabs' and 'itches' are concerned, Fumitory is used both internally and externally for skin complaints, including psoriasis, eczema and dermatitis. When made into a cream or an ointment it is effective for itchy rashes and helpful in case of the cradle cap on babies.

DOSAGE

Tisane – 1tsp/5g. Drink a half cup, 3 times per day.
Tincture – 1:5 25% – 1–4ml, 3 times per day – 20 drops = 1ml/1tsp = 5ml.

PRECAUTIONS

Avoid in those with fits and epilepsy. Contraindicated with glaucoma patients. Avoid during pregnancy and breast-feeding. Allopathic medication for high blood pressure – effects increased.

Fumitory recipes

Medicinal recipes

Fumitory tisane
Pour 250ml boiling water over 1tsp/5g of the herb and allow to steep for 10 minutes. Use as a laxative and diuretic, as a treatment for digestive disorders, and for colic pain.

Fumitory compress
Use for skin complaints, including psoriasis, eczema and dermatitis. Soak a cloth in a tisane of the dried flowers and apply it to the affected areas 2–3 times a day.

Fumitory infused tincture 1:5 25%
If you are using 40% alcohol, ie. vodka, then you will need to dilute this at the ratio of 60ml water to every 100ml of vodka to make a 25% medium and then cover 1 part herb to 5 parts fluid.

If you are using Everclear or other 100% proof, use the following method for a specific tincture:

- 100g dried Fumitory herb
- 125ml alcohol
- 375ml water

Take 100g of dried herb and split into two parts of 50g each. Place 50g in the alcohol and the other 50g in the boiled water. Steep/infuse in the water for 10 minutes. Strain thoroughly and top up if the water is less than 375ml. Add the infusion to the alcohol mix and leave for 14 days before straining. Use in cases of diarrhoea and as opposite. Use to stimulate the smooth muscles of the intestines to help with irritable bowel syndrome (IBS) and stomach cramps but also to promote the function of both the liver and the gallbladder and have an antispasmodic effect, thus normalising the bile flow.

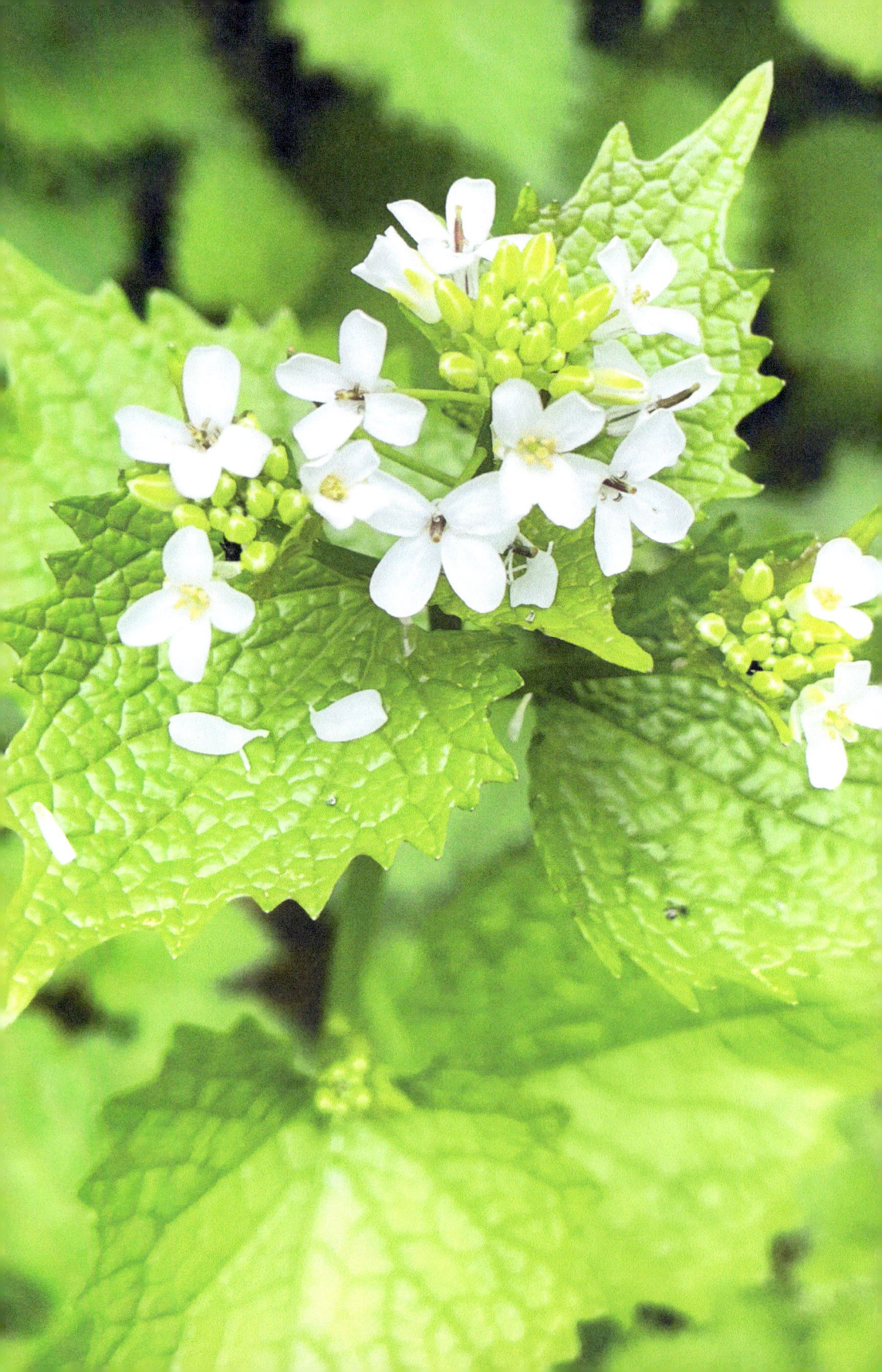

GARLIC MUSTARD
Alliaria petiolata

Alliaria petiolata, commonly known as Garlic mustard, is a plant species native to the UK. It belongs to the *Brassicaceae* family, which also includes Cabbage, Broccoli and Mustard. Garlic mustard is commonly found in woodlands, hedgerows, roadsides and disturbed habitats. It has been used as a culinary herb but also in traditional herbal medicine for various purposes.

HISTORICAL USES

Garlic mustard is one of the oldest herbs used in Europe. Remnants have been found in the pottery of the Ertebølle and Funnelneck Beaker culture in north-eastern Germany and Denmark, dating to 4100–3750 BCE.

Nicholas Culpeper's *Herbal* described its virtues as follows:

It warms also the stomach and causes digestion. The juice thereof boiled with honey is accounted to be as good as hedge mustard for the cough, to cut and expectorate the tough phlegm. The seed bruised and boiled in wine, is a singularly good remedy for the wind colic, or the stone, being drank warm. It is also given to women troubled with the mother, both to drink, and the seed put into a cloth, and applied while it is warm, is of singularly good use. The leaves also, or the seed boiled, is good to be used in clysters to ease the pains of the

ETYMOLOGY OF COMMON NAME
From the garlic fragrance that comes from rubbing the leaves.

PLANT LORE
Also known as 'Poor man's garlic' and 'Jack-by-the-hedge', with Jack denoting the common (or poor) man.

USE
The flowers, leaves and seeds.

EDIBILITY
The young leaves, raw or cooked as a potherb or as a flavouring. A good addition to salads especially early in the year.

HARVEST
Before the plant flowers.

MEDICINAL PROPERTIES
Anti-inflammatory, antioxidant, diaphoretic, anticancerogenic and antimicrobial.

ACTIVE CONSTITUENTS
Glucosinolates, flavonoids, phenolic compounds, essential oils.

stone. The green leaves are held to be good to heal the ulcers in the legs.

MODERN RESEARCH

Though it clearly has a history of use, Garlic mustard seems to be regarded more as a food than a medicine in modern times. It is worth noting that it has good amounts of vitamins A, C, E and some of the B group, potassium, calcium, magnesium, copper and iron. In fact, the leaves of the plant just prior to flowering have a higher vitamin C content than oranges and more vitamin A than spinach.

Garlic mustard, like many plants in the *Brassicaceae* family, may contain various phytochemicals, including glucosinolates. Glucosinolates are compounds that can be converted into bioactive substances, such as isothiocyanates, when the plant is damaged (eg during chewing or cooking). Isothiocyanates are known to have the following medicinal properties:

Diaphoretic

The leaves of Garlic mustard when eaten trigger the conversion of glucosinolates into isothiocyanates. One of the results of this is sweating, hence Culpeper's description of it as warming and digestive. Sweating has an important role in regulating human body temperature, expelling toxins and in the treatment of illnesses such as bronchitis, asthma and eczema. The leaves and stems are harvested before the plant comes into flower and they can be dried for later use. The roots are chopped up small and then heated in oil to make an ointment to rub on the chest in order to bring relief from bronchitis. The juice of the plant has an inhibitory effect on *Bacillus* and on gram-negative bacteria of the typhoid–paratyphoid–enteritis group, and could therefore be useful in reducing typhoid fevers.

Antioxidant and anti-inflammatory

Isothiocyanates have been shown to inhibit the activation of pro-inflammatory pathways and modulate the activity of enzymes involved in inflammation. Isothiocyanates also possess antioxidant properties, which means they can neutralise free radicals and reduce the oxidative stress that is often associated with inflammation. By mitigating this stress, isothiocyanates may contribute to a reduction in inflammation.

Anticancerogenic

Its isothiocyanates are also believed to be responsible for the plant's cancer prevention and treatment potential, which was first reported in 1977 by Professor Lee Wattenberg. In a 2022 review, isothiocyanates were noted to act across all stages of carcinogenesis and control early-stage cancer onset by demonstrating anti-proliferative, pro-apoptotic, anti-inflammatory, anti-migratory and anti-angiogenic effects against several cancers including cervical, liver, laryngeal, skin, lymph and brain.

Antimicrobial

The antimicrobial activity of isothiocyanates has been documented in several studies, suggesting use as natural antibiotic agent and/or pesticide. A 2018 study found that isothiocyanates exert a broad spectrum of action against gram-positive and gram-negative bacteria, such as *Escherichia coli* strains and *Staphylococcus aureus*, including multi-drug-resistance strains, which is why Culpeper may have found the leaves good for healing ulcers in the legs. Finally, isothiocyanates showed strong activity against *Helicobacter pylori*, which may again be why Culpeper saw some relief when using it for colic etc.

TOPICAL USES

Externally, the leaves, as Culpeper said, have been used as an antiseptic poultice on ulcers etc. and are effective in relieving the itching caused by bites and stings.

DOSAGE

Eaten or used externally.

PRECAUTIONS

Not suitable for children or those who are pregnant or lactating.

Garlic mustard recipes

Medicinal recipes

Garlic mustard honey

Pack a sterilised jar about two-thirds full of either fresh or dried herbs, then add a good-quality honey. Once the herbs are generously covered it's important to stir well to break any air bubbles (which could encourage bacterial growth). Then the jar can be sealed and left to steep/infuse for at least a month. To make the straining process easier, sit the sealed jar in a bowl of hot water. This will slightly loosen the honey, without overheating it, making it much easier to strain through a sieve. Store in a cool place. Use 1–2tsp of the mixture every hour as an expectorant for chesty coughs.

Garlic mustard poultice

- 1tsp fresh herb (if using dried you will need to moisten with water first)
- 2tsp coconut oil
- cheesecloth or cotton bandage

Finely chop the herb into a pulp and add the coconut oil to make a paste. Spread the paste evenly over the desired area and wrap with the cloth or bandage. Use as an antiseptic for wounds and ulcers.

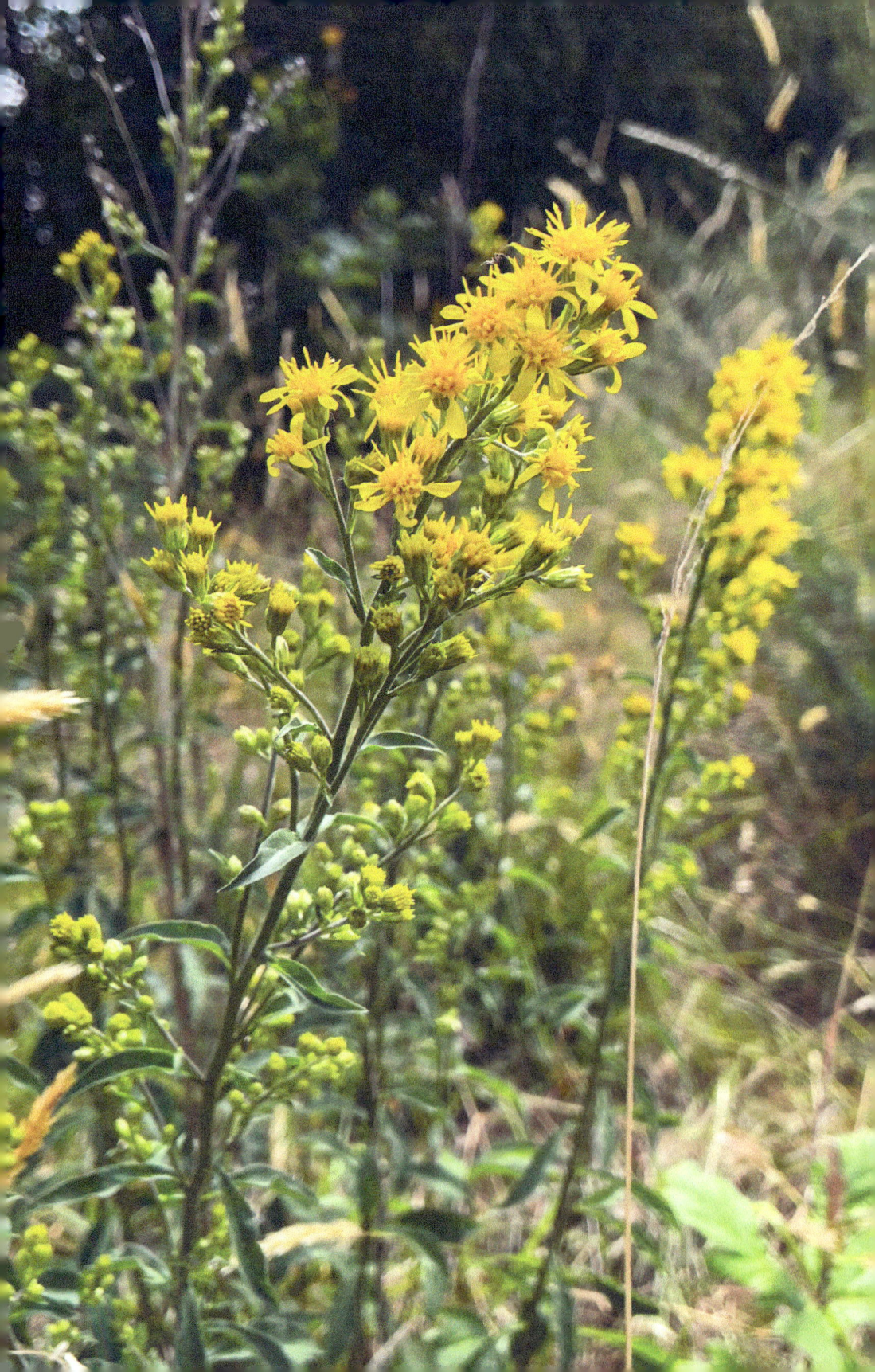

GOLDENROD
Solidago virgaurea

While there are several species of *Solidago* or Goldenrods found in the UK, including Canadian goldenrod (*Solidago canadensis*), only *Solidago virgaurea*, commonly known as European goldenrod, is native. It is a member of the large *Asteraceae* family, popularly referred to as the Aster, Daisy or Sunflower family, and is found in open, sunny habitats such as meadows, woodland edges, grasslands and disturbed areas. It has a history of use in traditional herbal medicine.

HISTORICAL USES

John Gerard said in his *Herball* that Goldenrod is: *extolled above all herbes for the stopping of blood in wounds.*

Nicholas Culpeper's *Herbal* described it as '*an excellent diuretic and few remedies can exceed it where there is gravel in the kidneys ... It is a sovereign wound herb, inferior to none, both for the inward and outward hurts; green wounds, old sores and ulcers, are quickly cured therewith. It also is of especial use in all lotions for sores or ulcers in the mouth, throat, or privy parts of man or woman. The decoction also helps to fasten the teeth that are loose in the gums.*'

In *Fray's Golden Recipes for the Use of All Ages* (1897) it was recommended as a remedy for backache '*used in the manner of tea, 1 ounce to a pint of water.*'

ETYMOLOGY OF COMMON NAME
Named from the 1560s, so called for its yellow heads.

PLANT LORE
Goldenrod is often seen as a symbol of good luck and prosperity. Abundant Goldenrod is said to be a sign of buried treasure.

USE
The leaves and flowers.

EDIBILITY
The flowers garnish salads while the leaves can be cooked like spinach or added to soups, stews or casseroles, and can also be blanched and frozen for later use.

HARVEST
In July/August.

MEDICINAL PROPERTIES
Anti-inflammatory, analgesic, diuretic, antihyperlipidemic and decongestant.

ACTIVE CONSTITUENTS
Gentianin, xanthones, flavonoids, phenolic acids, triterpenes, alkaloids.

LEFT: EUROPEAN GOLDENROD

MODERN RESEARCH

The following research has been carried out on the medicinal properties of Goldenrod:

Astringent

Goldenrod contains tannins, which are responsible for its astringent nature and the reason for Culpeper's use of it for wounds, sores and ulcers. The astringency would also explain the use of it 'to fasten the teeth that are loose in the gums'.

Decongestant

These tannins also make both Canadian and European goldenrod useful for drying itchy, watery or burning eyes and sinus congestion associated with allergies. Goldenrod is known as a premier decongestant, effectively alleviating upper respiratory congestion stemming from allergies, sinusitis, flu or the common cold. For this purpose it can be taken as a tea, syrup or tincture.

Antidiabetic

A 2020 study confirmed the use of European goldenrod as an antidiabetic and antihyperlipidemic in the management of diabetes, after it was shown to significantly reduce blood glucose levels, serum amylase activity and pancreatic levels while increasing the levels of serum insulin, liver glycogen and pancreatic action, and catalase activities in diabetic rats.

Anti-obesity

In vitro studies have shown that Goldenrod extracts can inhibit adipogenesis (the formation of fat cells) and promote lipolysis (the breakdown of fats), while inhibiting the activity of pancreatic lipase, an enzyme involved in fat digestion. Together these reduce fat absorption and accumulation in the body. Furthermore, the results of a 2017 study in mice showed that the extracts significantly reduced body weight gain, fat mass and improved lipid profiles without affecting food intake of the animals.

Diuretic and urological agent

As Culpeper said, Goldenrod is an excellent diuretic. This applies to both the Canadian and European species which, by increasing urine output, aid in the elimination of waste products and toxins from the body, which can benefit the kidneys and urinary tract. *In vitro* studies published in the journal *Planta Medica* examined the mechanisms behind the diuretic effects of Goldenrod and found that the activity is facilitated through the modulation of kidney function and electrolyte balance.

As a result, Goldenrod's main modern use is in the treatment of urinary tract infections. A 1996 study of 74 female patients with dysuria found that an extract of Goldenrod administered 3 times daily for 14 days decreased the frequency of urination in 69.2% of patients, as well as reducing other symptoms of cystitis in a greater number of patients.

Similarly, in another open study of 1,487 patients in 2002, a subgroup of 512 patients with chronic recurrent irritable bladder conditions were given Goldenrod 3 times daily, and 96% of these patients showed an improvement in the clinical global impression scale.

Antimicrobial and anti-inflammatory
Aiding with the above conditions is the fact that the Goldenrods also have anti-inflammatory and antimicrobial properties.

A 2006 study by Tkachev et al. showed that European goldenrod completely inhibited or killed *Aspergillus niger* and *Staphylococcus aureus*. Further research, published in the *Journal of Ethnopharmacology*, found that extracts from Goldenrod can be effective against various bacteria, including *Escherichia coli*, *Staphylococcus aureus* and *Pseudomonas aeruginosa*, as well as fungi such as *Candida albicans*.

In 2021, the anti-inflammatory effect of Goldenrod was tested in five rat groups. Rats from the control group were treated with saline solution while the animals from the reference group received orally a dose of 20mg/kg diclofenac. Goldenrod extract was administered to three rat groups by oral route in doses of either 125, 250 or 500mg/kg. Results for the highest dose showed significant anti-inflammatory effects, the effects being marginally inferior to those of diclofenac.

A 2022 study from Bulgaria confirmed the antimicrobial findings and revealed that 70% ethanol extracts had proved to be potentially effective against *Staphylococcus aureus* and *Pseudomonas aeruginosa* and could be an alternative to chemical antimicrobial agents.

Anti-hyperuricaemia
The same 2021 study that noted the anti-inflammatory effects of Goldenrod also evaluated its effects on hyperuricaemia (abnormally high levels of uric acid). Oral administration of Goldenrod extract in doses of 250 and 500mg/kg caused a significant decrease of uricaemia in rats and arterial hypertension usually resulting from elevated levels of uric acid. This, combined with the anti-inflammatory effects, means that Goldenrod is a very promising in the management of acute or chronic gout.

TOPICAL USE

Goldenrod, as Culpeper said, is also effective for topical ointments. It promotes wound-healing through its astringent and antiseptic properties while also helping in the contraction and closing of wounds and prevents infection, facilitating faster healing. Goldenrod's anti-inflammatory properties also contribute to pain relief and so can soothe sore muscles and joints, making it beneficial for conditions like arthritis and muscle strains.

An alcoholic extract of Goldenrod was claimed to exert anti-ageing effects, opening a door towards the possibility to use it as for anti-ageing purposes in topical or systemic preparations.

DOSAGE

Tisane – ½tsp. Drink a cup, 3 times per day.
Tincture – 1:5 45%, 3–6m 0.5–1ml, 3 times daily – 20 drops = 1ml/1tsp = 5ml.

PRECAUTIONS

It should be avoided in patients with cardiac or renal malfunction and should not be applied on open wounds. Not suitable for children or those who are pregnant or lactating.

Goldenrod recipes

Medicinal recipes

Goldenrod tisane

Pour 250ml boiling water over 1tsp/5g of the herb and allow to steep for 10 minutes. Use as an astringent, diuretic and anti-inflammatory for urinary tract infections and kidney stones as well as to ease gout.

Goldenrod infused tincture 1:5 45%

If you are using 40% aalcohol, ie. vodka, cover 1 part herb to 10 parts fluid.

If you are using Everclear or other 100% proof, use the following method for a specific tincture:

- 100g dried herb
- 225ml alcohol
- 275ml water

Take 100g of the dried herb and split into two parts of 50g each. Place 50g in the alcohol and the other 50g part in the boiled water. Steep/infuse in the water for 10 minutes. Strain thoroughly and top up if the water is less than 275ml. Add the infusion to the alcohol mix and leave for 14 days before straining. Use for infections of the urinary tract, allergies, kidney and bladder stones plus gout.

Goldenrod syrup

- 1 part Goldenrod tisane
- 1 part sugar

Simmer your strained tisane or decoction until reduced by half, and then add the sugar. You will always end up using double the amount of sugar to tisane. Stir until the sugar has dissolved and then continue cooking till the mixture has thickened to a syrup. Leave to cool. Pour into sterilised bottles closed with a cork. This will keep for a maximum of 3 months. Use to help ease allergies or to soothe a sore throat from sinus drainage. To fully preserve a syrup, it's wise to add 5% of your end volume with a tincture of the herb (or one of the herbs) in the syrup.

Goldenrod infused oil

- 100g dried herb
- 2tbsp alcohol, such as Everclear
- 1l grapeseed oil

Place the herb in the bottom of a jar with the Everclear. Allow to steep for 10 minutes and then add the oil. Allow the mix to steep/infuse for 4 weeks before using to reduce inflammation and pain in sore muscles.

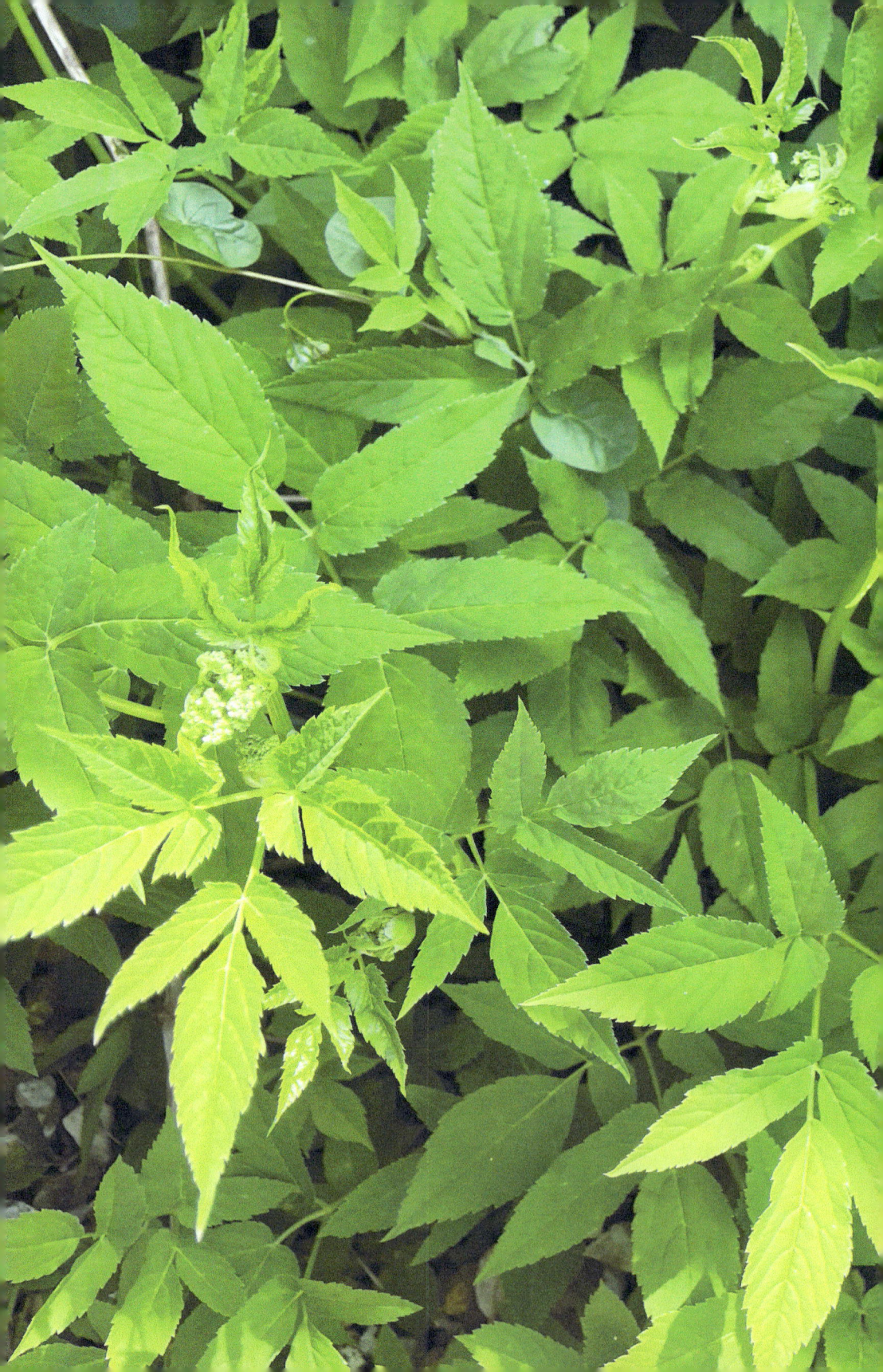

GROUND ELDER
Aegopodium podagraria

Aegopodium podagraria, commonly known as Ground elder, Goutweed, Herb Gerard or Bishop's weed, is a perennial plant species native to the UK. It has a history of traditional medicinal use as a diuretic and anti-inflammatory.

HISTORICAL USES

Hildegard of Bingen (1098–1179) called it *Herba gicht* or Goutweed, and advised that one who has pain in his stomach should drink it, warm and cooked in wine, but also that it should be drunk cold to prevent the stomach from becoming sick. She further said that one who is afflicted with 'gicht' (gout) should pound the herb with the seed and add bear fat and olive oil to make an unguent to anoint himself where it hurts.

In his *Herball*, John Gerard (1545–1612) described how *'with his roots stamped and laid upon members that are troubled or vexed with gout, swageth the paine, and taketh away the swelling and inflammation thereof, which occasioned the Germans to give it the name of Podagraria, because of his virtues in curing the gout.'*

Nicholas Culpeper, who called it Goutwort, wrote *'It is not to be supposed Goutwort hath its name for nothing, but upon experiment to heal the gout and*

ETYMOLOGY OF COMMON NAME
The name ground elder comes from the superficial similarity of the leaves and flowers to those of elder.

PLANT LORE
Also known as Herb Gerard after St Gerard, who was invoked to treat gout, which the plant is also known to cure.

USE
All parts.

EDIBILITY
The leaves, with their tangy flavour, can be used in salads, soups or as a vegetable.

HARVEST
In spring when it is in flower.

MEDICINAL PROPERTIES
Anti-inflammatory, antimicrobial, cytotoxic and diuretic.

ACTIVE CONSTITUENTS
Coumarins, flavonoids, phenolic acids, essential oil, polysaccharides.

LEFT: GROUND ELDER

sciatica as also joint-aches and other cold griefs. The very bearing of it about one ease the pains of the gout and defends him that bears it from the disease.'

Dr John Hill's *Family Herbal* of 1756 considered '*the root and fresh buds of the leaves as excellent in fomentations and poultices for pains; and the leaves, when boiled soft, together with the roots, for application about the hip in sciatica.*'

MODERN RESEARCH

Ground elder has a long history of medicinal use, particularly, as the above say, in the treatment of gout, sciatica and rheumatic diseases. The plant has been found to have the following properties:

Anti-inflammatory

Ground elder contains various bioactive compounds, including flavonoids, polyacetylenes and volatile oils, which are known to have anti-inflammatory effects. Studies of the plant showed that the flowers also contain high levels of falcarinol, a fatty alcohol, observed in flowers during blooming and related to the protective effect by its ability to inhibit the production of pro-inflammatory cytokines and enzymes.

Studies in 2016 showed that the administration of metformin, a diabetes drug, when combined with Ground elder tincture inhibited inflammation and activity of alanine aminotransferase (ALT), an enzyme found in the liver that acts as a damage indicator. The tincture also increased urea clearance in animals, confirming the benefits of combining the tincture with metformin when treating gout.

Antimicrobial

A 2020 review found that the rich compounds present in aerial parts and roots of Ground elder also showed antimicrobial activity against *Staphylococcus aureus, Escherichia coli,* and *Pseudomonas aeruginosa* and antifungal activity against *Candida albicans.* These organisms are common culprits in infections and can be resistant to multiple drugs, so this activity could indicate a natural and safe material that may be successfully used to treat or support the treatment of many diseases.

Cytotoxic

A 2023 study aimed at assessing the cytotoxic and antioxidant capacity of *Smilax excelsa* (Sarsaparilla) and Ground elder against human prostate, colorectal and lung carcinoma cell survival showed that the combination reduced cell viability in all cancer cells, and the most potent cytotoxic effects were noted on prostate cells. Results suggest that Sarsaparilla and Ground elder may contribute to the treatment of prostate cancer.

TOPICAL USES

As mentioned, it is applied externally as healing and soothing in the form of poultice.

DOSAGE

Tisane – 1–2tsp, 3 times per day.

PRECAUTIONS

Ground elder contains alkaloids and oxalates, and consuming large quantities should be avoided. Not suitable for children or those who are pregnant or lactating.

Ground elder recipes

Medicinal recipes

Ground elder tisane

Pour 250ml boiling water over 1–2tsp/ 5–10g of the herb and allow to steep for 10 minutes. Use to support detoxification and kidney function, as well as for the treatment of gout, haemorrhoids and inflammatory bladder conditions, and to improve metabolism.

Ground elder poultice

- 1tsp fresh roots and leaves (if using dried you will need to moisten with water first)
- 2tsp coconut oil
- cheesecloth or cotton bandage

Finely grate the root and chop the leaves into a pulp and add the coconut oil to make a paste. Spread the paste evenly over the desired area and wrap with the cloth or bandage. Use in cases of sciatica.

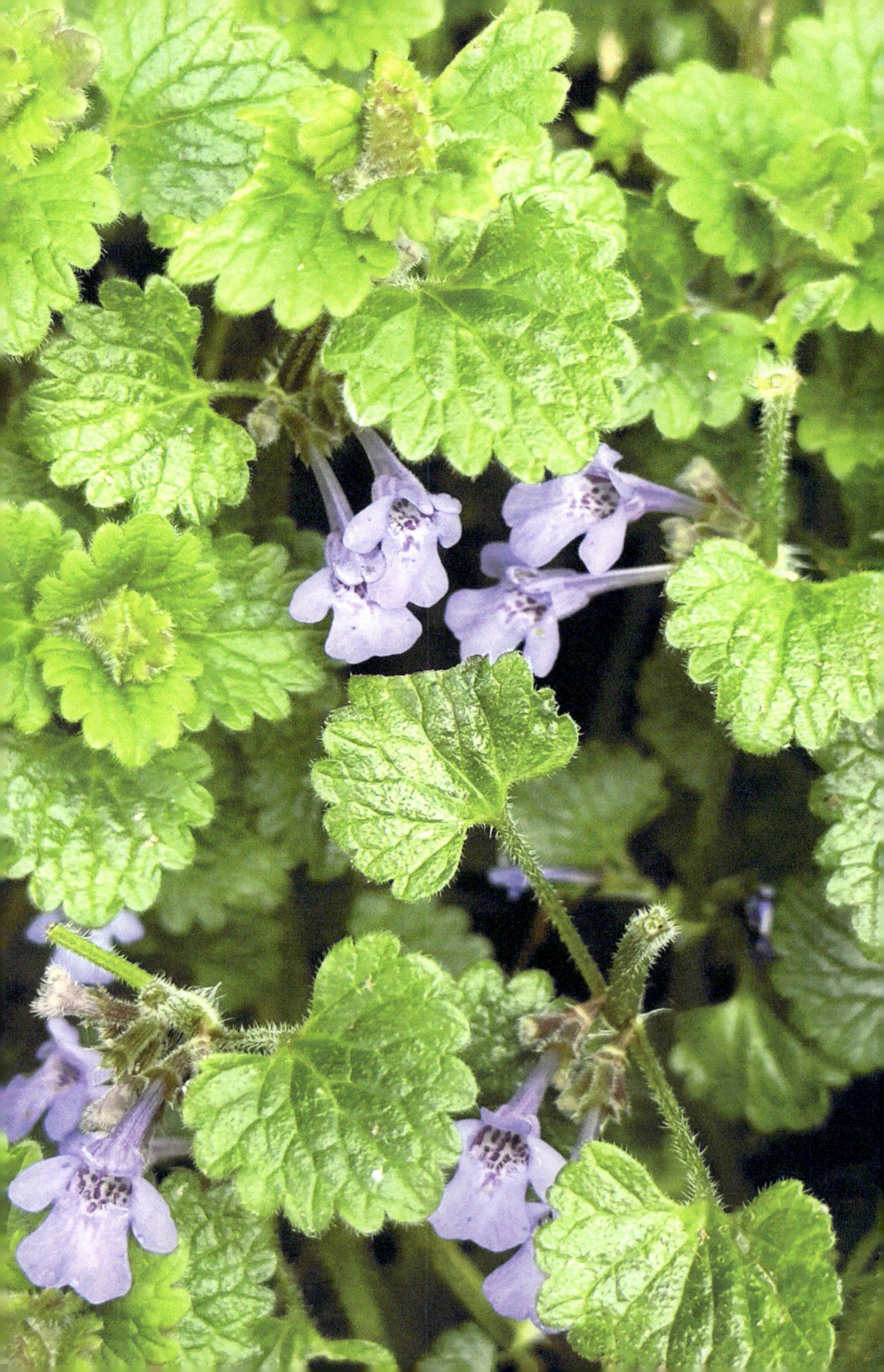

GROUND IVY
Glechoma hederacea

Glechoma hederacea, commonly known as Ground ivy, and historically as Creeping Charlie and Alehoof, is a plant in the mint family (*Lamiaceae*). It is abundant in shady, moist areas such as woodlands and hedgerows, and along stream banks. Ground ivy has been used in traditional herbal medicine for various purposes, including as a treatment for respiratory issues, digestive problems and as a mild sedative.

HISTORICAL USES

Hildegard of Bingen (1098–1179) recommended Ground ivy in her *Physica*, '*if bad humours trouble one's head, so that even his ears ring, boil ground ivy in water. When the water is squeezed out, place the warm ivy around his head. It diminishes the bad humour in his head and opens up his hearing.*'

John Gerard (1545–1612) recorded in his *Herball*, '*it is commended against the humming noise and ringing sound of the ears, being put into them, and for them that are hard of hearing.*'

Nicholas Culpeper's *Herbal* described it as '*a singular herb for all inward wounds, exulcerated lungs, or other parts, and being drank, in a short time it easeth all griping pains, windy and choleric humours in the stomach, spleen or belly; helps the yellow jaundice, by opening the*

ETYMOLOGY OF COMMON NAME
Its popular name is attributed to the resemblance borne by its foliage to that of the true Ivy.

PLANT LORE
Ground ivy has been associated with protection and healing. Some folklore suggested that it was able to protect cows against sorcery.

USE
All parts.

EDIBILITY
The leaves may be blended into salads to provide an aromatic essence. Alternatively, the young leaves can be cooked like spinach or added to soups and stews.

HARVEST
When in flower.

MEDICINAL PROPERTIES
Anti-inflammatory, analgesic, hepatoprotective, antioxidant, antibacterial and expectorant.

ACTIVE CONSTITUENTS
Gentianin, xanthones, flavonoids, phenolic acids, triterpenes, alkaloids.

stoppings of the gall and liver, and melancholy, by opening the stoppings of the spleen; expelleth venom or poison, and also the plague; it provokes urine and women's courses; the decoction of it in wine drank for some time together, procures ease to them that are troubled with the sciatica, or hip-gout: as also the gout in hands, knees or feet; if you put to the decoction some honey and a little burnt alum, it is excellently good to gargle any sore mouth or throat, and to wash the sores and ulcers in the privy parts of man or woman; it speedily helpeth green wounds, being bruised and bound thereto.'

William Fernie's 1897 edition of *Herbal Simples* specified that 'an infusion of the fresh herb, or, if made in winter, from its dried leaves, and drank under the name of Gill tea, is a favourite remedy with the poor, for coughs of long standing, accompanied with much phlegm. One ounce of the herb should be infused in 1 pint of boiling water, and a wineglassful of this when cool is to be taken three or four times in the day.'

MODERN RESEARCH

There isn't a huge amount of research material in relation to this plant, but Ground ivy has been found to possess the following properties:

Anti-inflammatory and analgesic

Culpeper was correct in saying that Ground ivy is both anti-inflammatory and pain-relieving. In a 2011 study, these effects were found to be related to phenolic compounds, which were noted to block inflammatory responses and impede the production of prostaglandin, which is often the cause of pain and swelling.

While I was unable to specifically find anything to substantiate Hildegard and Gerard's recommendation for its use in ringing or humming in the ears (tinnitus) it could be that the anti-inflammatory and analgesic properties described might theoretically offer some relief for certain underlying causes of tinnitus when related to inflammation.

Hepatoprotective

Again, Culpeper was correct that the plant helps jaundice, by opening the blockages of the gall and liver. Ground ivy is known to stimulate bile production, and its protective effects on the liver were studied in 2017 against cholestatic liver injury in rats. The effects are believed to potential of value to those with familial genetic disorders, autoimmune diseases, xenobiotic exposure, gallstones and tumours, the common causes of cholestasis.

Antioxidant

A 2018 study to evaluate the chemical composition and the antioxidant, anti-melanogenic and anti-inflammatory properties of Ground ivy essential oil demonstrated powerful antioxidative activity on lipid peroxidation, which will usually result in cell damage. It was also found that the oil may suppress the inflammatory responses of macrophage leukaemia cells, ie cells responsible for defending the body.

Antibacterial and vulnerary
A 2023 *in vivo* study on the wound-healing potential of Ground ivy hydrogels showed that a 5% infused hydrogel produced significant shrinkage of *Staphylococcus* colonies in comparison with standard Fucidin. Meanwhile, wound closure associated with full re-epithelisation and hair follicle production was noticed after 10 days of treatment.

Expectorant
While I was unable to find any studies on the expectorant effects of Ground ivy itself, significant amounts of eucalyptol, also known as 1,8-cineole, have been found to be among the dominant compounds of the plant. Eucalyptol is well known for its antiseptic and expectorant activity, and may well be the reason for use of the Gill tea described by Fernie.

TOPICAL USES

As mentioned above, the plant has antibacterial, anti-inflammatory and vulnerary properties. A poultice can therefore be employed to heal wounds, bruises, cuts and abscesses. A tisane of Ground ivy is said to soothe the eyes if cooled and used as an eye compress.

The anti-cancer activity of acids isolated from the plant were studied against Epstein Barr virus which produces skin tumours. The inhibition of tumours was successful and considered comparable to a known tumour promoter inhibitor, retinolic acid (1986).

DOSAGE

Tisane – 1–2tsp, 3 times per day.
Tincture – 1:5 25% – 1–2ml, 3 times per day – 20 drops = 1ml/1tsp = 5ml.

Externally, crushed leaves are placed on the affected areas.

PRECAUTIONS

Fatal poisonings were observed among horses following intake of large quantities of the fresh plant. Not suitable for children or those who are pregnant or lactating.

Ground ivy recipes

Medicinal recipes

Ground ivy tisane

Pour 250ml boiling water over 1-2tsp/ 5-10g of the herb and allow to steep for 10 minutes. Use for the treatment of arthritis, asthma, colds, coughs, flu, gastric issues, headaches and inflammation.

Ground ivy infused tincture 1:5 25%

If using 40% alcohol, ie. vodka, you will need to dilute this at the ratio of 60ml water to every 100ml of vodka to make a 25% medium and then cover 1 part herb to 5 parts fluid.

If using Everclear or other 100% proof, use the following method for a specific tincture:

- 100g dried Ground ivy herb
- 125ml alcohol
- 375ml water

Take 100g of the dried herb and split into two parts of 50g each. Place 50g in the alcohol. Take the other 50g part and place in the boiled water. Steep/infuse in the water for 10 minutes. Strain thoroughly and top up if the water is less than 375ml. Add the infusion to the alcohol mix and leave for 14 days before straining. Use for inflammation, sinusitis and inflammation-induced tinnitus.

Ground ivy poultice

- 1tsp fresh leaves (if using dried you will need to moisten with water first)
- 2tsp coconut oil
- cheesecloth or cotton bandage

Finely chop the leaves into a pulp and add the coconut oil to make a paste. Spread the paste evenly over the desired area and wrap with the cloth or bandage. Use in cases of wounds, bruises, cuts and abscesses.

Ground ivy infused oil

- 100g dried herb
- 2tbsp alcohol, such as Everclear
- 1l grapeseed oil

Roughly chop the herb and place in the bottom of a jar with the Everclear. Allow to steep for 10 minutes and then add the oil. Allow the mix to steep/infuse for 4 weeks and use topically to soothe sore muscles or as a general skin tonic

GROUNDSEL
Senecio vulgaris

Senecio vulgaris, Common groundsel, is a widespread plant found throughout the UK. It is a member of the *Asteraceae* family, along with Asters, Daisies and Sunflowers, and can thrive in a variety of habitats, including gardens, fields, waste areas and disturbed sites.

HISTORICAL USES

In the *Herball* of John Gerard (1545–1612), there is reference to the leaves of Groundsel, which, '*boiled in wine or water, and drunk, heal the paine and ach of the stomacke that proceeds of Choler. Stamped and strained into milk and drunk, they help the red gums and frets in Children.*'

Gerard also reported that Dioscorides said, '*That with the fine pouder of Frankincense it healeth wounds in the sinues. The like operation hath the down of the floures mixed with vineger. Boiled in ale with a little hony and vineger, it provoketh vomit.*'

Nicholas Culpeper's *Herbal* described the virtues of Groundsel as follows, '*It is cooling and digesting in inflammations; it is an easy emetic when made like tea. Taken in ale, it acts against the pains of the stomach, strangury, and jaundice; it destroys worms, and is useful in scrofulous tumours and inflammations of the breasts and scald head. Its juice is a good purgative,*

ETYMOLOGY OF COMMON NAME
From the Anglo-Saxon *Grondeswyle*, from *grund*, 'ground', and *swelgun*, 'to swallow', a reference to the speed at which the plant spreads.

PLANT LORE
Groundsel is often associated with themes of ageing and decay owing to its habit of growing in neglected or disturbed soils and was often worn as a charm to ward off evil.

USE
All parts.

EDIBILITY
Not edible – TOXIC.

HARVEST
In spring (particularly, May).

MEDICINAL PROPERTIES
Purgative, diuretic, anthelmintic, antifungal and anticancerogenic.

ACTIVE CONSTITUENTS
Alkaloids, sesquiterpene lactones, flavonoids, essential oils, phenolic acids.

but the dose should not exceed two ounces. The leaves bruised and applied outwardly to the stomach, produces the like effect, and there is no better application for the gripes and colic of infants. For the sore breasts of women, pick a handful of the fresh juicy leaves, bruise them, and make a poultice with a little bread boiled in milk, then lay the poultice on, and repeat as often as needful, and an effectual cure will be the result. The juice also provokes urine and expels the gravel in the reins and kidneys, when taken in wine. The distilled water performs everything that can be expected from its virtues, especially for inflammations or watering of the eyes, when proceeding from defluctions of rheum into them. An infusion of it taken inwardly cures staggers and bot-worms in horses.'*

In his 1897 edition of *Herbal Simples*, William Fernie recommended, 'A weak infusion of the whole plant with boiling water makes a simple and easy purgative dose, but a strong infusion will act as an emetic. For the former purpose two drachms by weight of the fresh plant should be boiled in four fluid ounces of water, and the same decoction serves as a useful gargle for sore throat from catarrh.'*

MODERN RESEARCH

Groundsel has a long history of herbal use, and when taken internally it has been found to be an effective purgative and emetic. Additionally, the toxic principles of the drug are the pyrrolizidine alkaloids and sesquiterpene lactones, which are believed to be hepatotoxic and carcinogenic with prolonged use.

Traditional use of Groundsel for worm infestation can be explained by the high toxicity of the drug. Modern research has however shown the following properties:

Diuretic

As Culpeper says, the plant 'provokes urine and expels the gravel in the reins (bladder) and kidneys'. This is now known to be a result of its content of flavonoids and alkaloids, which are diuretic and as a consequence are an aid to expelling kidney stones (Jin et al., 2018; Lin et al., 2018).

Antifungal

In 2004, a hexane extract of Groundsel was found to show significant activity against *Trichophyton tonsurans*, the cause of scalp ringworm, or as Culpeper called it, 'scald head'.

Anticancerogenic

In 2019, Groundsel was shown to have promising inhibitory activity against liver and prostate cancer cells. These early results demonstrate the potential of Groundsel essential oils for future cancer treatments.

TOPICAL USES

Groundsel is a common ingredient in cosmetics that promote skin conditioning and also in shampoos. It is also an old well-known remedy for chapped hands and, as Culpeper says, makes a great topical anti-inflammatory compress for the treatment of joint

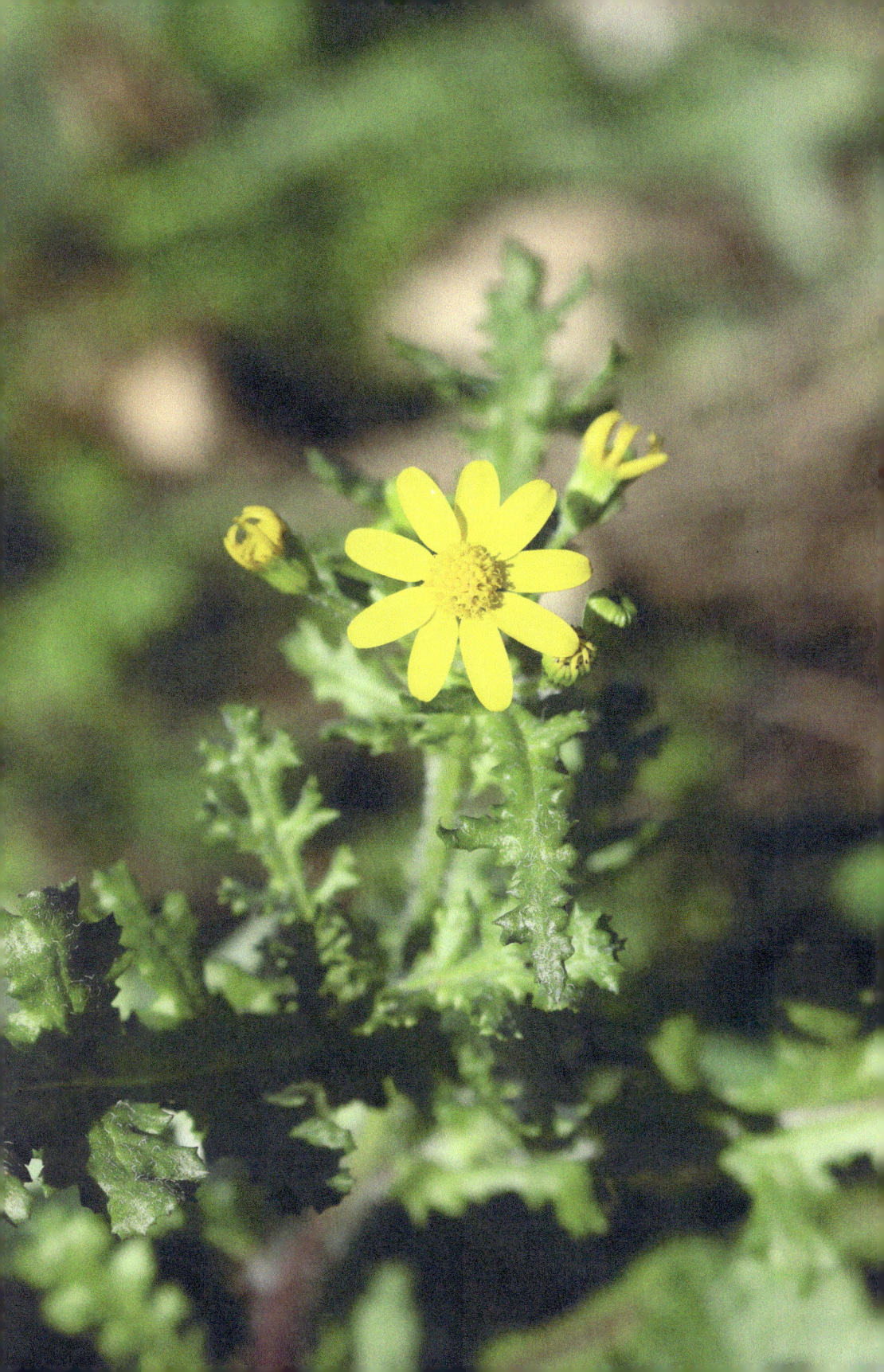

inflammation, boils and for an athlete's foot. Analysis in 2019 showed the presence of secondary metabolites with antimicrobial and antioxidant activity, while the essential oil reveals the presence of terpenes such as monoterpenes and diterpenes, which have great free-radical scavenger activity as well as antibacterial and antifungal capacity.

DOSAGE

Internal use of Groundsel is not advised. Note that the following are historical remedies and dosages.

Infusion – a weak infusion of the aerial plant will act as a laxative.

The same decoction serves as a useful gargle for a sore throat from catarrh.

Relief of biliary pains in 2-ounce doses of the 1 ounce to 1 pint infusion. A stronger infusion acts as a purgative and emetic (to cause vomiting).

PRECAUTIONS

Note the presence of pyrrolizidine alkaloids. Not suitable for children or those who are pregnant or lactating.

Groundsel recipes

Medicinal recipes

Groundsel infusion

A weak infusion of the aerial plant, 14g to 1 pint of boiling water, taken in doses of 28ml will act as a laxative; any stronger will act as an emetic (cause vomiting).

Groundsel poultice

- 1tsp fresh herb (if using dried you will need to moisten with water first)
- 2tsp coconut oil
- cheesecloth or cotton bandage

Finely chop the herb into a pulp and add the coconut oil to make a paste. Spread the paste evenly over the desired area and wrap with the cloth or bandage. Use for the treatment of fungal infections and chapped hands.

HAWKWEED, MOUSE-EAR
Pilosella officinarum

There are many native *Pilosella* or Hawkweed species in the UK, including *Pilosella officinarum*, the Mouse-ear hawkweed. This is found in various habitats across the country, including grasslands, meadows, heaths and woodland edges. Hawkweeds belong to the largest family of flowering plants, the *Asteraceae*, commonly referred to as the Aster, Daisy or Sunflower family. Given the astringency of Hawkweed, it was much employed as a medicine in the Middle Ages under the name of *Auricula muris*, from which the popular name is taken.

HISTORICAL USES

Nicholas Culpeper's *Herbal* stated:

Hawk-weed is cooling, somewhat drying and binding, and good for the beat of the stomach, and gnawing therein; for inflammations, and the hot fits of agues. The juice of it in wine helps digestion, dispels wind, hinders crudities abiding in the stomach, and helps the difficulty in making water. It is good against all poisonous bites. A scruple of the dry root given in wine and vinegar, is profitable for dropsy. The decoction of the herb taken in honey digests phlegm, and with hyssop helps the coughs. The decoction of the herb and wild succory with wine, helps the wind colic and hardness of the spleen, it procures rest

ETYMOLOGY OF COMMON NAME
Mouse-ear is named for the small leaves, which do somewhat resemble mouse ears.

PLANT LORE
Hawkweeds are so called following Pliny, who said that hawks drank from them 'to aid sight'. It consequently became a symbol of keen vision and strength in many cultures.

USE
All aerial parts.

EDIBILITY
The leaves and flowers, though they can be bitter.

HARVEST
In May and June, when in flower.

MEDICINAL PROPERTIES
Digestive, stomachic, tonic, antidiabetic and anticancerogenic.

ACTIVE CONSTITUENTS
Gentianin, xanthones, flavonoids, phenolic acids, triterpenes, alkaloids.

and sleep, cools heat, purges the stomach, increases blood, and helps diseases of the reins and bladder. Outwardly applied, it is good for the defects and diseases of the eyes, used with some women's milk; it may be used with success for healing spreading ulcers. The green leaves bruised, with a little salt, applied to burns and scalds, greatly helps them: as also St Anthony's fire, and all pushes and eruptions, and hot and salt phlegm. Applied with meal poultice, it eases and helps cramps and convulsions. The distilled water takes away wrinkles, freckles, spots, etc.

MODERN RESEARCH

Modern research has confirmed Culpeper and found the following:

Digestive

Culpeper tells us that the plant helps digestion, dispels wind and hinders crudities (undigested foods) remaining in the stomach. This is also a function of the astringent properties, which help in firming up loose stools and reducing gastrointestinal inflammation.

Expectorant

As Culpeper also states, Hawkweed is good for phlegm and coughs. It is regarded as a specific for whooping cough and all afflictions of the lungs owing to its astringency and the saponins it contains, which help to loosen and thin the mucus, making it easier to expel through coughing. It also contains umbelliferone, which reduces lung inflammation.

Diuretic

In Serbia, Hawkweed is traditionally recommended for intensifying urination and eliminating sand and small stones from the urinary tract and the kidneys. In fact, it was introduced in the European Union market of medicinal herbs in 1986 for its diuretic properties. Confirming the traditional uses, Mouse-ear has been observed to notably increase chlorides and nitrogenous substances in the urine; and this diuretic action is mainly related to flavonoids, particularly luteoloside (Becker et al., 2017).

Antimicrobial

A 2008 study of the antimicrobial activities of Hawkweed found that it had an inhibitory effect on *Staphylococcus aureus*, *Bacillus subtilis* and *Escherichia coli*. An ethyl acetate extract was also effective on the bacteria *Pseudomonas aeruginosa* and *Klebsiella pneumoniae* and the fungus *Aspergillus niger*.

Antioxidant

As part of the above research, the leaves and roots were also studied and found to have significant free-radical scavenging activity. Chlorogenic acid was detected in the highest quantities in all investigated extracts. Chlorogenic acid scavenges free radicals, which inhibits DNA damage and may protect against the induction of carcinogenesis.

RIGHT: HAWKWEED

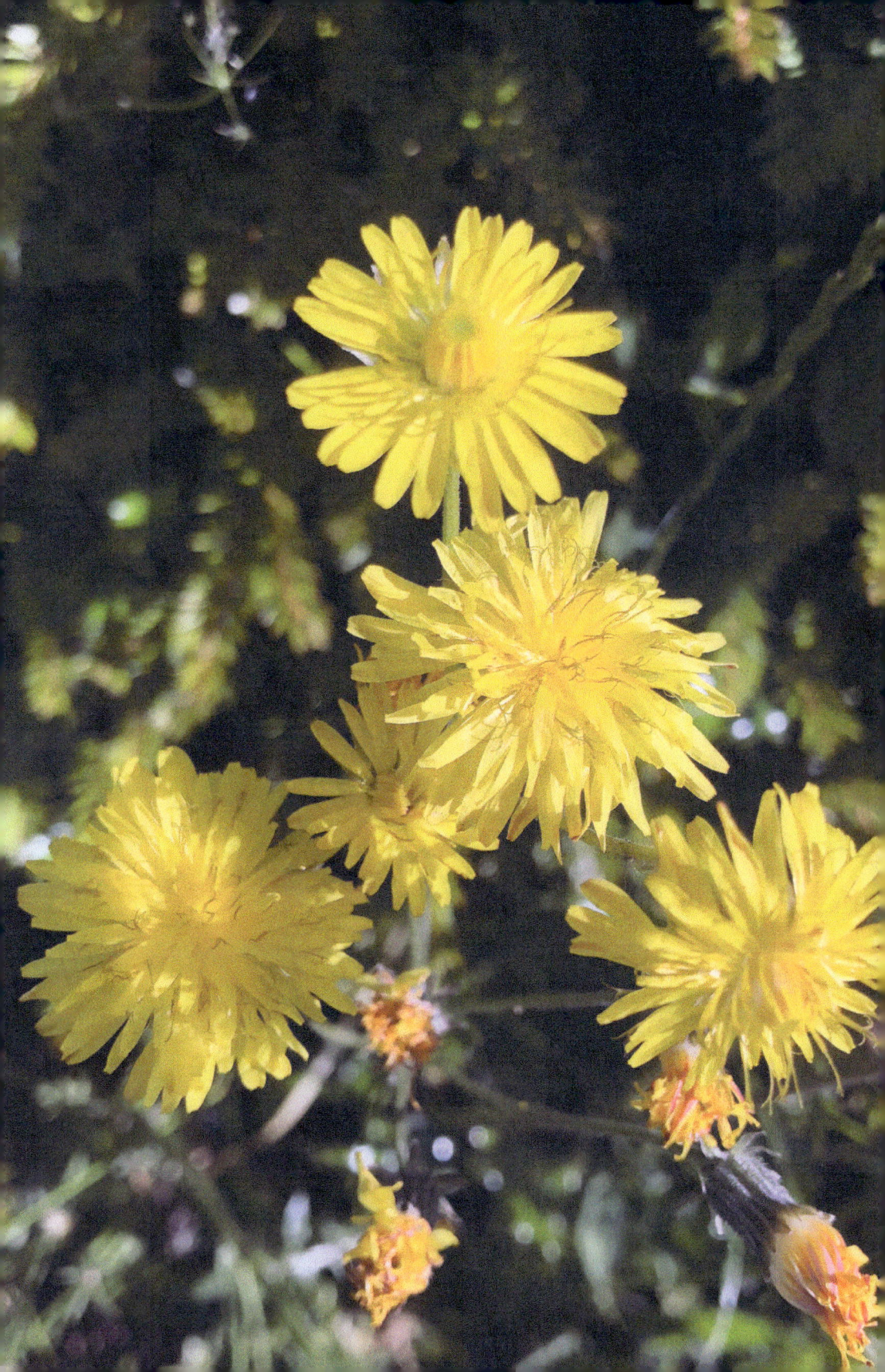

TOPICAL USES

Owing to the astringency, a powder prepared from the dried herb can be employed to stop nosebleeds and may also be employed externally in the form of a poultice to speed up the healing of wounds.

Results from a 2019 study demonstrated that an eye cream containing a proprietary blend of *Tephrosia purpurea* (Wild indigo) seed extract (1%–4%), *E. Cruſtaceum* plankton extract (1%–4%), *Hieracium pilosella* (a synonym for *Pilosella officinarum*) (1%-3%) and *Bellis perennis* (Daisy) flower (1%–3%) extracts achieved global skin rejuvenation by improving appearance of periorbital hyperpigmentation, puffiness, and fine and coarse wrinkles.

DOSAGE

Tisane – 1–2tsp, 3 times per day.
Tincture – 1:5 45%, 1–3ml, 3 times a day – 20 drops = 1ml/1tsp = 5ml.

PRECAUTIONS

Not suitable for children or those who are pregnant or lactating.

Hawkweed recipes

Medicinal recipes

Hawkweed tisane

Pour 250ml boiling water over 1–2tsp/5–10g of the herb and allow to steep for 10 minutes. Use for the treatment of diarrhoea and as a diuretic or expectorant.

Hawkweed tincture 1:5 45%

If you are using 40% alcohol, ie vodka, cover 1 part herb to 10 parts fluid.

If you are using Everclear or other 100% proof, use the following method for a specific tincture:

- 100g dried Hawkweed herb
- 225ml alcohol
- 275ml water

Take 100g of the dried herb and split into two parts of 50g each. Place 50g in the alcohol and the other 50g in the boiled water. Steep/infuse in the water for 10 minutes. Strain thoroughly and top up if the water is less than 275ml. Add the infusion to the alcohol mix and leave for 14 days before straining. Use to promote digestion, for diarrhoea and as an expectorant.

Hawkweed poultice

- 1tsp fresh Hawkweed herb (if using dried you will need to moisten with water first)
- 2tsp coconut oil
- cheesecloth or cotton bandage

Finely chop the herb into a pulp and add the coconut oil to make a paste. Spread the paste evenly over the desired area and wrap with the cloth or bandage. Use to speed up the healing of wounds.

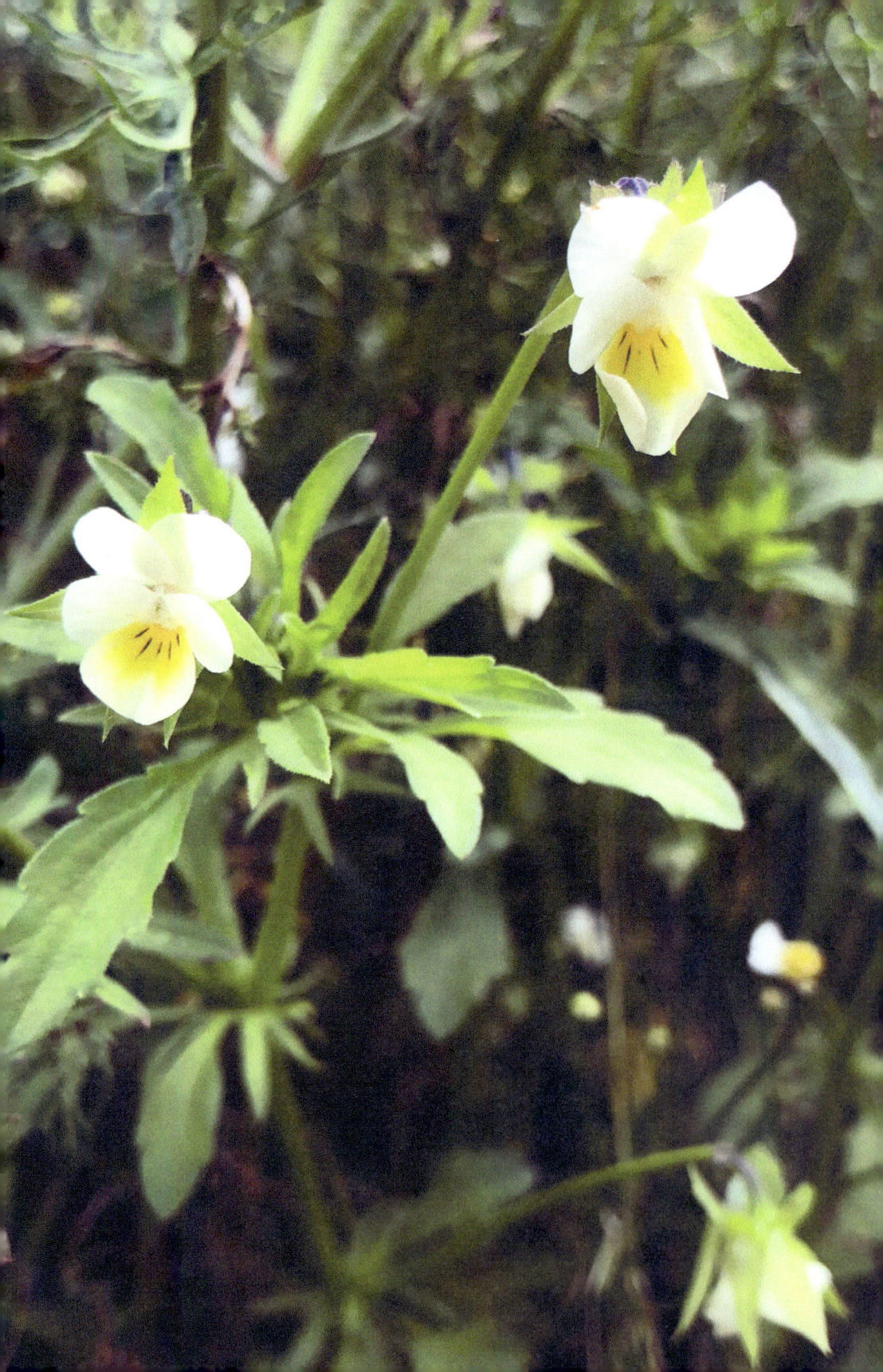

HEARTSEASE
Viola tricolor

Viola tricolor, also known as Heartsease, Johnny jump-up or Wild pansy, is a native member of the Violet family, the *Violaceae*. It grows in meadows, grasslands, open woodlands and disturbed areas, and has a long history of cultivation for use in medicine for respiratory ailments, skin conditions and inflammation as well as for edible decorations in salads or desserts.

HISTORICAL USES

John Gerard (1545–1612) wrote in his *Herball* 'It is good for such as are sick of ague, especially children and infants, whose convulsions and fits of the falling sickness it is thought to cure. It is commended against inflammation of the lungs and chest, and against scabs and itchings of the whole body and healeth ulcers.'

Nicholas Culpeper's *Herbal* recommended '*a strong decoction or syrup of the herb and flowers, is an excellent cure for the venereal disease. The spirit of it is excellent good for convulsions in children, and a remedy for falling sickness, inflammation of the lungs and breasts, pleurisy, scabs, itch. The flowers are cooling, Emollient* [moisturising], *and cathartic: it is best to make a syrup, as their virtues are lost by drying.*'

ETYMOLOGY OF COMMON NAME
In the period 1375–1425, *hertesese* signified a cordial, meaning it is comforting to the heart.

PLANT LORE
Heartsease was believed to have the power to soothe a broken heart and bring luck in matters of love. In some traditions, it was carried or worn as an amulet to attract love or protect against love spells.

USE
All parts.

EDIBILITY
The flowers are used in salads.

HARVEST
When in flower.

MEDICINAL PROPERTIES
Anticonvulsant, expectorant, anti-inflammatory, analgesic, anticancerogenic, cardioprotective and emollient.

ACTIVE CONSTITUENTS
Flavonoids, triterpene saponins, mucilage, anthocyanins, salicylic acid.

According to Harold Ward's *Herbal Manual* (1936):

> *The mildness of action makes it applicable in infantile skin eruptions, for which the ounce to pint infusion is given in doses according to age. It has been said that the medicine will ward off asthmatic and epileptic convulsions, but there would appear to be no reliable confirmation of this. The claim may have originated with Culpeper.*

MODERN RESEARCH

Research has now confirmed that Heartsease possesses many of the properties noted by the historical writers, such as:

Anticonvulsant

A 2019 study confirmed the anticonvulsant and anti-epileptic effects described by Gerard and Culpeper as the 'falling sickness', and noted that it prolonged the delay of grand mal seizures while decreasing the duration of seizures in mice. This could be related to the presence of flavonoids, which have been studied for their neuroprotective effects, and could theoretically contribute to anticonvulsant activity.

Anti-inflammatory and analgesic

In 2007, the anti-inflammatory activity of Heartsease was tested in acute inflammation in male Wistar rats, and showed a significantly reduced white blood cell response activation of immune cells. Then, in November 2013, the historical use of Heartsease for inflammatory disorders of the skin was confirmed in a study that showed that an aqueous extract contains bioactive cyclotides, which inhibit the triggering of the immune system response. These findings support the use of Heartsease in disorders related to an overactive immune system. In the same study the anti-inflammatory and pain-reducing effects of a gel containing Heartsease flowers were investigated on thermal burns, and found to have both pain-blocking and anti-inflammatory topical effects.

While I have not found any studies for the use of Heartsease for the venereal disease that Culpeper mentions, there is no doubt that it was used for this purpose as it was believed that its diuretic and purifying properties could help alleviate symptoms, though not the cause. Since the discovery of antibiotics and antivirals herbal remedies are no longer used for this purpose.

Expectorant

Heartsease contains saponins and mucilage, which are demulcent, and act as an expectorant for phlegm in the lungs, bronchitis and whooping cough. The anti-inflammatory properties indicated above further contribute to reduction of pulmonary inflammation and oedema, making it an excellent remedy for asthmatics as well as those with coughs.

Anticancerogenic

In 2014, the cytotoxic and apoptogenic properties of extracts of Heartsease were investigated in human breast cancer cells, and showed that an ethyl acetate extract was the most potent form in inducing apoptosis and inhibiting angiogenesis.

Cardioprotective

A 2020 study of the potential cardio-protective and anti-hypertensive effects of Heartsease showed vasodilator, cardio-depressant and anti-hypertensive effects during *in vitro* studies and displayed the potential role of Heartsease in cardiovascular disease.

Antibacterial

In 2016, the cyclotides in Heartsease were studied for their effects against several bacterial strains. The most susceptible bacterium to the extracts from Heartsease flowers were *Escherichia coli* and *Pseudomonas aeruginosa*.

TOPICAL USE

Heartsease has soothing, salve-like effects, and studies such as those mentioned above have shown that the anti-inflammatory and antimicrobial properties from the cyclotides make it a promising treatment for skin issues such as psoriasis. The saponin content also makes it a great herb to use in baths and in shampoos.

DOSAGE

Tisane – 2tsp/10g, 3 times per day.

PRECAUTIONS

Not suitable for children or those who are pregnant or lactating.

Heartsease recipes

Medicinal recipes

Heartsease tisane

Pour 250ml boiling water over 2tsp/10g of the fresh herb and allow to steep for 10 minutes. Use to ease asthma and coughs.

Heartsease compress

Soak a cloth in a tisane of the dried herb and use to soothe eczema and psoriasis.

Heartsease bath

- 50g Heartsease flowers
- 1l of water

Steep the herb in the water for 15 minutes, then strain and add to the bathwater to soothe itchy eczema-prone skin.

Heartsease infused oil

- 100g dried Heartsease herb
- 2tbsp alcohol, such as Everclear
- 1l grapeseed oil

Place the herb in the bottom of a jar with the Everclear. Allow to steep for 10 minutes and then add the oil. Allow the mix to steep/infuse for 4 weeks. Use to reduce inflammation and ease psoriasis.

Psoriasis salve

- 1 part Heartsease infused oil
- 1 part Chickweed infused oil
- 1 part Red clover infused oil

Combine the oils and use to soothe irritation or make into a salve by using a 1:4 ratio of melted beeswax to oil. Melt the wax pellets in the oil in a double boiler or bain-marie. Remove from the heat and allow to cool and set completely before using topically.

HEDGE PARSLEY
Torilis japonica

Torilis japonica, also known as Japanese Hedge parsley, has a history of traditional medicinal uses, primarily in East Asian countries where it is native, such as Japan, Korea and China. It was introduced to the UK, probably accidentally, and like many of its other relatives in the Carrot family (*Apiaceae*), can now be found in disturbed habitats such as roadsides, waste areas and cultivated fields.

HISTORICAL USES

This plant was introduced after the time of Nicholas Culpeper's writings but has a long history of use by humans in its native range and in the traditional medicine of China and eastern Asia, where it is used as treatment for dysentery, fever, haemorrhoids, spasms and uterine tumours (Duke and Ayensu, 1985).

MODERN RESEARCH

While Hedge parsley is not as widely studied or documented as some other medicinal plants, its major component is torilin, a bioactive sesquiterpene lactone with some very promising properties attributed to it, as follows:

Anti-inflammatory
The anti-inflammatory activity of torilin was found to be triggered by inhibition

ETYMOLOGY OF COMMON NAME
As with cultivated Parsley, it is based on the Greek *petroselinon*, from *petra*, 'rock' + *selinon*, 'parsley', but with this species' favoured habitat added.

PLANT LORE
In some folklore traditions, plants resembling parsley, including Hedge parsley, were believed to have protective qualities. They were sometimes hung or placed around homes to ward off evil spirits or negative energies.

USE
Flowers, leaves and seeds (the seeds are the main source of torilin).

EDIBILITY
The leaves can be eaten raw and the root cooked.

HARVEST
In spring and summer.

MEDICINAL PROPERTIES
Antiparasitic, antimicrobial, anti-inflammatory, anticancerogenic and expectorant.

ACTIVE CONSTITUENTS
Coumarins, flavonoids, phenolic acids, polysaccharides, essential oils.

of pro-inflammatory cytokines and mediators, which trigger inflammation.

Anticancerogenic

Medical studies have also shown that torilin has potentially cancer-combating properties (Kim et al., 2000; Park et al., 2003, 2006) and, additionally, has an inhibitory effect on angiogenesis or the growth of blood vessels, which is a critical phase in the change of tumours from benign to malignant (Kim et al., 2000).

Torilin also inhibits the transformation of testosterone into androgen, which may be useful in the treatment of androgen-dependent cancers, such as prostate cancer (Park et al., 2003). A June 2016 study evaluated the apoptotic (cell death) effects of Hedge parsley and showed that it could be of great value in cancer treatment. It inhibits melanin production in hormone-activated melanoma cells, and it may have a strong ability to suppress tumour growth. It reverses multidrug-resistance in cancer cells and can increase the cytotoxicity of medications against drug-resistant carcinoma cells. The study results show that this plant may even provide a substitute for chemotherapeutic drugs and so has great potential as an anticancer agent.

One of the other effects of the above conversion of testosterone to androgen is the potential to promote hair growth linked to androgenetic alopecia and suggests its potential use in hair loss treatments.

Antibacterial

The spread of antibiotic-resistant strains of *Staphylococcus aureus* has increased following the frequent use of antibiotics. Torilin has demonstrated antimicrobial activity against a variety of pathogens and can disrupt the cell membrane of microbes to reduce their harm. In a 2022 study, Hedge parsley was found to suppress biofilm formation and virulence factor-related gene expression in MSSA and MRSA strains. The extract may therefore be used to develop treatments for infections caused by antibiotic-resistant *Staphylococcus aureus*.

Antiparasitic

Hedge parsley has been used as a human antiparasitic in Asian countries for many years, and studies have shown it inhibits *Toxoplasma gondii* proliferation by 99.3% and 98.7%, *in vitro*. This means that the plant could be used to enhance the effects of conventional antimicrobials, which will probably decrease costs and improve the treatment quality with fewer side effects.

TOPICAL USES

A 2009 study showed that torilin contributes to hypopigmenting and suggests its potential in hyperpigmentation disorders.

A 2023 study of Hedge parsley extract aimed to verify the use of the plant against atopic inflammation. The findings of the study affirmed the regenerative properties of the plant,

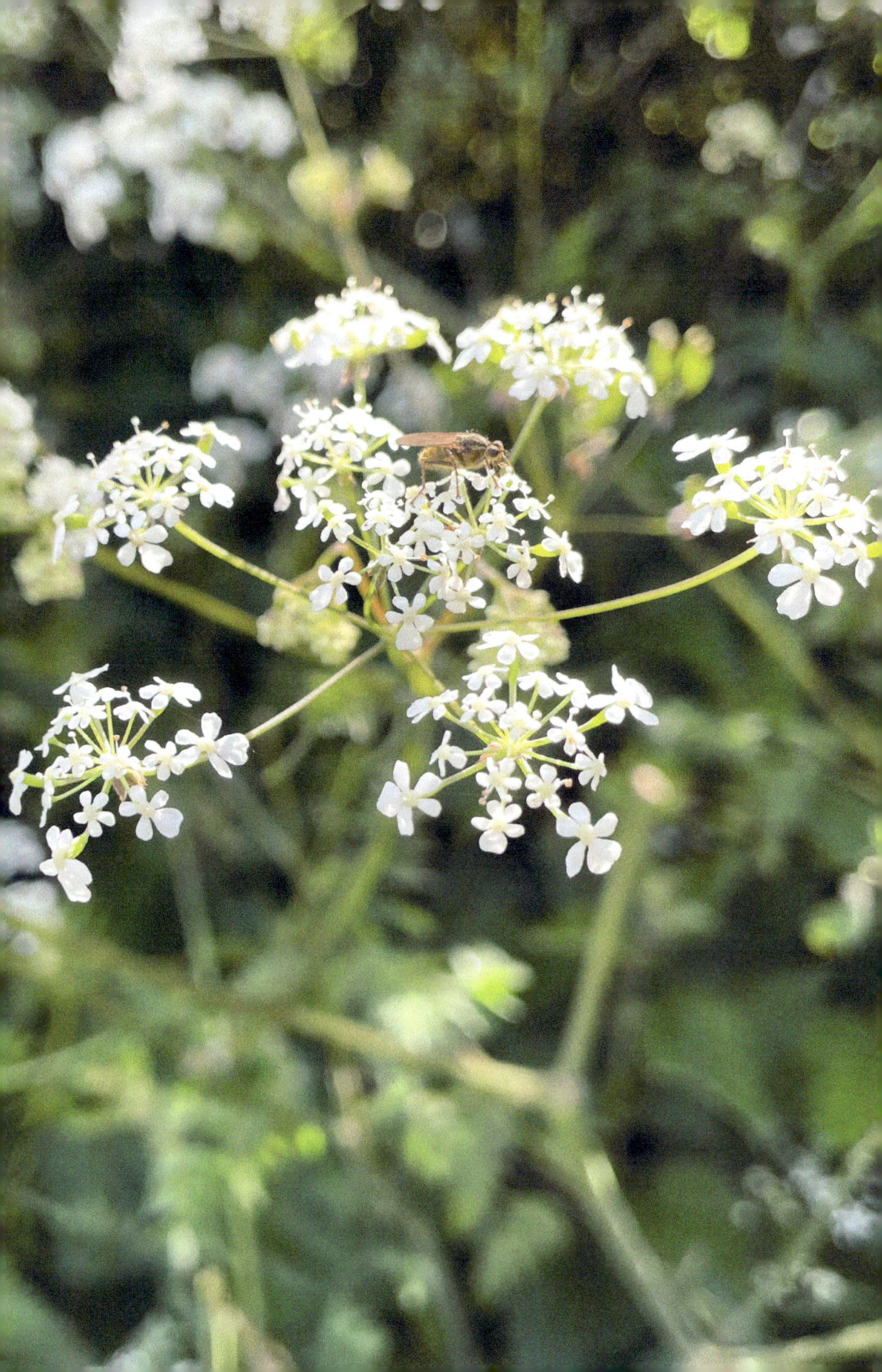

demonstrating its ability not only to alleviate surface-level symptoms but also to eliminate the underlying causes. The results indicated that the plant contributes to the restoration of healthy and smooth skin, going beyond mere superficial symptom relief.

DOSAGE

Decoction – 1tsp/5g, 2 times per day.

PRECAUTIONS

Not suitable for children or those who are pregnant or lactating.

Hedge parsley recipes

Medicinal recipes

Hedge parsley seed decoction

Simmer 1tbsp/15g of the flowering tops or seeds in 1 cup water for 15 minutes. Use as a general tonic, for inflammation, diarrhoea and for internal parasites.

Hedge parsley compress

Soak a cloth in a tisane of the dried herb and use to soothe atopic dermatitis.

Hedge parsley infused oil

- 100g dried Hedge parsley herb
- 2tbsp alcohol, such as Everclear
- 1l grapeseed oil

Place the herb in the bottom of a jar with the Everclear. Allow to steep for 10 minutes and then add the oil. Allow the mix to steep/infuse for 4 weeks. Use to reduce inflammation and eczema.

Hedge parsley poultice

- 1tsp fresh leaves (if using dried you will need to moisten with water first)
- 2tsp coconut oil
- cheesecloth or cotton bandage

Finely chop the leaves into a pulp and add the coconut oil to make a paste. Spread the paste evenly over the desired area and wrap with the cloth or bandage. Use to soothe rashes, insect bites, or minor wounds.

HEMLOCK
Conium maculatum

Conium maculatum, commonly known as Poison hemlock, is a native, highly toxic plant belonging to the *Apiaceae* family, which includes other well-known and benign plants such as Chervil, Carrot and Parsley. Despite its toxic properties, Hemlock has a long history of use.

HISTORICAL USES

This plant is mentioned in early Greek literature and is the plant that Socrates is said to have chosen to drink for his execution.

It was also used in Anglo-Saxon medicine and is mentioned as early as the 10th century in *Bald's Leechbook*, which recommended, '*If a knee is sore, pound hemlock and henbane, foment with it and lay it on.*'

Hildegard of Bingen (1098–1179) advised that '*one who has fallen from a high altitude so that his flesh and limbs are crushed, should cook hemlock in water and then place the water over the limbs that are injured to dissipate the humours that have collected there.*'

Nicholas Culpeper's *Herbal* stated, '*It may be safely applied to inflammations, tumults and swellings, to St Anthony's fire* [ergot poisoning] *wheals and creeping ulcers.*' He also said that the root, roasted and applied to the hands would help gout.

ETYMOLOGY OF COMMON NAME
From the Anglo-Saxon words *healm*, 'straw', and *leac*, 'a plant', because of the dry, hollow stalks that remain after flowering is done.

PLANT LORE
Hemlock is famously known for its poisonous properties, which have led to its association with death and mortality in folklore. The purple spotting on the stem has been known as the 'mark of Cain'.

USE
If at all, the leaves and fruit from second-year plants.

EDIBILITY
Not edible – HIGHLY POISONOUS.

HARVEST
When in flower, avoiding direct contact.

MEDICINAL PROPERTIES
Analgesic, anti-inflammatory, anticancerogenic and antimicrobial.

ACTIVE CONSTITUENTS
Aalkaloids, γ-lactones, volatile oils, resins.

In his 1897 *Herbal Simples*, William Fernie advised that:

> *The dried leaves of the plant, if put into a small bag, and steeped in boiling water for a few minutes, and then applied hot to a gouty part, will quickly relieve the pain and help to soften the hard concretions which form about gouty joints.*

MODERN RESEARCH

Hemlock belongs to the same family as Carrot, Chervil and the Dropworts, and is well-known for its extreme toxicity. All parts of the plant contain alkaloids such as coniine and γ-coniceine, which can cause respiratory failure and death in relatively small amounts. It should not be handled, and care must be taken not to confuse it with other non-toxic plants that look similar. Like many other poisonous plants, when cut and dried, Hemlock loses many of its poisonous properties, and I have included it as some historical uses have been confirmed as follows:

Analgesic and anti-inflammatory

All of the above writers, including the unfortunate Socrates, discovered that the plant has the ability to relieve pain. We now know that it does this by paralysing muscles and blocking receptors in the central nervous system. In 2012, Hemlock was evaluated pharmacologically to validate the claims for analgesic and anti-inflammatory activities. Test doses were evaluated and shown to exhibit significant anti-inflammatory activity in paw oedema in rats. The anti-inflammatory properties reduced the paw volume by a quarter, and it is suggested that alkaloids are responsible for both the pain-relieving and anti-inflammatory activities of the plant.

Anticancerogenic

A 2014 study noted that extracts of Hemlock had also been used as an anti-inflammatory for diseases of the prostate gland, swelling of the testes and in homeopathy, as a remedy for breast cancer and cancer of the cervix. The study aimed to evaluate the mechanism of the drug and found that extracts have the potential to reduce cancer cell viability and colony formation, and inhibit cell proliferation, thereby providing support for its use in traditional systems of medicine.

Antimicrobial

In 2019, the leaves of the plant were studied against two gram-negative bacterias, *Escherichia coli* and *Pseudomonas aeruginosa*, and were found to inhibit the growth of *P. aeruginosa* at a rate almost comparable to the antibiotic colistin, though *E. coli* proved resistant.

Further studies in 2023 showed that extracts had bactericidal activity against *Staphylococcus aureus*, *Enterococcus faecalis* and *Klebsiella pneumoniae* at a very low concentration of 25mg/ml of extract. This is promising as the leaf extracts of Hemlock may have the potential to be used as antibacterial agents for new medicines.

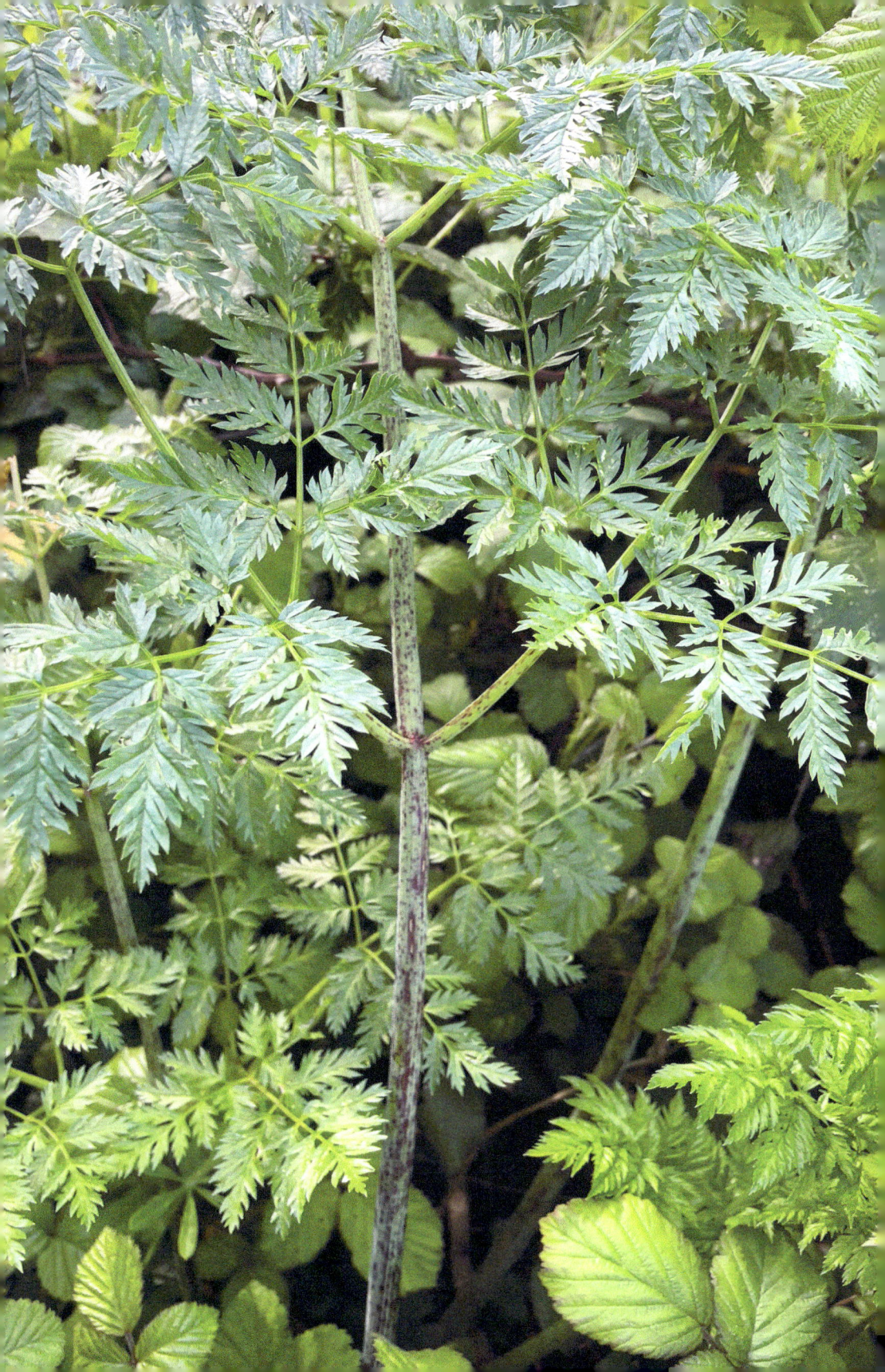

TOPICAL USES

Hemlock is reported to be still used externally, in the form of ointments and oils, in the treatment of mastitis and malignant tumours. But please note that touching any part of the plant with bare hands can be dangerous, and especially if sap gets into a cut on your skin, or into your eyes or nostrils you could suffer deadly impacts to your nervous system.

DOSAGE

Use of Hemlock is highly discouraged, and internal use must be avoided.

PRECAUTIONS

In poisonous doses, Hemlock produces complete paralysis, with loss of speech, depression and ultimate failure of the respiratory system, and death resulting from asphyxia. In Hemlock poisoning, the antidotes are tannic acid, stimulants and coffee, emetics of zinc, or mustard and castor oil, and, if necessary, artificial respiration. It is essential to keep up the temperature of the body.

Hemlock recipes

Medicinal recipes

In view of the highly poisonous nature of this plant, this recipe is given for interest purposes only. Readers should consider whether remedies using other plants are more suitable.

Hemlock poultice

- 1tsp dried herb, moistened with water
- 9tsp coconut oil
- cheesecloth or cotton bandage

Finely chop the herb into a pulp, without touching it and being mindful of its high toxicity levels, and add the coconut oil to make a paste. Spread the paste evenly over the desired area and wrap with the cloth or bandage. Use to relieve the pain of rheumatism or gout.

In his 1814 *Family Herbal* Robert Thornton provided a recipe to treat open cancerous wounds as follows:

Take of the dried herb hemlock, chamomile flowers, of each one ounce; boiling water, a pint: Boil for ten minutes, and add to the strained juice linseed meal, as much as may be sufficient to make a cataplasm [poultice], to be applied warm to the affected part, passing over it a little oil, and renewed twice a day.

HEMP AGRIMONY
Eupatorium cannabinum

Eupatorium cannabinum, commonly known as Hemp agrimony, is a plant native to the UK and belongs to the *Asteraceae* family, which includes Asters, Daisies and Sunflowers. Historically, various parts of the plant have been used in herbal medicine for treating ailments such as fevers and digestive issues.

HISTORICAL USES

Written accounts of the beneficial effects of agrimony date back as far as the 4th to 5th centuries; the herb was also mentioned in the Old English Herbarium from the 10th century (Cameron 2006, Voights 1979, Watkins *et al.* 2012).

Though it is native to the UK, I have been unable to find any description of use by either Gerard or Culpeper, but it may be that they knew the plant by a different name. St John's herb, Holy rope, Dutch agrimony and Thoroughwort have been suggested as alternative names, but these failed to yield any information.

William Fernie's 1897 edition of *Herbal Simples*, however, told us that a Hemp agrimony tincture, prepared from the whole plant '*may be confidently given in frequent small well-diluted doses with water for influenza, or for a similar feverish chill, with break bone pains, prostration, hot dry skin, and some bilious vomiting.*

ETYMOLOGY OF COMMON NAME

As with cultivated Parsley, it is based on the Greek *petroselinon*, from *petra*, 'rock' + *selinon*, 'parsley', but with this species' favoured habitat added.

PLANT LORE

In some folklore traditions, plants resembling parsley, including Hedge parsley, were believed to have protective qualities. They were sometimes hung or placed around homes to ward off evil spirits or negative energies.

USE

Flowers, leaves and seeds (the seeds are the main source of torilin).

EDIBILITY

The leaves can be eaten raw and the root cooked.

HARVEST

In spring and summer.

MEDICINAL PROPERTIES

Antiparasitic, antimicrobial, anti-inflammatory, anticancerogenic and expectorant.

ACTIVE CONSTITUENTS

Coumarins, flavonoids, phenolic acids, polysaccharides, essential oils.

Likewise, a tea made with boiling water poured on the dried leaves will give prompt relief if taken hot at the onset of a bilious catarrh, or of influenza.'

MODERN RESEARCH

Despite the paucity of historical references, modern research has so far confirmed the following properties of Hemp agrimony:

Antioxidant and febrifuge

As pointed out by Fernie, Hemp agrimony can be used for fevers, colds, flu and other viral infections. This may be because it contains flavonoids and sesquiterpene lactones. These promote sweating, which helps to lower body temperature during a fever, and which seem to have antiviral properties.

A 2016 study confirmed these uses and concluded that the plant has a moderate number of flavonoids, but a high number of phenols, which are potential antioxidants.

Antimicrobial

In 2015, three different extracts of Hemp agrimony were tested for their antimicrobial activity. Inhibitory activity was demonstrated against *Escherichia coli* and *Bacillus cereus* while the fungus *Candida albicans* was inhibited by the chloroformic and hydro-alcoholic extracts only.

Anti-inflammatory

A 2018 study in mice with endotoxemia demonstrated that Hemp agrimony increased the survival times of mice and led to inhibition of immune responses. Endotoxemia causes a state of low-grade inflammation, which is a feature of a range of conditions including type-2 diabetes, non-alcoholic fatty liver disease, chronic kidney disease and atherosclerosis.

Cytotoxic

A study in 2021 of isolated eucannabinolide from Hemp agrimony showed cytotoxicity and an ability to induce apoptosis (programmed cell death) in breast cancer cells. Considering the results of this study eucannabinolide is now regarded as a promising candidate for developing and producing new anticancer treatments for human breast cancer studies.

Pyrrolizidine alkaloids

As with Coltsfoot and Comfrey, Hemp agrimony contains pyrrolizidine alkaloids, particularly echimidine. This plant has not been studied as extensively as Coltsfoot or Comfrey but a report on the former in 2020 concluded that, *'Based on these case reports, the evidence of harm caused by these plants is weak. These cases are up to thirty years old and insufficient detail and inconsistent information make it difficult for clear assessments of causality; nor is it possible to make such judgements with insufficient information about concomitant medication and without full relevant medical history.* As with Comfrey and Coltsfoot, therefore, a risk/benefit

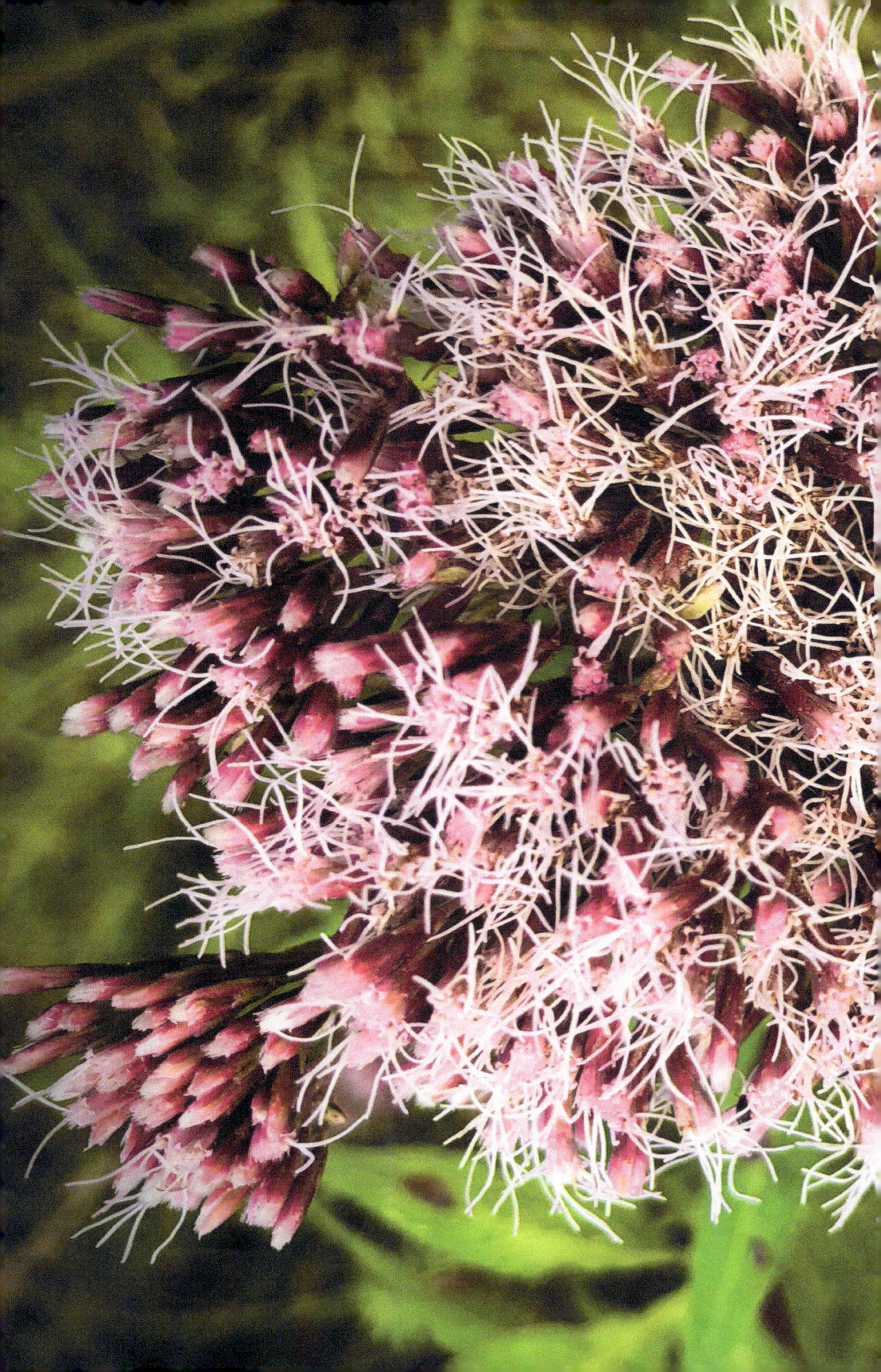

analysis should be made before use and the potential benefits weighed against the risks and the weakness of the evidence, including dietary and supplementary recommendations to support protective liver function during treatment. In the case of Hemp agrimony, unlike the others, it is likely that there are safer alternatives that provide the same benefits.

TOPICAL USAGE

In 2023, a study was undertaken on the wound-healing activity of antimicrobial ointment with Hemp agrimony extract in order to validate use for the treatment of wounds. Results showed that the epithelium was restored with dry, pink, natural tissue earlier than in the control groups treated with a control ointment for an average of 6–8 days.

DOSAGE

The herb is generally unsafe to take as an infusion but is used as an inhalation for the treatment of colds. Single-dose toxicity testing proved that the extract is non-toxic at the dose of 125mg and it is safe to use.

PRECAUTIONS

Because of the pyrrolizidine alkaloid content, hepatotoxicity and carcinogenicity are possible consequences of prolonged internal use. Sensitisation after skin contact with the plant has been reported. Not suitable for children or those who are pregnant or lactating.

Hemp agrimony recipes

Medicinal recipes

Hemp agrimony steam

- 1tbsp/15g of dried leaves and flowers
- 500ml boiling water

Add the herb to a bowl and cover with the water. Place a towel over the head and inhale the vapour to treat colds and fevers. Repeat as necessary.

Hemp agrimony poultice

- 1tsp fresh leaves and flowers (if using dried, moisten with hot water)
- 2tsp coconut oil
- cheesecloth or cotton bandage

Finely chop the herb and add the coconut oil to make a paste. Spread the mix onto a clean cloth or piece of gauze. Fold the cloth or gauze over the herbs to form a small packet and place the poultice directly onto the affected skin area. Ensure that the herb paste is in contact with the skin and secure the poultice in place with a bandage, wrap or medical tape to keep it from moving. Do not use on broken skin.

HERB ROBERT
Geranium robertianum

Geranium robertianum, commonly known as Herb Robert, is a native of the UK and, as the name suggests, is part of the Geranium family, which also includes its cousins, the Cranesbills. Herb Robert is commonly found in woodlands, hedgerows, meadows and disturbed areas such as roadsides and urban green spaces. Herb Robert has a long history of use in traditional herbal medicine.

HISTORICAL USES

Herb Robert was the 'Geranium' of the Middle Ages and was a plant highly valued by medieval apothecaries. If a person was plagued by mosquitos, traditional herbalism suggested that you rub crushed Herb Robert leaves on the skin as a bug repellent. This remedy is still used, particularly in parts of Scotland and the Orkneys, to avoid mosquito bites.

Hildegard of Bingen mentioned in *Physica* that this herb, when powdered and mixed with Feverfew and Nutmeg, was *'the best powder for a healthy heart.'* She went on to recommend the use of the powder for coughs and constrictions of the chest as it *'gently and tenderly weakens the cough and chest wound bringing them to an end.'*

Nicholas Culpeper's *Herbal* stated

ETYMOLOGY OF COMMON NAME
Some writers believe it to be named after Robert Molesme, an 11th-century monk who cured many people using the plant.

PLANT LORE
Often associated with Robin Goodfellow, a hobgoblin also known as Puck in a *Midsummer Night's Dream*.

USE
All aerial parts.

EDIBILITY
Great as an addition to pesto.

HARVEST
When in flower.

MEDICINAL PROPERTIES
Astringent, diuretic, anticancerogenic, antimicrobial.

ACTIVE CONSTITUENTS
Phenolic acids, flavonoids, terpenoids, tannins, alkaloids, anthocyanins.

'Herb Robert is commended not only against the stone, but to stay blood, where or howsoever flowing, it speedily heals all green wounds, and is effectual in old ulcers in the privy parts, or elsewhere ... All geraniums are vulnaries, but this one particularly so.'

The 1756 *British Herbal: a History of Plants and Trees* by Dr John Hill held that *'This plant is an astringent of a very powerful kind; but is not enough known to those who might make its virtues a benefit to, mankind. The farmers give it their cattle when they make bloody urine or have bloody stools; and this with certain success: it should be brought into use in the shops on the same occasions.'*

MODERN RESEARCH

Much like its other Cranesbill cousins, Herb Robert is a useful astringent and haemostatic owing to its high tannin content. Modern research confirms and supports the historical use of the plant for the following:

Astringent and diuretic

The astringency of tannins is attributed to healing of wounds and inflamed mucous membranes, so would indeed provide relief as described by Hildegard. Tannins also act as a diuretic by stimulating blood flow and vasodilation and their drying effects are used to treat diarrhoea and inflammation of the mouth (Ofokansi et al., 2005), which confirms Culpeper's use of the herb.

Anticancerogenic and antioxidant

This small plant has also been found to have great potential as a cancer preventative. Dr Otto Warburg, twice a Nobel Prize winner, said in 1966, *'The prime cause of cancer is lack of oxygenation of the cells.'* He discovered that cancer cells could not exist in the presence of abundant oxygen, but only in an anaerobic state. Because oxygen plays such an important role in cell health and immune function, using Herb Robert regularly is something very practical we can do, for our own general wellbeing.

Phytochemical studies of Herb Robert indicate that it has high flavonoid content and therefore acts as a potent antioxidant, resulting in strong anticancer activity (Salah et al., 1995; Del-Rio et al., 1997; Okwu, 2004). A 2017 study analysed its compounds, finding that the concentrated samples had the highest content of total polyphenols and the strongest antioxidant effect, thereby having also the biggest impact upon cell viability, meaning they could be considered potential chemotherapeutic agents.

Anti-inflammatory and analgesic

Studies of Herb Robert have also confirmed the presence of the tannin geraniin, which has been found to dramatically reduce pain following an outbreak of shingles (Ericksen, 2000). In tests on mice in 2017, geraniin was able to exhibit analgesic effects without any dependency or withdrawal effects.

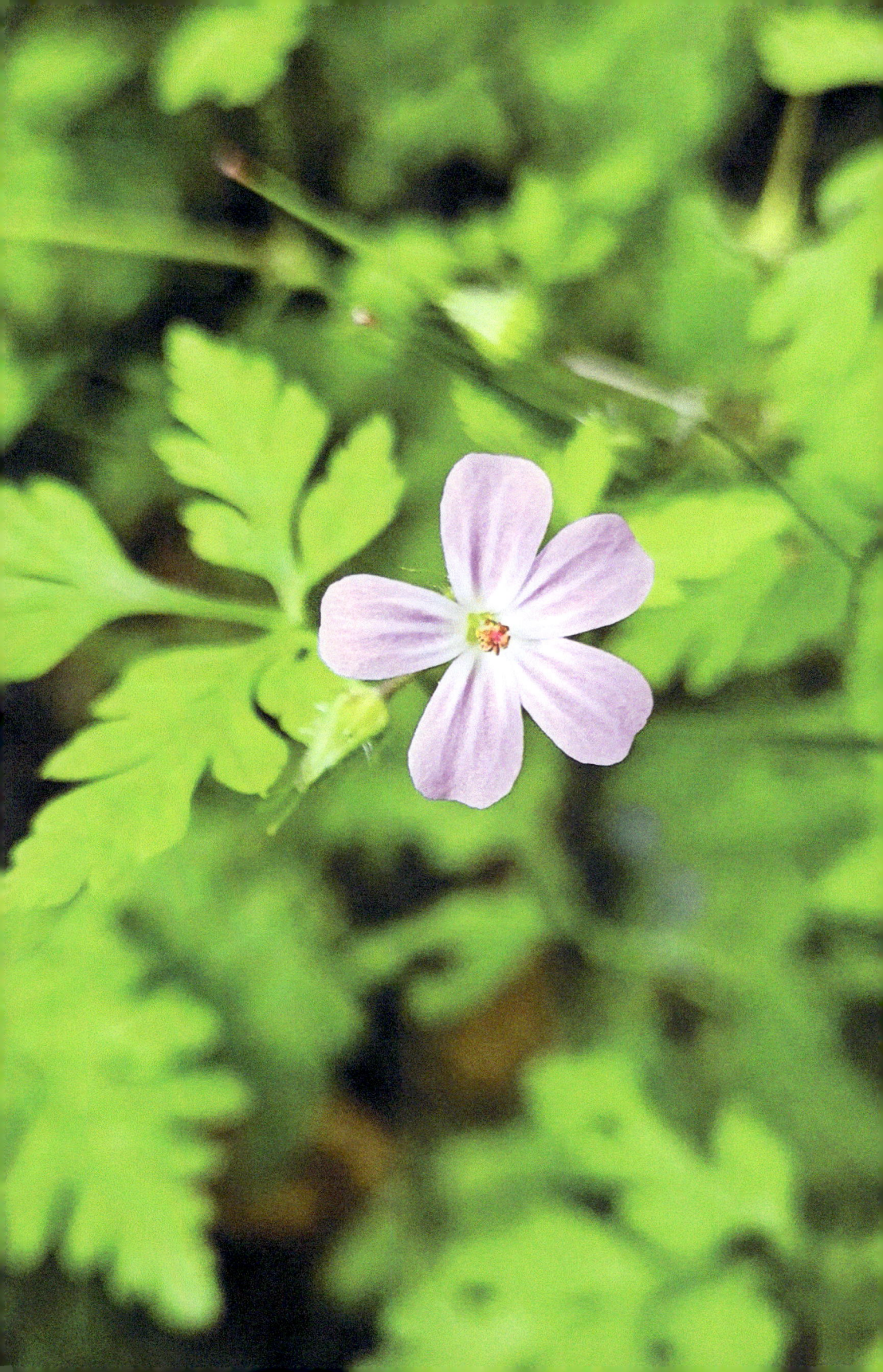

In another 2017 study, the decoctions of leaf and stem were analysed for their anti-inflammatory potentials, and results confirmed again that the plant is particularly rich in tannins and displayed strong scavenging effects. This suggested that its anti-inflammatory activity may partially result from its antioxidant actions towards nitric oxide, a pro-inflammatory'.

Antimicrobial

Yet another 2017 study showed that the leaves were found to be effective against all tested microorganisms (human, animal and plant pathogens), though gram-negative bacteria were more resistant than gram-positive bacteria. The microbiological activity is an indication that the plant can be a source of substances that could possess a broad spectrum of antibacterial activity.

TOPICAL USES

Herb Robert has quite a distinctive smell and has been traditionally used as an insect repellent when rubbed on the skin or placed in a pet's bed to deter fleas. It can also be applied topically to reduce inflammation in conditions such as eczema, dermatitis and insect bites.

DOSAGE

Tisane – 28g in 500ml. Drink freely.

PRECAUTIONS

Not to be taken with blood-thinning medications. Not suitable for children or those who are pregnant or lactating.

Herb Robert recipes

Medicinal recipes

Herb Robert tisane

Pour 500ml boiling water over 6tsp/30g of the herb and allow to steep for 15 minutes. Use as a digestive tonic, immunity booster and anti-inflammatory. The infusion can also serve as a mouthwash to treat oral infections and inflammations.

Herb Robert poultice

- 1tsp fresh leaves (if using dried you will need to moisten with water first)
- 2tsp coconut oil
- cheesecloth or cotton bandage

Finely chop the leaves into a pulp and add the coconut oil to make a paste. Spread the paste evenly over the desired area and wrap with the cloth or bandage. Use for its antimicrobial and anti-inflammatory properties to promote healing of skin issues and as an analgesic.

Herb Robert infused oil

- 100g dried herb
- 2tbsp alcohol, such as Everclear
- 1l grapeseed oil

Place the herb in the bottom of a jar with the Everclear. Allow to steep for 10 minutes and then add the oil. Allow the mix to steep/infuse for 4 weeks. Use as a massage oil for sore muscles and joints or apply it to the skin for its soothing and healing properties on skin irritations, cuts and bruises. Also works well as a repellent for mosquitos.

HOGWEED
Heracleum sphondylium

Heracleum sphondylium, commonly known as Hogweed, is a herbaceous plant species native to the UK, found in a variety of habitats, including meadows, woodland edges, riverbanks and roadside verges. In traditional herbal medicine, Hogweed has been used for various purposes, including as a diuretic and expectorant.

HISTORICAL USES

Hogweed was enjoyed by virtually all native people throughout north-western North America, where it was gathered before flowering. Gorman (1896) noted that Cow parsnip was '… *pre-eminently the fresh vegetable of the* [Alaskan] *natives, who gather and eat the succulent leaf stalks and young stems in enormous quantities, the Kloochmen* [Chinook jargon for women] *and children gathering it most of the day when it is in the proper condition.*'

Nicholas Culpeper's *Herbal* said '*The seed thereof is of a sharp and cutting quality, and therefore is a fit medicine for a cough and shortness of breath, the falling sickness and jaundice. It also helps the running scab and shingles. The juice of the flowers dropped into the ears, cleanses and heals them.*'

In the Isle of Man, the seeds and roots have been traditionally boiled and the

ETYMOLOGY OF COMMON NAME
Seemingly simply because it is said that the flower gives off a pig-like odour!

PLANT LORE
Also known as Cow parsnip (particularly in North America), because cows eat it, and it is related to parsnip.

USE
Leaves, flowers and roots. Other uses – the seeds can be dried and used as a spice, with a flavour similar to that of cardamom.

EDIBILITY
Young hogweed shoots can be cooked and make a tasty soup.

HARVEST
In spring and summer.

MEDICINAL PROPERTIES
Antimicrobial, antihypertensive, aphrodisiac, anti-inflammatory, analgesic, expectorant.

ACTIVE CONSTITUENTS
Phenolic acids, flavonoids, furanocoumarins, polyacetylenes, volatile oils.

liquid drunk for treating jaundice and other liver troubles. In addition, Hogweed juice has featured as a wart cure, while the tender shoots, stripped of the outer skin, enjoyed a reputation as a digestive (Allen and Hatfield, 2004).

In Italian folk medicine, the essential oil from the fruits was used as sedative and in general against depression (Gastaldo, 1987) while, in Abruzzo, the plant decoction was used to clean healing wounds, and the infusion of leaves and stems as stomachic, digestive and aphrodisiac (Tammaro, 1984). In Romania and Morocco, the extract of aerial parts is reputed to be aphrodisiac and antihypertensive, and used to treat male and female sterility, impotence, frigidity, hypertension etc. (Eddouks et al., 2002).

MODERN RESEARCH

Young Hogweed leaves are high in vitamin C, which is no doubt why it was popular with the Alaskan native peoples. The genus has also been found to have great potential to produce novel furanocoumarins, such as xanthotoxin and bergapten with several important pharmacological properties:

Antimicrobial

Extracts of Hogweed have shown antimicrobial activity against *Staphylococcus aureus, Enterococcus feacalis, Escherichia coli, Pseudomonas aeruginosa Listeria monocytogenes,* and many other forms of bacteria (Ergene et al., 2006). A 2017 study highlighted that the leaves and flowers are a source of antioxidant flavonoids and antibacterial agents, which could be used in pharmaceuticals, particularly against *Staphylococcus aureus* strains. *Staphylococcus* grows in warm moist environments, which may be the reason that Culpeper found this herb so useful in treating ear problems.

Anti-inflammatory and analgesic

Hogweed possesses notable anti-inflammatory properties, making it useful for treating various conditions. This again is primarily on account of its furanocoumarins (Hajhashemi et al., 2009; Panahi et al., 2015), which inhibit the production of pro-inflammatory cytokines and enzymes, thereby reducing inflammation while modulating the immune response to minimise tissue damage.

Expectorant

As Culpeper said, the plant is useful for coughs and chest complaints. Again, this is related to its furanocoumarins, but also its flavonoids and essential oils, which work together to reduce mucus viscosity, stimulate production and reduce inflammation in the respiratory tract, making it easier to expel mucus and alleviate symptoms of respiratory conditions such as bronchitis, coughs and colds.

Antihypertensive

With regard to its traditional use in Romania and Morocco as an antihypertensive, this was proven in a 2013

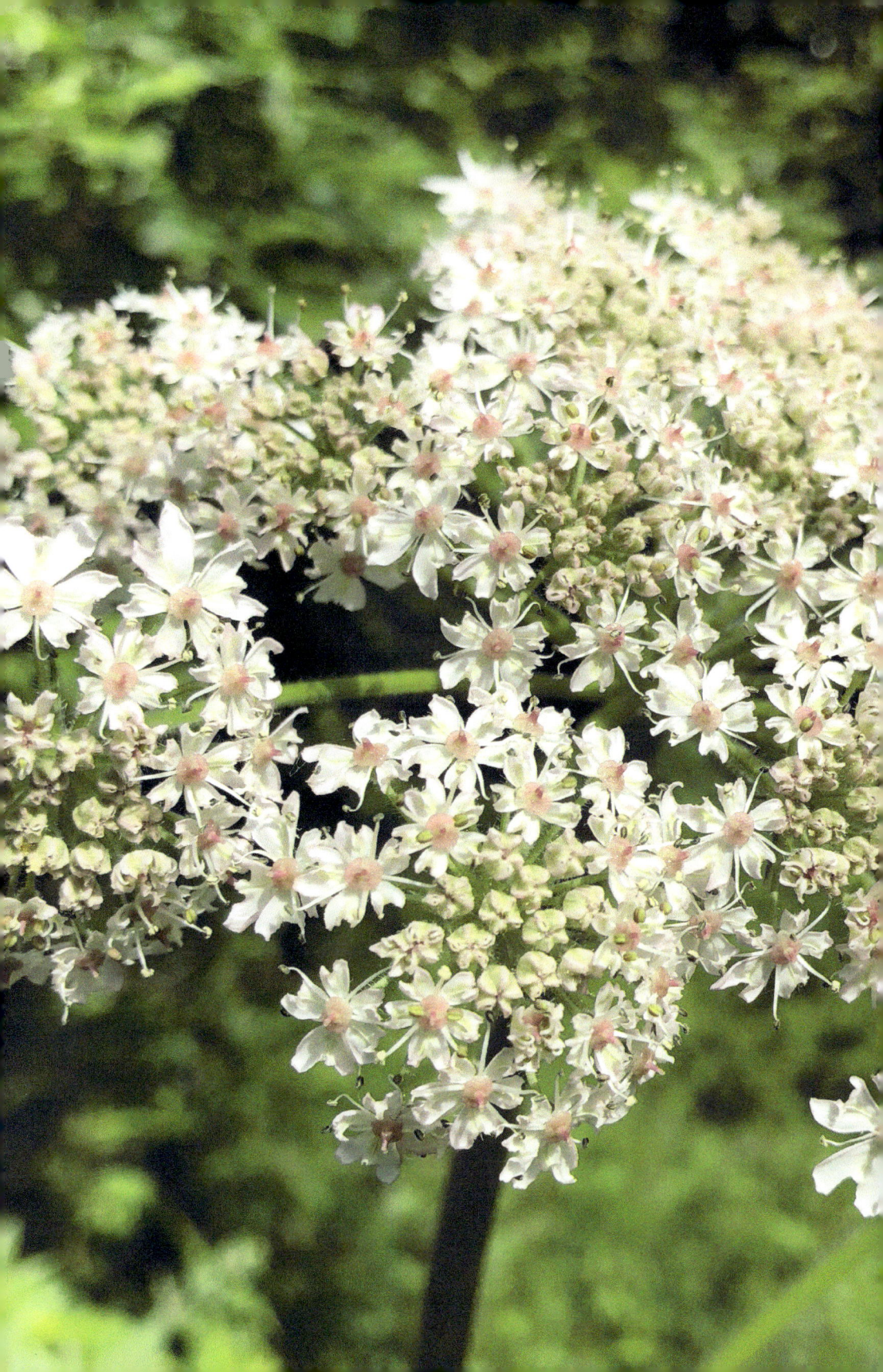

study that showed that extracts exhibit vasorelaxant properties, providing a good argument for its use in treatment of high blood pressure.

Aphrodisiac

In addition, in many parts of the world, as mentioned, Hogweed is considered a natural aphrodisiac. Many companies sell tablets made from the extract of this plant to boost sexual energy, and in Romania it is used pretty much like Ginseng for strength and vitality. While I have been unable to verify this via scientific study, the effects are likely to be attributed to antioxidant, anti-inflammatory and vasodilatory actions of flavonoids, which lead to improved circulation and reduced stress.

TOPICAL USE

The furanocoumarins in Hogweed, as well as other *Apiaceae* herbs, are phototoxic (Carroll et al., 2000). It is not therefore recommended for topical use as these chemicals in the sap can cause photodermatitis.

DOSAGE

Tisane – 3tsp/15g to 2 glasses of cold water and allow to draw for 8 hours.

PRECAUTIONS

Not suitable for children or those who are pregnant or lactating.

Hogweed Recipes

Be sure not to confuse Hogweed with the rather similar-looking but poisonous or toxic Giant hogweed, Poison hemlock or Hemlock water dropwort.

Medicinal recipes

Hogweed tisane

Pour 250ml boiling water over 1tsp/5g of the dried leaf and stem and allow to steep for 10-15 minutes. Use as a tonic or for coughs, colds, inflammation of the joints, digestive issues and sore throats. Inhalation of the steam from boiling hogweed leaves or stems may provide respiratory anti-inflammatory benefits for conditions such as bronchitis or sinusitis.

Hogweed cold infusion

Pour 2 glasses of cold water over 3tsp/15g of the leaves and flowers, then allow to infuse for 8 hours. Drink in small amounts throughout the day to help with digestion and relieve mild digestive issues like bloating and gas.

Hogweed poultice

- 1tsp fresh leaves (if using dried you will need to moisten with water first)
- 2tsp coconut oil
- cheesecloth or cotton bandage

Finely chop the leaves into a pulp and add the coconut oil to make a paste. Spread the paste evenly over the desired area and wrap with the cloth or bandage. Use to soothe joint pain, muscle aches or minor wounds.

HONEYSUCKLE
Lonicera spp.

In the UK, several species of *Lonicera*, commonly known as Honeysuckles, can be found. These include the native Honeysuckle, *Lonicera peryclymenum*, also known as Common honeysuckle or Woodbine, with its white or yellow flowers with a pink or red flush. The garden escapee, *Lonicera japonica* or Japanese honeysuckle, has become naturalised and can also be found in disturbed habitats, such as roadsides, waste areas and woodland edges, where it displays its vigorous, twining vine and fragrant yellow flowers.

HISTORICAL USES

In his *Herball*, John Gerard called the plant Wood-binde or Hony-suckle, and said '*The floures steeped in oile, and set in the Sun, are good to annoint the body that is benummed, and growne very cold.*'

Nicholas Culpeper also called it Woodbine and wrote, '*The leaves are the only parts used and are put into gargarisms for sore throats. Some recommend a decoction for a cough and the phthisic, and to open obstructions of the liver and spleen. The oil made by infusion of the leaves, is healing and warming and good for the cramps and convulsions of the nerve.*'

The Japanese honeysuckle was

ETYMOLOGY OF COMMON NAME
From Old English *hunigsūce*, 'honey suck', referring to the tubular flowers, which are sucked for their nectar.

PLANT LORE
It was believed that fairies would use the vines of honeysuckle to weave their magic and create enchanted bowers or hideaways.

USE
The leaves and flowers.

EDIBILITY
The flowers are edible.

HARVEST
In spring and summer.

MEDICINAL PROPERTIES
Anti-inflammatory, antimicrobial, anticancerogenic, antidiabetic and hepatoprotective.

ACTIVE CONSTITUENTS
Flavonoids, phenolic acids, triterpenoid saponins, iridoids, tannins.

employed in Ancient China as a healthy beverage to improve body and prevent ills. In the Qing dynasty, according to *Yan Shou Dan Fan*, it was used to moisturise and rejuvenate the skin (Chen, 2008).

MODERN RESEARCH

Both Japanese honeysuckle and Common honeysuckle have been traditionally used in herbal medicine for their antioxidant, anti-inflammatory and antimicrobial properties. However, unlike the native Honeysuckle, Japanese honeysuckle has been extensively studied. As mentioned above, it has historically been used in East Asian countries to treat fever, headache, upper respiratory tract infections, urinary disorders, rheumatoid arthritis and diabetes mellitus$_3$ and the modern research confirms the following:

Anti-inflammatory

Common honeysuckle and Japanese honeysuckle both contain flavonoids such as quercetin and kaempferol, which exhibit anti-inflammatory properties. In 1998, Lee et al. evaluated the anti-inflammatory activity of *Japonica* and found that it showed anti-inflammatory activities comparable to aspirin, making it a safe and mild anti-inflammatory agent. These properties, as Culpeper points out, are useful for inflammations of the mucous membranes.

Anticancerogenic

Yip et al. in 2006 demonstrated that the compounds of Japanese honeysuckle could be a useful ally against cancer after extracts were seen to trigger cell death in human liver cancer cells. In addition, luteoin and kaempferol, which are the major active constituents of both Common honeysuckle and Japanese honeysuckle, were observed to induce cell death in various cancers.

Antimicrobial

In 2002, Ma et al. selected 44 medicinal herbs that are used for the treatment of respiratory tract infectious diseases in China and tested the antiviral activities against respiratory viruses. Japanese honeysuckle showed potent antiviral activities in the study and confirmed its use in upper respiratory tract infections.

Then, in 2009, Rahman et al. evaluated the antibacterial potential of essential oil from *Japonica* flowers and ethanol extracts from the leaf. A remarkable antibacterial effect of the oil and extracts was revealed against *Listeria, Bacillus subtilis, Bacillus cereus, Staphylococcus aureus,* and *Salmonella enteritidis* and *Escherichia coli.* Furthermore, Papageorgiou et al. in 2010 found that both Common honeysuckle and Japanese honeysuckle extracts have excellent activity against *Staphylococcus* aureus, *Pseudomonas aeruginosa, Escherichia coli, Candida albicans* and *Aspergillus niger.*

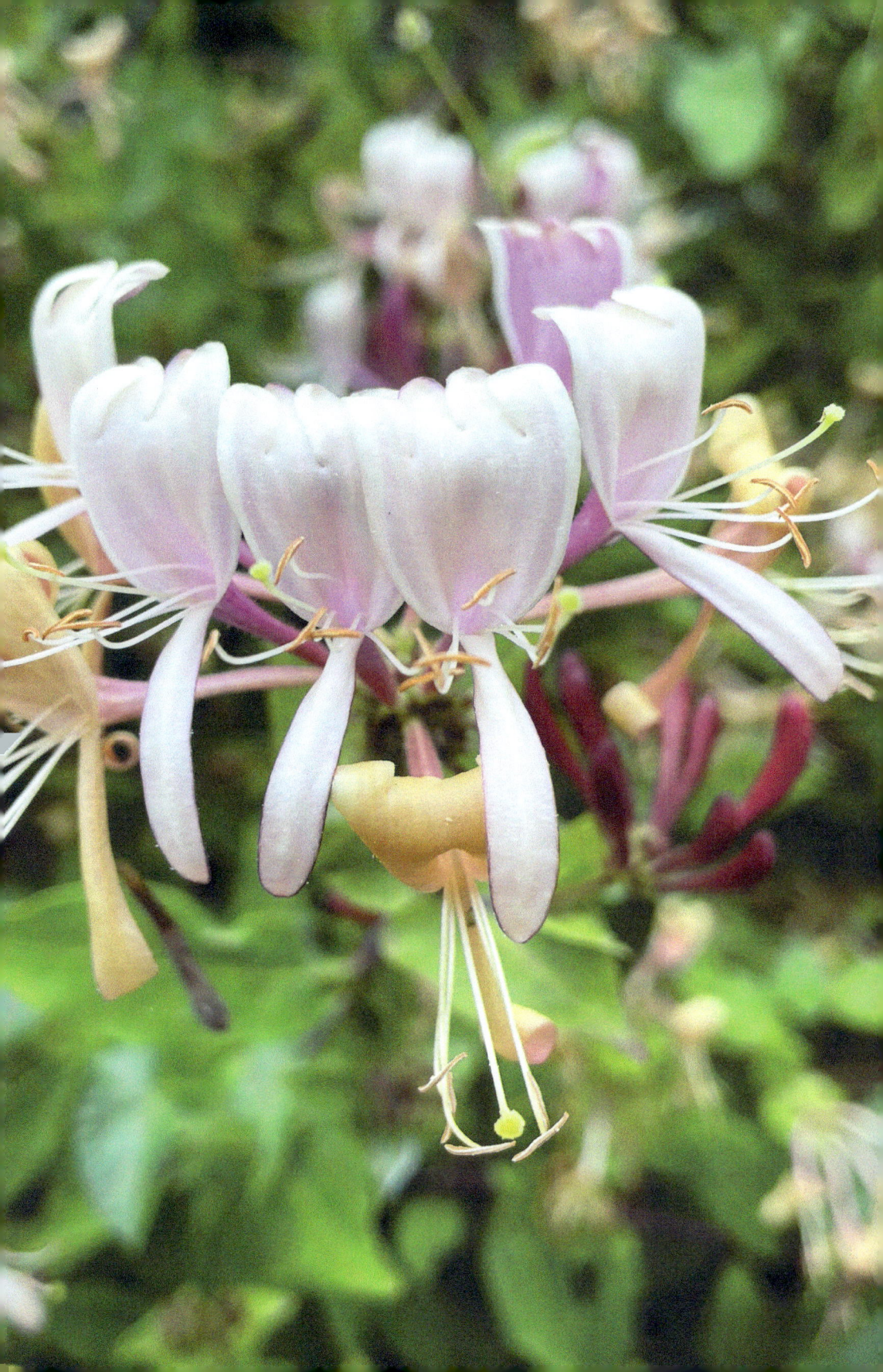

Antidiabetic and anticancerogenic

A 2015 study found that Japanese honeysuckle given to diabetic rats for four weeks at dose of 100mg/kg decreased high blood glucose levels and insulin resistance after four weeks. Then, in 2018, one of four new flavonoids, japoflavone, was isolated and found to show significant hepatoprotective activity against cervical cancer and hepatoma cells.

Hepatoprotective

The anti-inflammatory properties of Japanese honeysuckle make it a potential medicine for the treatment of non-alcoholic fatty liver disease (NAFLD). A 2021 study revealed a total of 17 active components related to NAFLD, and showed that *Japonica* reduced the necrosis and hepatocellular death to protect the normal function of the liver in an NAFLD cell model.

TOPICAL USE

Honeysuckle leaves and flowers have been traditionally used in herbal medicine for treating skin irritations, such as minor cuts, burns and rashes. The anti-inflammatory and soothing properties may help alleviate discomfort and promote healing. The berries meanwhile when studied in topical gel form were found to make a good antioxidant barrier against free radicals that damage and age the skin. The plant's antiseptic abilities also make it a natural way to cleanse skin while evening out skin tone.

DOSAGE

Tisane – 20-40g of dried herb in two cups of boiled water, 3 times a day.

PRECAUTIONS

Honeysuckle is not intended for long-term use. While the flowers are low in toxicity, the fruits, leaves and stems are more toxic. Not suitable for children or those who are pregnant or lactating.

Honeysuckle recipes

Medicinal recipes

Honeysuckle tisane
Pour 500ml boiling water over 4–8tsp/ 20–40g of Honeysuckle flowers and allow to steep for 10 minutes. Use for soothing sore throats, reducing fever and alleviating cold symptoms.

Honeysuckle compress
Use for skin irritations, rashes and minor wounds to benefit from the antibacterial and anti-inflammatory properties. Soak a cloth in a tisane of the dried flowers and apply it to the affected areas 2–3 times a day.

Honeysuckle sore throat honey
Fill a jar about two-thirds full of fresh Honeysuckle flowers, then pour over a good-quality honey. Once the flowers are covered, stir well, seal and leave to infuse for 4 weeks. Loosen the contents a little in a bowl of hot water and then strain. Store in a cool place. Use 2 dessertspoons every 2 hours to ease sore throats, infections, cold/flu, etc.

Honeysuckle infused oil
- 100g fresh Honeysuckle berries, mashed
- 2tbsp alcohol, such as Everclear
- 1l grapeseed oil

Place the berries in the bottom of a jar with the Everclear. Allow to steep for 10 minutes and then add the oil. Infuse for 4 weeks and then use topically to reduce inflammation and protect against ageing.

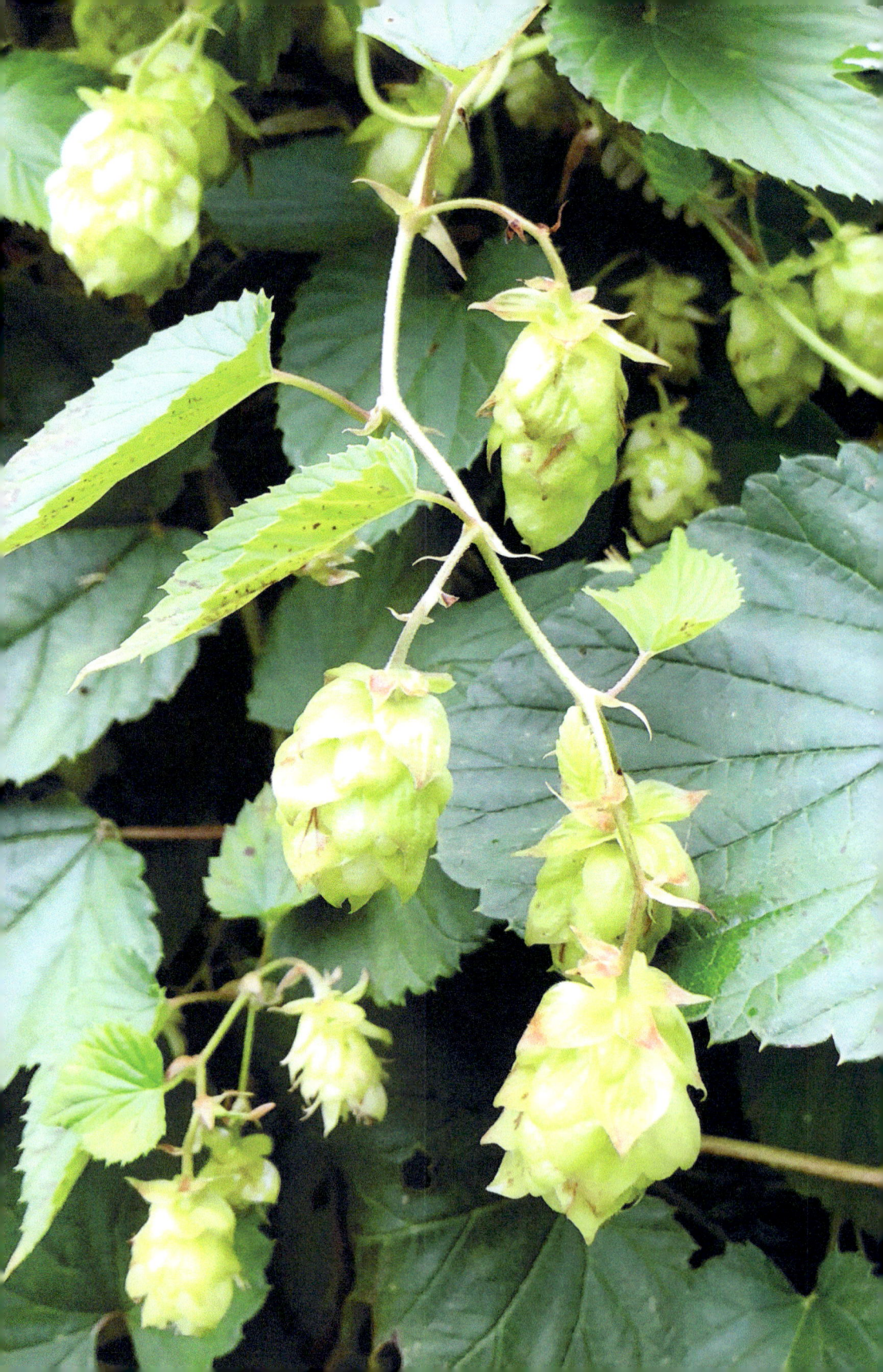

HOPS
Humulus lupulus

Humulus lupulus, Common hops, is a species of flowering plant in the Hemp family (*Cannabaceae*), and is native to West Asia, Europe and North America. In the UK Hops are cultivated as a key ingredient in beer production, contributing bitterness, flavour and aroma to the finished product. They also have a long history of use in traditional herbal medicine for their sedative and calming properties.

HISTORICAL USES

Hops were first brought to the UK from Flanders, in 1524. Before Hops were used for improving and preserving beer, the Saxons used Ground ivy and the Picts used Heather in their ales. However, according to Martyn Cornell's blog Zythophile, under *A short history of hops*, Hildegard von Bingen recorded in her *Physica* that the bitterness of hops *'keeps some putrefactions from beverages, to which it may be added, so that they may last longer.'*

Nicholas Culpeper's *Herbal* stated *'The decoction of the tops of Hops, as well of the tame as the wild, works the same effects. In cleansing the blood, they help to cure the French diseases* [syphilis]*, and all manner of scabs, itch, and other breakings-out of the body, as also all tetters, ringworms and spreading sores, the morphew and all*

ETYMOLOGY OF COMMON NAME
From the Anglo-Saxon *lioppan*, 'to climb'.

PLANT LORE
In Celtic mythology Hops are associated with wolves, winter, the Underworld, Brigid and the Imbolc celebration.

USE
The female flowers.

EDIBILITY
Young leaves and shoots can be eaten in salads before the end of May.

HARVEST
In September with careful handling on drying to prevent loss of pollen.

MEDICINAL PROPERTIES
Tonic, oestrogenic, diuretic, antimicrobial and sedative.

ACTIVE CONSTITUENTS
Bitter acids, flavonoids, essential oils, tannins, polyphenols, resins.

LEFT: HOPS

discolouring of the skin. The decoction of the flowers and hops do help to expel poison that any one hath drank. Half a dram of the seed in powder taken in drink, kills worms in the body, brings down women's courses, and expels urine. A syrup made of the juice and sugar, cures the yellow jaundice, eases the headache that comes of heat, and tempers the heat of the liver and stomach, and is profitably given in long and hot agues that rise in choler and blood.'

In his *History of Plants*, published in 1657, William Coles related the virtues of Hops as follows, *'They are good to cleanse the kidneys from gravel, and to provoke urine; they likewise open obstructions of the liver and spleen, cleanse the blood, and loosen the belly; and as they cleanse the blood, so consequently they help to cure eruptions of the skin, … half a drachm of the seeds powdered, and taken in drink, will kill worms … the expressed juice will cure the jaundice.'*

In his book *The General Dispensatory*, published in 1753, Dr R.B. Brookes wrote of Hops, *'Lupulus, hops, the leaves. They help digestion, open obstructions of the viscera, especially the spleen, promote urine, and loosen the belly; they are good in the hypochondriac passion, the scurvy, and diseases of the skin, if given as an alterative* [healing] *in whey or broths. The depurated juice may be given from two to four ounces, the decoction of the tops from one to two handfuls, and half a drachm of the seeds may be given against worms.'*

William Fernie's *Herbal Simples* edition of 1897 noted that *'a pillow stuffed with newly dried Hops was successfully prescribed by Dr Willis for George the Third, when sedative medicines had failed to give him sleep; and again, for the Prince of Wales at the time of his severe typhoid fever, 1871.'*

MODERN RESEARCH

As can be seen from the numerous references by the historical writers, Hops have been much used in traditional medicine. Modern research has both confirmed the traditional uses and discovered new properties as follows:

Diuretic

Culpeper's assertion (along with William Coles and Dr Brookes) that Hops act as a diuretic is borne out in scientific studies. In fact, in a study on obesity in mice, the extract enhanced water excretion while inhibiting the increase in adipose tissue weight and may therefore be a candidate in the fight against human obesity.

Antimicrobial

While I have not been able to substantiate Culpeper's assertion that the plant cures the 'French diseases' or syphilis as we now know it, lupulone, a component of Hops, can control bacterial growth, while other compounds such as humulone and xanthohumol are also now being shown to exert antimicrobial effects.

As far as the antiparasitic effects that were noted by the historic writers are concerned, the humulones and lupulones in Hops are a natural acaricide, and are still used to control mites in the shipment of bees and establishment of new colonies in the spring (DeGrandi-Hoffman et al., 2012, 2014).

Oestrogenic

In Germany, Hops baths were traditionally used to treat gynaecological disorders, and the presence of oestrogenic substances in hops was firstly suggested by Koch and Heim (1953). In a 2001 study by Liu et al., this oestrogenic activity was demonstrated, and was then confirmed by Overk et al. in 2005 when Hops showed a potency equivalent to that of Red clover. In a clinical study of menopausal women by Heyerick et al. in 2006, the daily administration of a Hops extract for 6 weeks decreased the incidence of hot flushes and other discomforts associated with oestrogen deficiency (sweating, insomnia, heart palpitation, irritability). Vaginal dryness in postmenopausal women was also significantly reduced by the topical application of a gel containing hyaluronic acid, liposomes, vitamin E and hops extract (Morali et al., 2006).

Anticancerogenic

Hops have also been studied for their anticancer potential. Several *in vitro* studies have shown that xanthohumol seems to inhibit the initiation, promotion and progression stages of carcinogenesis, meaning that it could be a broad-spectrum chemopreventive agent (Stevens and Page, 2004; Gerhauser, 2005; Colgate et al., 2007).

Sedative

Hops are probably best known as a sedative. A 2019 article on plants with sedative effects found that this is related to the alpha bitter acids and beta acids contained in them. Hops appear to interact with melatonin receptors, which play a role in sleep. A study by Shishehgar et al. in 2012 showed that Hops had superior sedation and anxiolytic effect when compared to diazepam.

Metabolic and anti-inflammatory

A 2021 review found that the bitter molecules within Hops also have a beneficial effect on weight gain, lipid metabolism, glucose homeostasis, insulin sensitivities and inflammation, by acting on different targets. They have also been shown to reduce cortisol levels and improve gastrointestinal mucosal integrity in mice. Furthermore, they appear to be safely able to reduce inflammation without the toxic impact on the cardiovascular system and gastrointestinal tract commonly seen in NSAIDs. Similarly, they mitigate insulin resistance and hyperglycaemia without side effects such as weight gain or oedema. All these aspects make these acids excellent candidates to treat metabolic syndrome disorders.

TOPICAL USES

Hops extract showed antibacterial activity against *Propionibacterium acnes*, a gram-positive bacterium that forms part of the normal flora of the skin, oral cavity, large intestine, the conjunctiva and the external ear canal. Although primarily recognised for its role in acne this makes it a promising topical ingredient to treat acne-prone skin and to reduce the application of antibiotics in mild forms of acne.

DOSAGE

Tisane – 1tsp/5g. Drink half a cup, 3 times per day.
Tincture – 1:5 60% – 1–2ml, 3 times per day – 20 drops = 1ml/1tsp = 5ml.

PRECAUTIONS

Skin contact with Hops can cause dermatitis in sensitive people. Consumption should be avoided during pregnancy and breastfeeding as well as by people who suffer from chronic depression and those with hormone-dependent cancers.

Hops recipes

Medicinal recipes

Hops tisane

Pour 250ml boiling water over 1tsp/5g of Hops flowers and allow to steep for 10 minutes. Drink 30 minutes before bedtime for peaceful sleep. Can also be used for menopausal symptoms, hypertension, ADHD, dyspepsia and bladder inflammation as well as being externally applied to inflamed areas for pain relief from arthritis.

Hops infused tincture, 1:5 60%

If you are using 40% alcohol, ie vodka, cover 1part herb to 10 parts fluid.

If you are using Everclear or other 100% proof, use the following method for a specific tincture:

- 100g dried Hops flowers
- 300ml alcohol
- 200ml water

Take 100g of dried Hops herb and split into two parts of 50g each. Place 50g in the alcohol. Take the other 50g part and place in the boiled water. Steep/infuse in the water for 10 minutes. Strain thoroughly and top up if the water is less than 200ml. Add the infusion to the alcohol mix and leave for 14 days before straining. Use for anxiety and digestion.

Hops honey

Fill a sterilised jar about two-thirds full with either fresh or dried Hops herbs, then pour over a good-quality honey. Once the herbs are generously covered it's important to stir well to break any air bubbles (which could encourage bacterial growth). Then the jar can be sealed and left to steep/infuse for at least a month. To make the straining process easier, sit the sealed jar in a bowl of hot water. This will slightly loosen the honey, without overheating it, making it much easier to strain through a sieve. Store in a cool place and use as an alternative to the tisane.

Hops herbal bath blend

A blend of Lavender oil, Lemon balm, Oat extract and Hops exhibited a relaxing effect, documented by electroencephalographic analysis, in healthy volunteers (Dimpfel et al., 2004).

Hops hair wash

- 1tbsp/15g of Hops
- 250ml boiling water

Allow the mix to steep overnight, then add 3 litres of warm water for a hair rinse once a week.

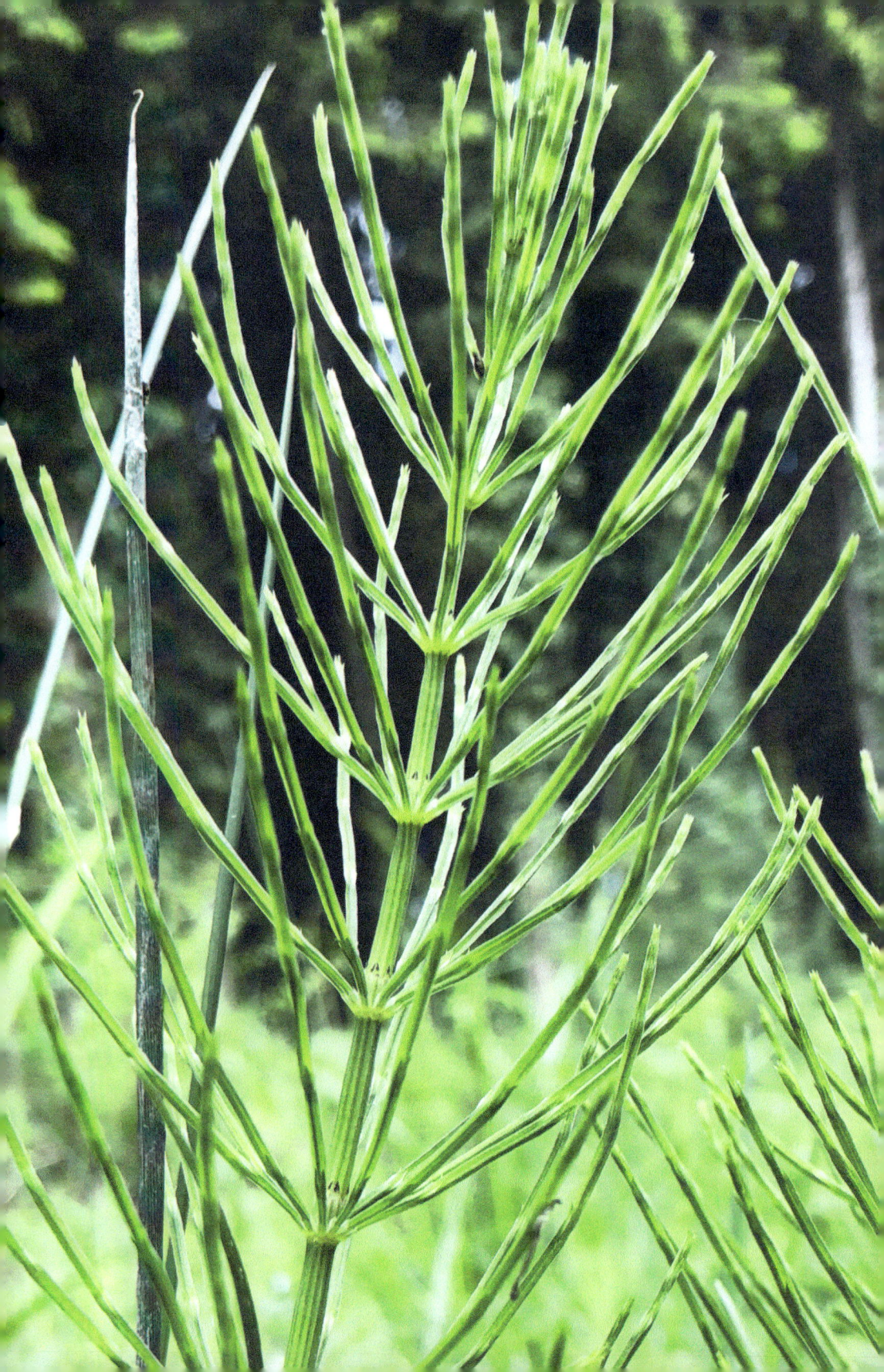

HORSETAIL
Equisetum arvense

Equisetum arvense, generally known as Field or Common horsetail, is one of a number of Horsetail plants native to the UK. Horsetails are ancient plants that have persisted since the time of the dinosaurs, and the Field horsetail is one of the most common and widespread species. It is often found in damp habitats such as meadows, marshes, riverbanks and disturbed areas like road verges.

HISTORICAL USES

In his *Herball*, John Gerard related that '*Dioscorides saith, that Horse-taile being stamped and laid to, doth perfectly cure wounds, yea although the sinues be cut' in sunder, as Galen addeth. The herb drunke either with water or wine, is an excellent remedy against bleeding at the nose. Horse-taile with his roots boiled in wine is very profitable for difficultie of breathing.*'

Nicholas Culpeper's *Herbal* explained, '*It is very powerful to stop bleeding, either inward or outward, the juice or the decoction being drunk, or the juice, decoction or distilled water applied outwardly ... It also heals inward ulcers. ... It solders together the tops of green wounds and cures all ruptures in children. The decoction taken in wine helps stone and strangury; the*

ETYMOLOGY OF COMMON NAME
From the bristly appearance of the jointed stems of the plants, which resemble horses' tails.

PLANT LORE
Traditionally, Horsetail plays a role in ceremonies and spiritual practices. It is seen as a protector and is often associated with affirmations and commitments.

EDIBILITY
The young shoots are edible. Use the barren stems only after the fruiting stems have died down, cut them off just above the root.

HARVEST
In spring and early summer.

MEDICINAL PROPERTIES
Diuretic, antihypertensive, vulnerary and astringent.

ACTIVE CONSTITUENTS
Flavonoids, alkaloids, phenolic acids, silica, saponins, alkaloids.

diſtilled water drunk two or three times a day eases and ſtrengthens the inteſtines and is effectual in a cough that comes by diſtillation from the head. The juice or diſtilled water used as a warm fomentation is of service in inflammations and breakings-out in the skin.'

MODERN RESEARCH

This chapter concentrates on Field horsetail, for which the following properties have been identified:

Diuretic

Horsetail's silica content likely contributes to its diuretic effect and is why we see Culpeper saying a 'decoction taken in wine helps stone and strangury' (ie bladder blockage). As further confirmation, literature suggests that Horsetail is specifically indicated as a diuretic in inflammation of the renal pelvis as it increases the irrigation of the urinary tract (Pallag et al., 2018).

A 2014 clinical trial reported that the diuretic effect of Horsetail was equivalent to that of hydrochlorothiazide, a medication used to treat fluid retention, without significant changes in electrolyte excretion, signs of toxicity or significant adverse effects, suggesting that Horsetail is effective and safe for acute use.

Antihypertensive

A 2022 study assessed the antihypertensive effect of Horsetail, again as compared to hydrochlorothiazide, on systemic arterial hypertension sufferers. A Horsetail dry extract was administered for 3 months after which the Horsetail treatment demonstrated a significant antihypertensive effect, decreasing blood pressure to the normal ranges, and demonstrating a well-tolerability profile similar to hydrochlorothiazide intervention.

Vulnerary

The other use championed by Culpeper and Gerard was the effectiveness of Horsetail on wound treatments. A topical Horsetail ointment was found to promote wound-healing and relieve pain during a 10-day period after episiotomy, and it was proposed that this resulted from the silicea, silicic acid, silicon and saponin content in the extracts. The results support the traditional use of the water decoction in wound-healing.

TOPICAL USES

In a clinical trial, the effect of a water-soluble nail polish containing Horsetail on nail psoriasis showed superiority over a placebo. Horsetail is a source of organic silicon, and since nails contain 16mg of silicon dioxide per 100g, it seems to contribute to their strength and hardness while maintaining stability among keratin fibrils.

DOSAGE

Tisane – ½ to 1tsp/2.5g. Drink a half cup 2–3 times per day.

PRECAUTIONS

Aqueous preparations should be avoided by patients with health problems that demand fluid restriction (heart or kidney failure). Not suitable for children or those who are pregnant or lactating.

Horsetail recipes

Medicinal recipes

Horsetail tisane

Pour 250ml boiling water over 1tsp/5g of Horsetail herb and simmer 5 minutes; then infuse 30 minutes. Allow to cool completely and drink cold. Use for minor oedema in blood spotting in urine/stool, stomach ulcers, urinary tract inflammations and for treating various prostate and lung conditions. Owing to the high silica, selenium and zinc content this treatment is best staggered to avoid kidney strain. Use for one month, followed by one week's break. The tisane can also be used externally in the treatment of various skin conditions such as acne and eczema. Adding the herb to a bath also benefits slow-healing sprains and fractures.

Horsetail poultice

- 1tsp fresh Horsetail stems (if using dried you will need to moisten with water first)
- 2tsp coconut oil
- cheesecloth or cotton bandage

Finely chop the stems into a pulp and add the coconut oil to make a paste. Spread the paste evenly over the desired area and wrap with the cloth or bandage. Use to heal wounds such as ulcers, sores and chilblains.

Horsetail juice

- A big handful of stems, roughly chopped

Put everything through a juicer (or use a blender and then strain through muslin) and drink 5–10ml of this juice 3 times daily for treatment of urinary disorders and long-term lung damage. The juice can also be used for the treatment of nosebleeds. Dip a cotton bud in place into the nostril to stop the bleeding.

Horsetail hair rinse

- Fresh horsetail
- Apple cider vinegar

Fill a jar approximately three-quarters full of fresh Horsetail. Top up the jar with the vinegar, ensuring that all plant parts are covered. Infuse for 6 weeks shaking every few days and then strain. To use, rinse through your hair either after washing or between washes. I like to rinse and leave it in, combing it through my hair. But you can also comb the rinse through your hair and then rinse it outrightly with water. Do not follow with any conditioner or any other products.

KNAPWEED
Centaurea nigra/scabiosa

The *Centaurea* are a genus of flowering plants in the *Asteraceae*, the Daisy and Sunflower family. The Common knapweed (*Centaurea nigra*) and Greater knapweed (*Centaurea scabiosa*) are both native to the UK and can be found in a variety of habitats, including grasslands, meadows, road verges and waste areas. Both plants have a history of traditional use in herbal medicine.

HISTORICAL USES

Knapweed was included in the 14th-century ointment known as 'Save', to treat wounds, bruises and sores, and was mixed with pepper to treat loss of appetite (Grieve, 1931).

Nicholas Culpeper's *Herbal* said *'Knapweed helps to stay fluxes, both of blood at the mouth or nose, or other outward parts, and those veins that are inwardly broken, or inward wounds, as also the fluxes of the belly. It stays distillation of thin and sharp humours from the head upon the stomach and lungs; it is good for those that are bruised by any fall, blows or otherwise, and is profitable for those that are bursten, and have ruptures. It is singularly good in all running sores, cancerous and fistulous, drying up of the moisture, and healing them up so gently, without sharpness; it doth the like to running sores or scabs of*

ETYMOLOGY OF COMMON NAME
Late Middle English, originally *knopweed*, because of the hard, rounded 'head'.

PLANT LORE
It was believed that rubbing the flowerheads on warts could cure them, leading to the alternative name.

USE
The roots and seeds.

EDIBILITY
The flower petals can be eaten raw, especially added to salads.

HARVEST
In autumn.

MEDICINAL PROPERTIES
Diaphoretic, diuretic, antimicrobial and vulnerary.

ACTIVE CONSTITUENTS
Flavonoids, phenolic acids, polysaccharides, coumarins, tannins.

the head or other parts. It is of special use for the soreness of the throat, swelling of the uvula and jaws, and excellently good to stay bleeding, and heal up all green wounds.'

In her 1894 *Occult Family Physician and Botanic Guide to Health*, Antonette Matteson agreed with Culpeper, *'It is a good remedy for bloody flux, bleeding at the nose and inward bleedings. It is also good in catarrhal affections, restraining distillations of thin and sharp humors from the head upon the stomach and lungs. It is used also for cuts and sores, as it soon dries them up and heals them gently. It may be made into an ointment for outward application.'*

The Herbal Manual by Harold Ward, 1936, noted, *'Knapweed as a general tonic for most of the purposes for which Gentian is used. Knapweed is held in some quarters to equal Gentian in all-round efficacy, but the latter is much more frequently prescribed. The ounce to pint infusion is taken in wineglass doses.'*

MODERN RESEARCH

There isn't a huge amount of modern research so far into these plants, but they do have the following properties noted:

Vulnerary and astringent

The astringent properties make it useful for wound-healing and, as Culpeper says, to stay bleeding of 'the mouth or nose, or other outward parts, and those veins that are inwardly broken, or inward wounds, as also the fluxes of the belly'. The sesquiterpene α-bisabolol, which is found in Knapweeds, is also believed to be responsible for the anti-inflammatory and wound-healing effects seen by the historical authors.

Antimicrobial

Common knapweed was studied in 2003 by Kumarasamy et al., who found significant antimicrobial activity against penicillin-resistant *Escherichia coli*. Krasnov et al. (2012) showed the water extract of Greater knapweed to be markedly active against the gram-positive bacterias *Staphylococcus aureus* and *Mycobacterium smegmatis*. This was confirmed in a study in 2021 in which the greatest antimicrobial activity was detected in freshly harvested flowers. This activity is also thought to be related to the presence of sesquiterpene lactones.

TOPICAL USES

As can be seen above, Knapweed can be used as an ointment for treating wounds and skin infections. The α-bisabolol found in it is a versatile and beneficial compound widely used in skincare and cosmetic formulations for its anti-inflammatory, antimicrobial,

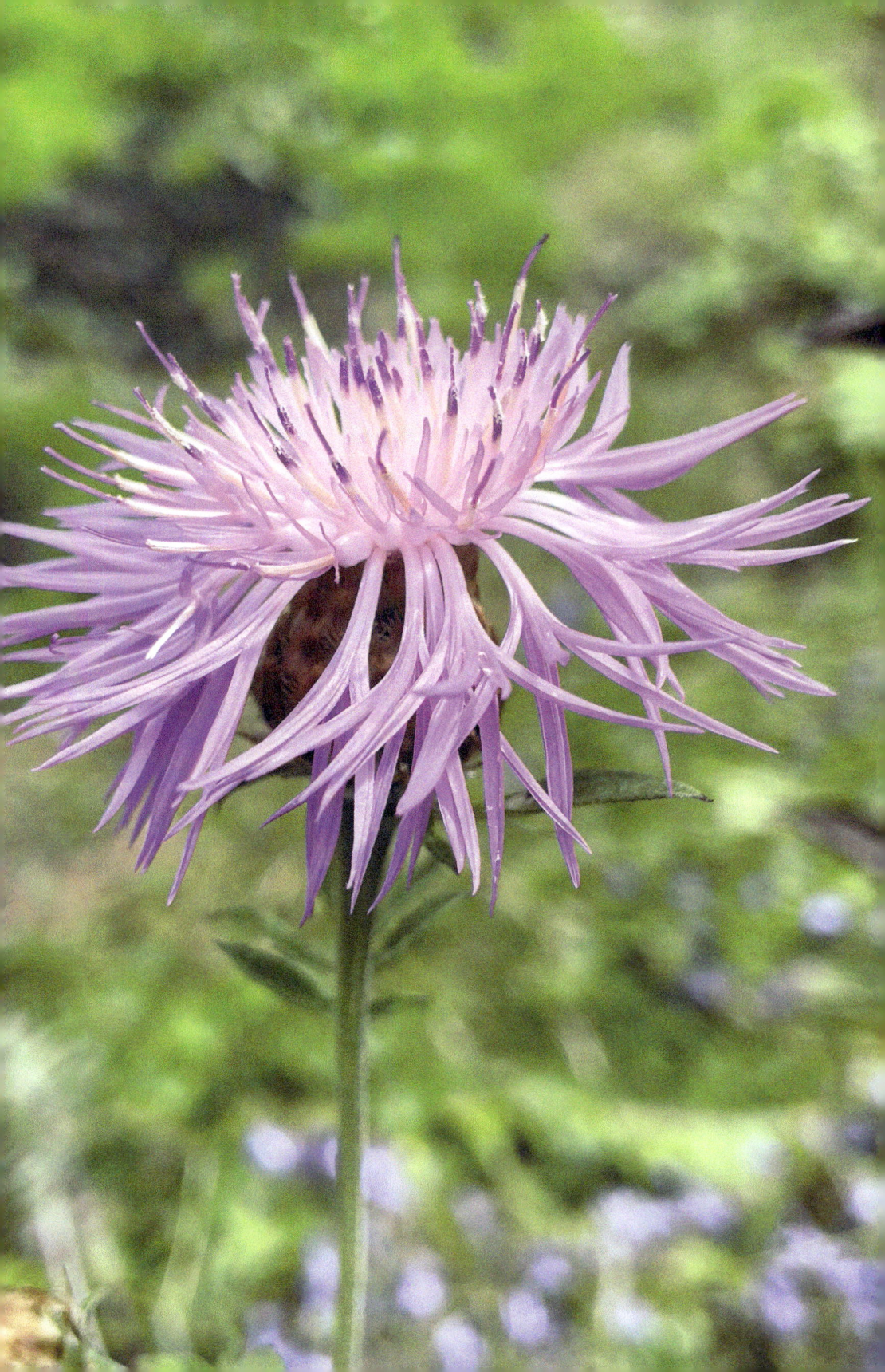

healing and soothing properties. Its ability to enhance the penetration of other active ingredients further adds to its value in topical applications.

DOSAGE
External use.

PRECAUTIONS
Overuse leads to irritation of the digestive system, with consequent of diarrhoea and vomiting. Not for use during pregnancy or breastfeeding.

Knapweed recipes

Medicinal recipes

Knapweed infusion for skin conditions

- 1 tablespoon fresh or dried Knapweed flowers
- 1 cup boiling water

Pour the boiling water over the flowers and allow to infuse for 20–30 minutes. Strain and, once cooled, use as a wash or compress for skin irritations, rashes and minor wounds to benefit from the plant's anti-inflammatory and astringent properties.

Knapweed poultice

- 1tsp fresh root (if using dried you will need to moisten with water first)
- 2tsp coconut oil
- cheesecloth or cotton bandage

Finely grate the root into a pulp and add the coconut oil to make a paste. Spread the paste evenly over the desired area and wrap with the cloth or bandage. Use to heal wounds and skin infections.

Knapweed infused oil

- 100g dried root or seeds
- 2tbsp alcohol, such as Everclear
- 1l grapeseed oil

Place the finely grated root in the bottom of a jar with the Everclear. Allow to steep for 10 minutes and then add the oil. Allow the mix to steep/infuse for 4 weeks before using to reduce inflammation and heal wounds.

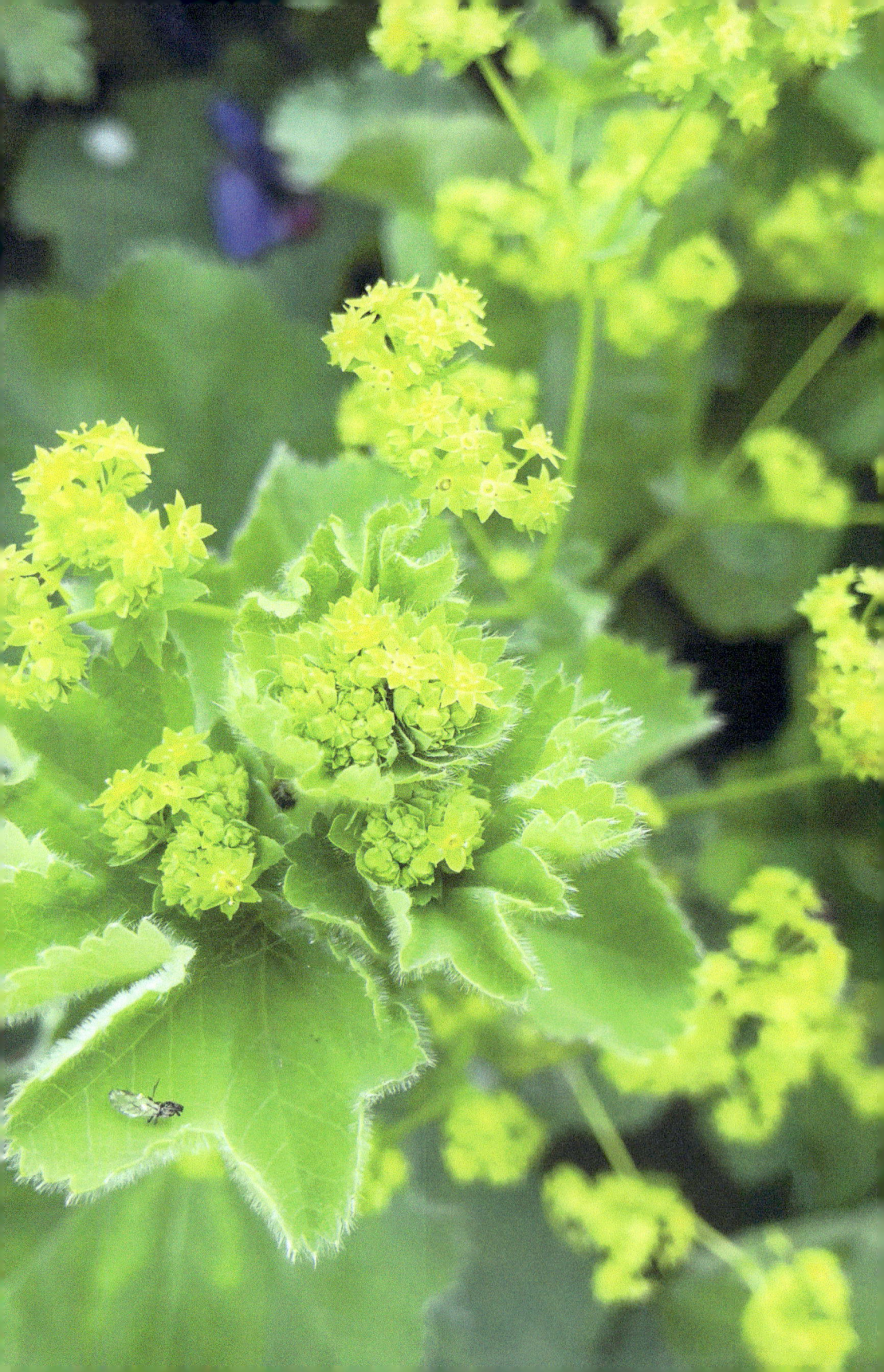

LADY'S MANTLE
Alchemilla vulgaris

Alchemilla vulgaris, commonly known as Lady's mantle, is a native of the UK and is commonly found in meadows, woodland edges, hedgerows and gardens. It has a long history of use in traditional herbal medicine and folklore, being used to treat a range of ailments, including menstrual disorders, digestive issues and wounds.

HISTORICAL USES

Nicholas Culpeper's *Herbal* stated, '*It is proper for those wounds that have inflammations, and is effectual to stay bleedings, vomiting and fluxes of all sorts, bruises by fails or otherwise, and helps ruptures. The distilled water drank for twenty days together, helps conception, and to retain the birth, if the woman does sometimes sit in a bath made of the decoction of the herb. It is also a good wound-herb both inwardly and outwardly, by drinking a decoction, or bathing and fomenting, for it dries up the humidity of the sores, and heals inflammation. It draws the corruption from, and heals green wounds; it cures all old sores, though fistulous and hollow.*'

Harold Ward's *Herbal Manual*, 1936, noted, '*In excessive menstruation, as well as spasmodic nervous complaints, a 1 ounce to 1 pint infusion may be taken internally in teacupful doses as required.*'

ETYMOLOGY OF COMMON NAME
From the lobes of the leaves being supposed to resemble the scalloped edges of the Virgin Mary's mantle (a cape or cloak).

PLANT LORE
In some folklore, Lady's mantle is associated with fairies. The plant's ability to collect dew was thought to attract fairies, and its leaves were sometimes used in rituals to communicate with them.

EDIBILITY
Young leaves, raw or cooked can be mixed with the leaves of Bistort and Lady's thumb in making a bitter herb pudding called 'Easter ledger'.

HARVEST
In June and July when in flower.

MEDICINAL PROPERTIES
Diaphoretic, diuretic, antimicrobial and vulnerary.

ACTIVE CONSTITUENTS
Flavonoids, phenolic acids, polysaccharides, coumarins, tannins.

LEFT: LADY'S MANTLE

MODERN RESEARCH

According to phytochemical studies, the aerial part of the plant contains mostly phenolic compounds, a large amount of tannins (the main one being agrimoniin), phenolcarboxylic, acids (ellagic, gallic and caffeic acid) and flavonoids (quercetin and kaempferol, and their glycosides) (Shilova et al. 2020). These give the plant the following properties:

Astringent and emmenagogue

Lady's mantle has been traditionally used, as Culpeper says, in wound-healing, where it acts as a styptic in minor cuts and wounds, as a result of the tannin content. It is also reported that the aerial parts of this plant are used traditionally in Montenegro, internally to treat mild and nonspecific diarrhoea and dysmenorrhea, and ulcers, eczema and skin rashes externally (Ergene et al., 2010).

Lady's mantle is also considered an all-round 'women's herb' as it will address both menorrhagia and scanty periods alike (Hoffman, 2003). It improves regulation of the cycle (Chevallier, 1996) and it is a uterine tonic (Menzies-Trull, 2003). The tannins act on the uterus in cases of excess menstrual bleeding, postpartum bleeding and conditions of abnormal tissue growth such as fibroids. It is also an emmenagogue and, as such, will help to stimulate the menstrual flow if suppressed, though this is paradoxical to its astringent effects. It stimulates production of progesterone, which can help to reduce the occurrence of hot flushes, night sweats and other menopausal symptoms such as anxiety and mood swings.

Antimicrobial and anti-inflammatory

A 2017 study of the antiviral activity of the roots of Lady's mantle showed the highest activity towards Vaccinia and Ectromelia pox viruses, while a 2018 study found remarkable antioxidant and anti-inflammatory activities. Additionally, the extract demonstrated antibacterial activity against *Agrobacterium tumefaciens*, *Serratia marcescens* and *Acinetobacter johnsoni*. It also showed antifungal activity against *Rhizoctonia solani*, *Penicillium italicum* and *Fusarium oxysporium*.

Anticancerogenic

Studies in 2022 looked at the possibility of the herb preventing and suppressing tumour development, finding that it strongly suppressed the growth of human cell lines derived from different types of tumours (breast, skin, lung and colon). A further study of the cytotoxic activity showed strong antiproliferative activity on prostate cancer cells.

TOPICAL USE

The use of the plant in wound-healing was confirmed in several scientific studies (Choi et al., 2018; Tasić-Kostov et al., 2019). Healing may be attributed to phenolic compounds found the plant and its antioxidant activity.

After removal of teeth, Lady's mantle tisane is recommended as one of the best remedies. Within a day the wounds heal after several rinses.

DOSAGE

Tisane – 1–2tsp/5–10g, 3 times per day.

PRECAUTIONS

Not suitable for children or those who are pregnant or lactating.

Lady's mantle recipes

Medicinal recipes

Lady's mantle tisane

Pour 250ml boiling water over the 1–2tsp/5–10g of the dried leaf and allow to steep for 10–15 minutes. Use for excessive menstruation, diarrhoea, colitis with bleeding, fibroids, menopausal symptoms and ulcers. Also beneficial as a mouthwash after dental surgery and for mouth ulcers and sore throats.

Lady's mantle compress

Soak a cloth in a tisane of the dried herb and apply 2–3 times a day to skin irritations, rashes and minor wounds to benefit from the plant's astringent and anti-inflammatory properties.

Lady's mantle vaginal douche

- 60g Lady's mantle herb
- 1l boiling water

Infuse herb for 30 minutes. Inject warm for leucorrhoea, Candida, inflammation, or as a lotion for pruritus.

Lady's mantle salve

- 100g grated dried root or seeds
- 2tbsp alcohol, such as Everclear
- 1l grapeseed oil

Place the finely grated root in the bottom of a jar with the Everclear. Allow to steep for 10 minutes and then add the oil. Allow the mix to steep/infuse for 4 weeks. Make into a salve by using a 1:4 ratio of melted beeswax to your oil mix, ie 1 part wax to 4 parts liquid. Melt the wax pellets in the oil in a double boiler or bain-marie. Remove from the heat and allow to cool and set completely before using on cuts, scrapes and other minor wounds to promote healing.

Menopause tea

- 1 part Raspberry (fruit and leaf)
- 1 part Red clover
- 1 part Lady's mantle
- 1 part Sage

Mix the herbs and pour 250ml boiling water over 1 tsp/5g of them and allow to steep for 10–15 minutes. Drink up to 3 cups per day to assist with perimenopausal periods and hot flushes.

LADY'S SMOCK
Cardamine pratensis

A beautiful early spring flower, *Cardamine pratensis* is a native of the UK and also known as Lady's smock or Cuckoo flower. It is a member of the Cardamine family, which also includes its relatives, the Mustards and Bittercresses.

HISTORICAL USES

Nicholas Culpeper's *Herbal* described how '*It provokes the urine, breaks the stone and effectually warms a cold and weak stomach, restores lost appetite and helps digestion.*'

In 1767, Lady's smock was recommended to the Trial of Physicians as an anti-convulsive remedy after physician Sir George Baker saw it administered and bring relief to a patient suffering from a '*hysteric affection in consequence of an interruption to menstrual discharge.*'

In his 1814 *Family Herbal*, Robert Thornton wrote, '*It is a warm plant, and has been esteemed to be a powerful diuretic. Galen and many authors allege that it possesses the same virtues as the watercresses. Dale, in his* Pharmacologia, *mentions that its flower is recommended in convulsive disorders in a manuscript of Dr Tailored Robinson's; and Sir George Baker, president of the College of Physicians, has mentioned, in the first volume of* Medical Transactions, *some*

ETYMOLOGY OF COMMON NAME
Named Lady's smock in honour of the Virgin Mary, because it comes first into flower about Lady Day.

PLANT LORE
Also known as Cuckooflower as it appears when the cuckoo starts to sing and its appearance was used to predict the arrival of spring.

EDIBILITY
All aerial parts.

HARVEST
In spring.

MEDICINAL PROPERTIES
Diuretic, antioxidant, anti-inflammatory and stimulant.

ACTIVE CONSTITUENTS
Glucosinolates, flavonoids, saponins, tannins, phenolic acids.

nervous and hysteric cases in which he administered the flowers with good effect.'

MODERN RESEARCH

While there is little research on Lady's smock itself, the Cardamine family is known to contain high levels of antioxidant phytochemicals (Raiola et al., 2018). I have found nothing to corroborate the use of the plant as an anticonvulsant, which is not surprising given its lack of scientific attention. However, it may contain bioactive compounds, such as flavonoids and glucosinolates, which could potentially have neurological effects, and its relative Black mustard has been found to reduce the intensity and duration of seizures (Kiasalari et al., 2012). Nevertheless, modern research has found the following properties for Lady's smock or its compounds so far:

Diuretic and bitter

Culpeper is right to say that this herb 'warms the stomach' and 'provokes the urine' as the leaves and aerial parts are rich in phenolic acids, which have been shown to be potent diuretics in rodent studies (Hailu and Engidawork, 2014; Chilo and Raju, 2021). The phytochemicals in the plant are also known to stimulate the production of digestive juices, including saliva, gastric acid and bile.

Antioxidant

While not on Lady's smock directly, various experiments have demonstrated that compounds such as flavonoids, phenolic acids, etc. are potential antioxidants and that the activity of these compounds is through their ability to scavenge free radicals. Accumulation of free radicals can cause pathological conditions such as asthma, arthritis, inflammation, neurodegeneration, heart disease, ageing effect, etc.

Anti-inflammatory

Also related to the high levels of flavonoids and phenolic acids, the anti-inflammatory properties of Cardamine species were evaluated in 2022, and results showed that oedema was significantly reduced in the later stage, which occurs after 2–6 hours, and it was theorised that this might be owing to the suppression of prostaglandins.

TOPICAL USES

In addition to high levels of vitamin C, Lady's smock also contains mustard oil compounds, which stimulate blood flow to the outer layer of skin. It may therefore be applied topically to promote blood flow to the skin, which can soothe the pain of arthritis and rheumatism and aid in the healing of skin irritations and eruptions.

DOSAGE

Tisane – 1tsp/5g, 2–3 times per day.

PRECAUTIONS

Not suitable for children or those who are pregnant or lactating.

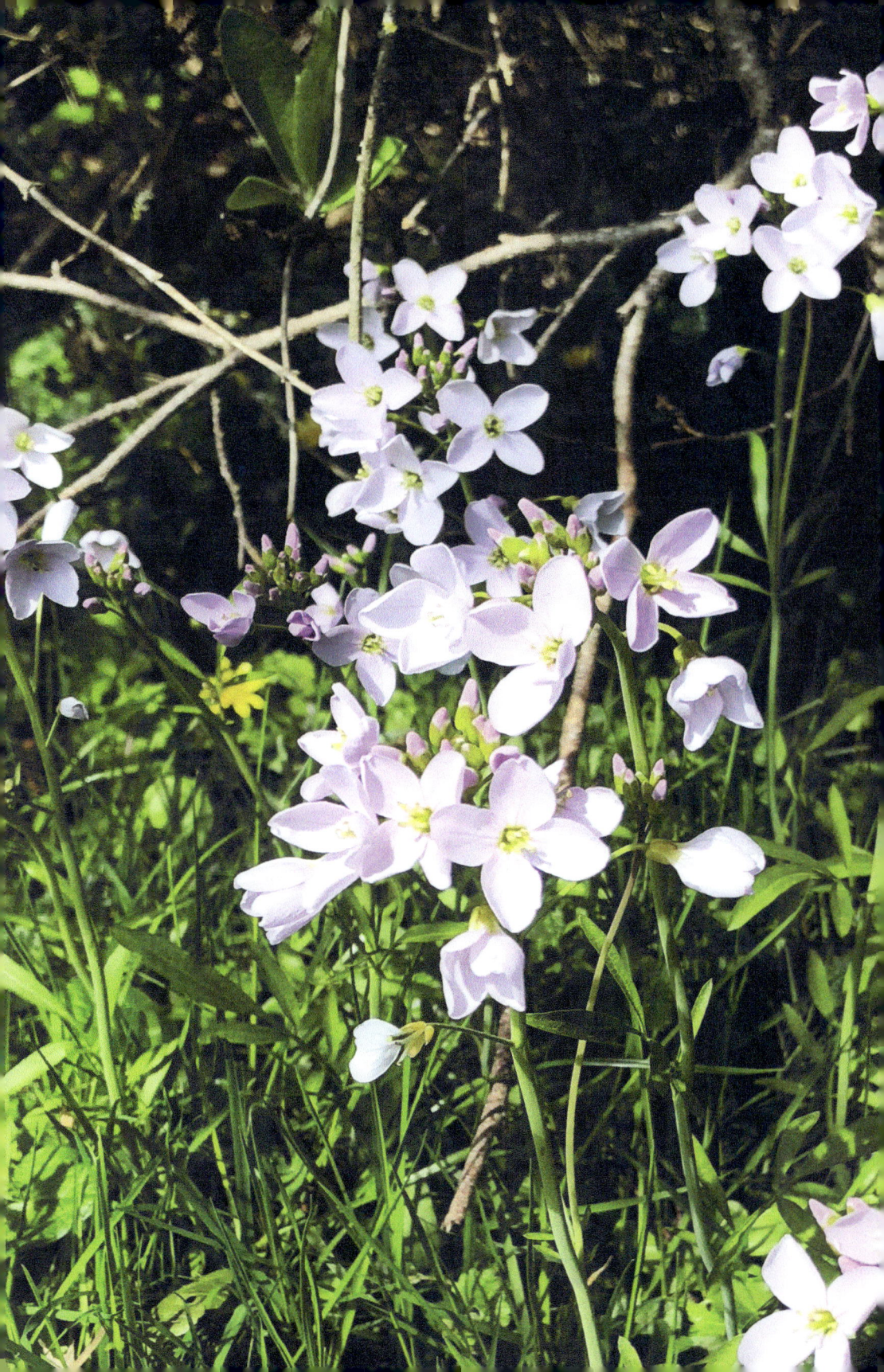

Lady's smock recipes

Medicinal recipes

Lady's smock tisane

Pour 250ml boiling water over 1tsp/5g of the dried flowering herb and allow to steep for 10–15 minutes. Use as a diuretic and for indigestion, as a spring tonic.

Lady's smock syrup

- 1 part Lady's smock tisane
- 1 part sugar

Simmer your strained tisane or decoction until it has reduced by half and then add the sugar. You will always end up using double the amount of sugar to tisane. Stir until the sugar has dissolved and then continue cooking till the mixture has thickened to a syrup. Leave to cool. Pour into sterilised bottles closed with a cork. This will keep for a maximum of 3 months. Use as above.

Lady's smock poultice

- 1tsp fresh herb (if using dried you will need to moisten with water first)
- 2tsp coconut oil
- cheesecloth or cotton bandage

Finely chop the herb into a pulp and add the coconut oil to make a paste. Spread the paste evenly over the desired area and wrap with the cloth or bandage. Use to promote blood flow and soothe the pain of arthritis and rheumatism as well as in the healing of skin irritations and eruptions.

LOOSESTRIFE (YELLOW)
Lysimachia vulgaris

Lysimachia vulgaris or Yellow loosestrife is native to the UK and can be found in various habitats, including wetlands, marshes and gardens. It belongs to the Primrose family and was traditionally used for medicinal purposes as well as a yellow dye for textiles, and a culinary herb or added to salads.

HISTORICAL USES

Despite many herbal writers noting that Yellow loosestrife has been used for thousands of years, the historical references are surprisingly few. One was Nicholas Culpeper whose *Herbal* stated:

> *This herb is good for all manner of bleeding at the mouth, nose, or wounds, and all fluxes of the belly, and the bloody-flux, given either to drink or taken by clysters; it stays also the abundance of women's courses; it is a singular good wound-herb for green wounds, to stay the bleeding, and quickly close together the lips of the wound, if the herb be bruised, and the juice only applied. It is often used in gargles for sore mouths, as also for the secret parts. The smoak hereof being bruised, drives away flies and gnats, which in the nighttime molest people inhabiting near marshes, and in the fenny countries.*

ETYMOLOGY OF COMMON NAME
After the belief that the plant would appease strife, originating from the Old English *luris trife*, which roughly translates to 'strife-liar' or 'trouble-deceiver'.

PLANT LORE
In Celtic mythology it was associated with the goddess Brigid, who was said to have used the plant to heal wounds.

EDIBILITY
The young leaves are edible.

HARVEST
In July.

MEDICINAL PROPERTIES
Astringent, antibacterial, expectorant, hepatoprotective and anti-inflammatory.

ACTIVE CONSTITUENTS
Flavonoids, saponins, tannins, phenolic acids, anthocyanins, polysaccharides.

MODERN RESEARCH

There is also a purple variety of Loosestrife, which is not related to the yellow variety but, surprisingly, has many of the same properties. Modern research has so far found and confirmed the following:

Astringent

Much like the purple variety, Yellow loosestrife is astringent and, as Culpeper says, is used in the treatment of diarrhoea, dysentery, internal and external bleeding, and to cleanse wounds (Chevallier, 1996). Its astringent properties help reduce intestinal inflammation and promote the normalisation of bowel movements.

Antibacterial

In a 2017 study, the antibacterial activities of the plant were investigated. Gram-positive bacteria such as *Streptococcus pyogenes*, *Staphylococcus aureus* and *Staphylococcus epidermidis* were more susceptible to the effects of Loosestrife than gram-negative bacteria, while field-grown plants exhibited better antibacterial activities than *in vitro*-grown plants. The study also noted anti-tumour and antioxidant properties and reported that the plant may be a suitable source for drugs that could improve the treatment of infections caused by gram-positive bacteria.

Hepatoprotective and anti-inflammatory

A 2021 study showed that lipid accumulation and inflammation in the liver were alleviated by feeding Loosestrife extract to mice with non-alcoholic steatohepatitis (NASH), a liver disease caused by a non-alcoholic fatty liver. Moreover, the extract strongly prevented liver fibrosis and showed sufficient potency for use as a therapeutic agent against NASH.

Antidiabetic

The anti-diabetic properties of Loosestrife were studied in 2022 in terms of the antioxidant properties found. The results showed that the root has a significantly higher ability to inhibit enzymes involved in the digestion of carbohydrates in comparison with the aerial extract. Furthermore, when compared to acarbose, a drug used for many years to treat diabetes, Loosestrife root had approximately ten times higher inhibition activity on the production of glucose. The obtained results confirmed that the root may significantly reduce the postprandial increase of blood glucose.

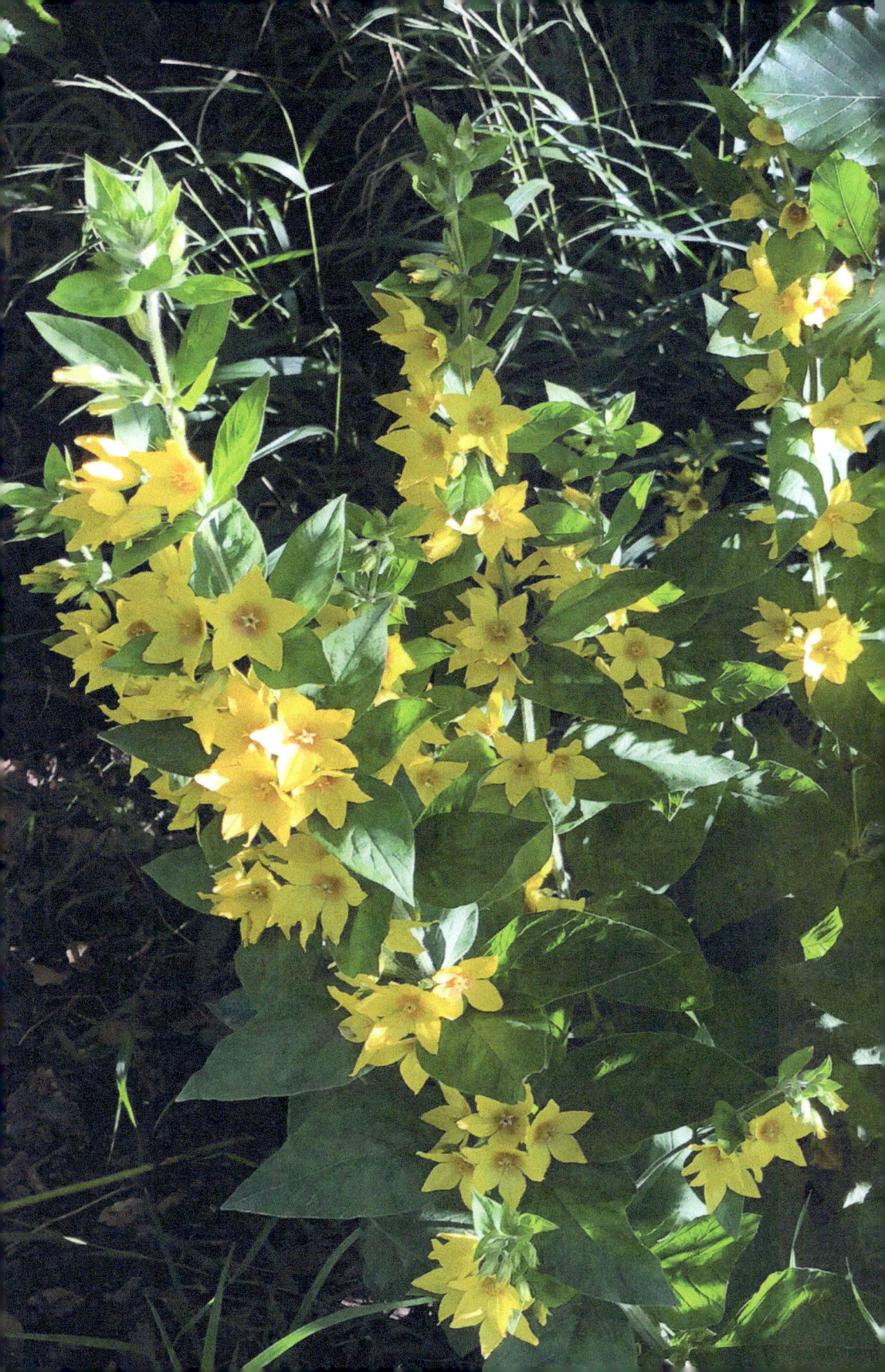

TOPICAL USES

The anti-inflammatory and astringent properties of Loosestrife make it useful for treating wounds, cuts and sores. It can help stop bleeding, reduce inflammation and promote healing. It can also be applied topically to treat various skin conditions such as eczema, rashes and insect bites.

DOSAGE

As a tea – add 1 or 2 teaspoons of the dried herb to a cup of steaming hot water. Allow to soak for about 10–15 minutes and then strain and drink.

PRECAUTIONS

None found, but if used for prolonged periods tannins contained in the plant may cause deficiency of essential minerals within the body. Not suitable for children or those who are pregnant or lactating.

Yellow loosestrife recipes

Medicinal recipes

Loosestrife tisane

Pour 250ml boiling water over 1tsp/5g of the dried flowering herb and allow to steep for 10–15 minutes. Use to treat gastrointestinal conditions such as diarrhoea as well as bleeding of the mouth and mouth ulcers.

Loosestrife skin compress

Soak a cloth in a tisane of the dried herb and apply 2–3 times a day to skin irritations, rashes and minor wounds to benefit from the astringent and anti-inflammatory properties.

Loosestrife eye compress

Add ½tsp of salt into 2 cups of steaming water. Subsequently, put in 1–2tsp of the dried herb or 1–2tbsp of the fresh herb. Allow the mixture to soak for about 10–15 minutes and then strain the solution. Use the solution when it is cool. If you want to use the medication as eyewash, it should be kept covered with a view to prevent contamination. It is regarded as being useful as a relief for sore eyes and is considered to be of equivalent or maybe greater value than Eyebright.

Loosestrife balm

- 100g Loosestrife
- 2tbsp alcohol, such as Everclear
- 1l grapeseed oil

Place the herbs in a jar with the alcohol and allow to steep for 10 minutes before adding the oil. Leave for 4 weeks and then strain. Make into a salve by using a 1:3 ratio of melted beeswax to oil. Melt the wax pellets in the oil in a double boiler or bain-marie. Remove from the heat and allow to cool and set completely before using as a topical balm for injuries, bruises and cuts.

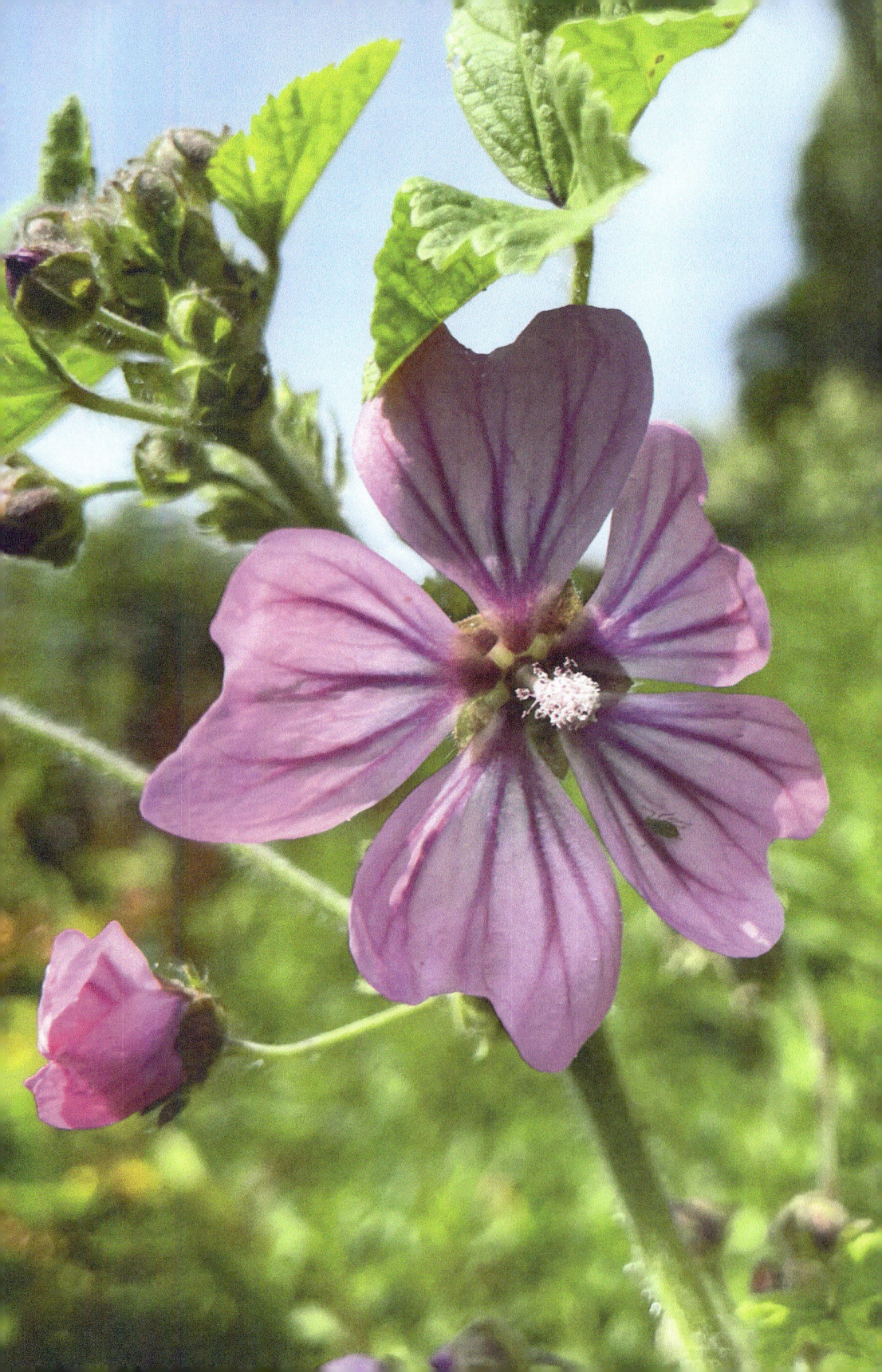

MALLOW
Malva sylvestris

Malva sylvestris, Common mallow or High mallow, is native to the UK and can be found in various habitats, including grasslands, roadsides and waste areas. While it's not commonly used in culinary recipes, Common mallow has historically been used in herbal medicine for its soothing properties.

HISTORICAL USES

Nicholas Culpeper's *Herbal* stated, '*It not only voids hot, choleric, and other offensive humours, but eases the pains and torments of the belly coming thereby. The decoction of the seed of any of the Mallows made in milk or wine, doth marvellously help excoriations, the phthisic pleurisy, and other diseases of the chest and lungs, that proceed of hot causes, if it be continued taking for some time together. The leaves and roots work the same effects. They help much also in the excoriations of the bowels, and hardness of the mother, and in all hot and sharp diseases thereof. The leaves bruised or rubbed upon any place stung with bees, wasps, or the like, presently take away the pain, redness, and swelling that rise thereupon.*'

Many of the historical remedies refer to the related Marshmallow. However, as Robert Thornton (1814) pointed out, '*The common mallow*

ETYMOLOGY OF COMMON NAME
Mallow is derived from the Greek *malasseiii*, 'to soften', which alludes to the demulcent qualities of these mucilaginous plants.

PLANT LORE
Owing to its hardy nature and ability to grow in various conditions, Mallow was often associated with fertility, growth and resilience. Consequently, Mallow flowers were used to promote fertility and successful harvests.

USE
All aerial parts.

EDIBILITY
Young leaves can be a substitute for Lettuce, whereas older leaves are better cooked as a leafy green vegetable. The buds and flowers can be used in salads.

HARVEST
The leaves from June to September and flowers from July to October.

MEDICINAL PROPERTIES
Anti-inflammatory, analgesic, antitussive, antiulcerogenic.

ACTIVE CONSTITUENTS
Mucilage, tannins, flavonoids, coumarins, phenolic acids, pectins.

(Malva sylvestris) *has somewhat similar virtues*', and William Fernie (1897, second edition) advised that '*All the Mallows* [Malvacece] *to the number of a thousand, agree in containing mucilage freely, and in possessing no unwholesome properties.*'

Harold Ward's *Herbal Manual* (1936) reported that a 1oz to 1pt infusion made a popular cough and cold remedy.

MODERN RESEARCH

The Mallows are best known for their mucilage content (and of course their excellent confectionery). However, modern research has confirmed the following uses to date:

Anti-inflammatory and analgesic

Culpeper's findings of Mallow as an anti-inflammatory agent were proven in mice when an extract was shown to significantly reduce inflammation in ear oedema. His use of the plant as an analgesic has also been shown in studies conducted in mice. In a formalin-induced pain test, the treatment reduced intensive licking activity by 61.8% in the neurogenic phase and 46.6% in the inflammatory phase of the model. In a capsaicin-induced test, the amount of time that the animals spent licking the injected paw was reduced by 62.9%.

Antitussive

The traditional use of the plant for coughs was also proven in animal and clinical studies, which specifically confirmed the efficacy of Common mallow extracts in the treatment of dry coughs, while a combination of Common mallow, Thyme and Ginger increased the efficacy and improved all kinds of cough.

Antiulcerogenic

The anti-ulcerogenic effect of Common mallow was demonstrated in recent work on rats with induced gastric ulcers. After a month of treatment, a maximum protection of 37% was achieved. This level of antiulcerogenic activity was similar to that of cimetidine, a drug that inhibits stomach acids.

Antioxidant

A 2022 study of the potential plants for COVID-19 resistance revealed that Common mallow has significant amounts of antioxidant potential, which appears promising in the prevention and treatment of SARS-CoV-2. The current finding is expected to aid future research into the development of a drug(s) from Common mallow.

TOPICAL USES

Mallow is most often linked to the maintenance of skin integrity, and several cosmetic products, topical compounds and moisturisers use Mallows for the prevention of skin ageing, particularly for its efficacy in relieving skin irritation, enhancing mucus production and scavenging free radicals.

DOSAGE

Tisane – 1tsp/5g. Drink a half cup, 3 times a day.
Tincture – 1:5 45% – 30–60 drops in water.

PRECAUTIONS

Caution – water-based preparations of Mallow are high in mucilage and therefore shouldn't be taken before a dose of any prescribed medication as it may reduce absorption. Not suitable for children or those who are pregnant or lactating.

Mallow recipes

Medicinal recipes

Mallow tisane

Pour 250ml boiling water over 1tsp/5g of the dried leaf and flower and allow to steep for 10-15 minutes. Use for respiratory ailments and to soothe the common cold, coughs and sore throats.

Mallow root decoction

Boil 1tsp/5g of the dried root for 10-15 minutes in 250ml of water. Drink up to 3 cups a day for respiratory ailments. Use also in the bath for soothing itchy, dry skin, including eczema.

Mallow infused tincture – 1:5 45%

If you are using 40% alcohol, ie. vodka, make a simple tincture by covering 1 part herb to 5 parts fluid.

If you are using Everclear or other 100% proof, use the following method for a specific tincture:

- 100g Mallow herb
- 225ml alcohol
- 275ml water

Split the herb into two parts, each 50g and place one part in the alcohol. Take the remaining part and place in the boiled water. Steep/infuse in the water for 10 minutes. Strain thoroughly and top up if the water is less than 275ml. Add the infusion to the alcohol mix and leave for 14 days before straining. Use for respiratory ailments and the common cold, coughs and irritation of the bronchi, or inflammation of the mouth or throat.

Mallow root cough syrup

- 1 part Mallow root decoction
- 1 part sugar

Simmer your strained decoction until it is reduced by half and then add the sugar. You will always end up using double the amount of sugar to tisane. Stir until the sugar has dissolved and then continue cooking till the mixture has thickened to a syrup. Leave to cool. Pour into sterilised bottles closed with a cork. This will keep for a maximum of 3 months. Use for coughs in doses of 1-2tsp at a time.

Mallow gel

Add water gradually to powdered root until a gel consistency is achieved, then apply to irritated skin.

MEADOWSWEET
Filipendula ulmaria

Filipendula ulmaria, commonly known as Meadowsweet, is native to the UK and can be found growing in damp meadows, riverbanks, marshes and woodland edges. Meadowsweet has a long history of use in traditional herbal medicine and culinary applications, with its fragrant flowers used to flavour beverages.

HISTORICAL USES

John Gerard said in his *Herball* that the leaves and flowers of Meadowsweet *'far excel all other strewing herbes'* but also that: *'the distilled water of the floures dropped into the eies, taketh away the burning and itching thereof, and cleareth the sight.'*

Nicholas Culpeper's *Herbal* stated, *'The flowers are alexipharmic* [antidotal] *and sudorific, and good in fevers, and all malignant distempers; they are likewise astringent, binding and useful in all fluxes. An infusion of the freshly gathered tops promote sweating. It is a good wound herb taken inwardly or externally applied.'*

Salicin was extracted from meadowsweet flowers by the Swiss pharmacist Johann Pagenstecher, in 1835. He then passed it to the German chemist Carl Jacob Löwig, for oxidation, which yielded salicylic acid (Fluckinger, 1888; Rainsford, 1984).

ETYMOLOGY OF COMMON NAME
From the Anglo-Saxon *meodu-swete*, meaning 'mead sweetener'.

PLANT LORE
Meadowsweet held a special place in Druidic and Celtic traditions. It was considered a sacred herb and was used in various rituals and ceremonies. Druids used it as a ritual incense and as an ingredient in love potions.

USE
The flowers, leaves, root.

EDIBILITY
The dried leaves are used as a flavouring and a sweetener, and the flowers are used as a flavouring in alcoholic beverages and stewed fruits.

HARVEST
When in flower.

MEDICINAL PROPERTIES
Antacid, antiulcerogenic, anti-inflammatory and analgesic.

ACTIVE CONSTITUENTS
Salicylates, flavonoids, phenolic compounds, volatile oil, tannins.

MODERN RESEARCH

While Gerard appreciated the wonderful scent of Meadowsweet in the home, it is, as Culpeper suggests, a useful astringent and has had many other properties confirmed or discovered as follows:

Antacid and antiulcerogenic

Meadowsweet contains mucilage that coats and protects the stomach lining. This action helps to provide a soothing barrier against stomach acid, reducing irritation and discomfort. A study published in the *Journal of Ethnopharmacology* in 2017 found that Meadowsweet exhibited significant antiulcer activity in rats with gastric ulcers, which was attributed to its antioxidant and anti-inflammatory properties. While this study did not specifically investigate gastric acid regulation, it suggests that Meadowsweet may have beneficial effects on the gastrointestinal tract.

Anti-inflammatory, antimicrobial and analgesic

As per the historical findings, Meadowsweet also contains salicylic acid, from which the drug aspirin can be synthesised. Unlike the extracted aspirin, however, which can cause gastric ulceration at high doses, the combination of constituents in Meadowsweet acts, as mentioned above, to protect the inner lining of the stomach while still providing the anti-inflammatory and sudorific benefits associated with salicylic acid. It also works well in conditions associated with mild-moderate pain/inflammation and arthritic and rheumatic problems, including gout, and in genitourinary tract disorders such as cystitis.

In 1997, the immunomodulatory activity of Meadowsweet flowers was shown to play a role in the inflammatory process. Extracts from the seeds and flowers of Meadowsweet indicated anticoagulant activity, which was believed to be associated with the salicylate compounds, while the rhizomes, stems and flowers showed antimicrobial activity against five strains of bacteria.

Anticancerogenic

Meadowsweet flower decoctions have been reported to show anticarcinogenic activity against tumours in rats and mice and also against transplanted tumours in mice (Bespalov et al., 2019; Halkes, 1998).

In a 2019 study on Lewis lung carcinoma in mice, a statistically significant 1.5 times decrease of the metastasis area was demonstrated. Increasing the dose then further reduced the number of lung metastases (by 1.3 times) and their area (by 1.7 times).

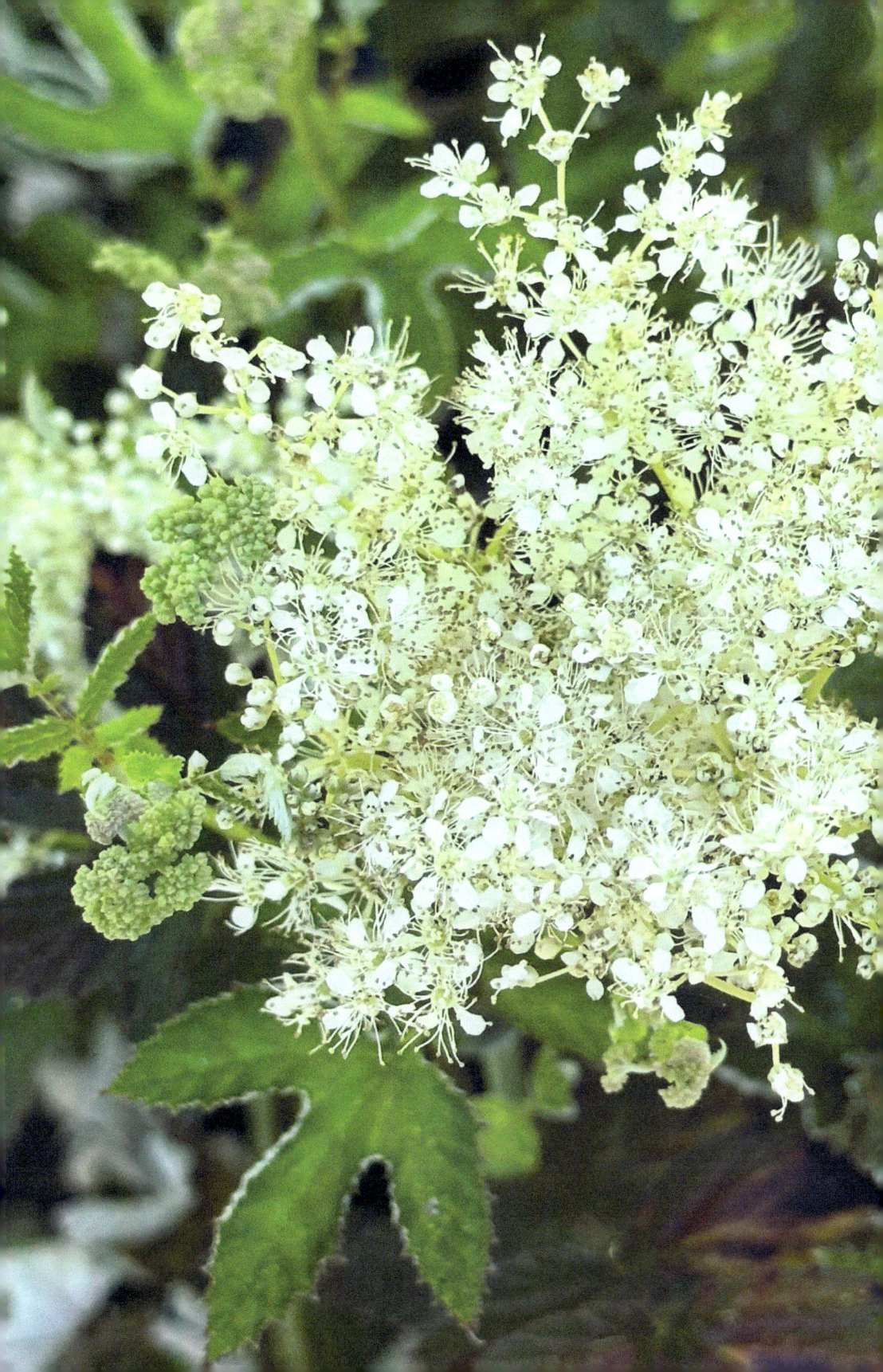

TOPICAL USES

In a clinical study, Meadowsweet was applied topically in 48 patients with known cervical dysplasia, a pre-cancerous condition where abnormal cell growth occurs on the surface lining of the cervix. Complete remission was seen in 25 cases, and in 32 patients beneficial results were conclusive. In addition, no reappearance of the cervical dysplasia occurred over a 12-month period in 10 of the patients in complete remission.

DOSAGE

Tisane – 1–2tsp/10–15g. Drink a half cup, 2–3 times per day.
Tincture – 1:5 25%, 2–4ml, three times per day – 20 drops = 1ml/1tsp = 5ml.

PRECAUTIONS

This remedy should not be given to people who are hypersensitive to aspirin or those who take anticoagulants. Not suitable for children or those who are pregnant or lactating.

Meadowsweet recipes

Medicinal recipes

Meadowsweet tisane

Pour 250ml boiling water over 1tsp/5g of dried leaf and flower, and allow to steep for 10–15 minutes. Use for symptomatic relief of indigestion and other upper gastrointestinal conditions associated with flatulence and hyperacidity as well as to ease pain and inflammation.

Meadowsweet infused tincture 1:5 25%

If you are using 40% alcohol, ie. vodka, you will need to dilute this at the ratio of 60ml water to every 100ml of vodka to make a 25% medium and then cover 1 part herb to 5 parts fluid.

If you are using Everclear or other 100% proof, use the following method for a specific tincture:

- 100g dried Meadowsweet herb
- 125ml alcohol
- 375ml water

Take 100g of dried herb and split into two parts of 50g each. Place 50g in the alcohol and the other 50g in the boiled water. Steep/infuse in the water for 10 minutes. Strain thoroughly and top up if the water is less than 375ml. Add the infusion to the alcohol mix and leave for 14 days before straining. Use to relieve pain and inflammation, as well as to support digestive health.

Meadowsweet bath

- 50g Meadowsweet
- 1l water

Steep the herb in the water for 15 minutes, then strain and add to the bathwater to ease aching joints and back, etc.

Meadowsweet poultice

- 1tsp fresh leaves and flowers (if using dried you will need to moisten with water first)
- 2tsp coconut oil
- cheesecloth or cotton bandage

Finely chop the herb and add the coconut oil to make a paste. Spread the paste evenly over the desired area and wrap with the cloth or bandage. Use to ease joint pain.

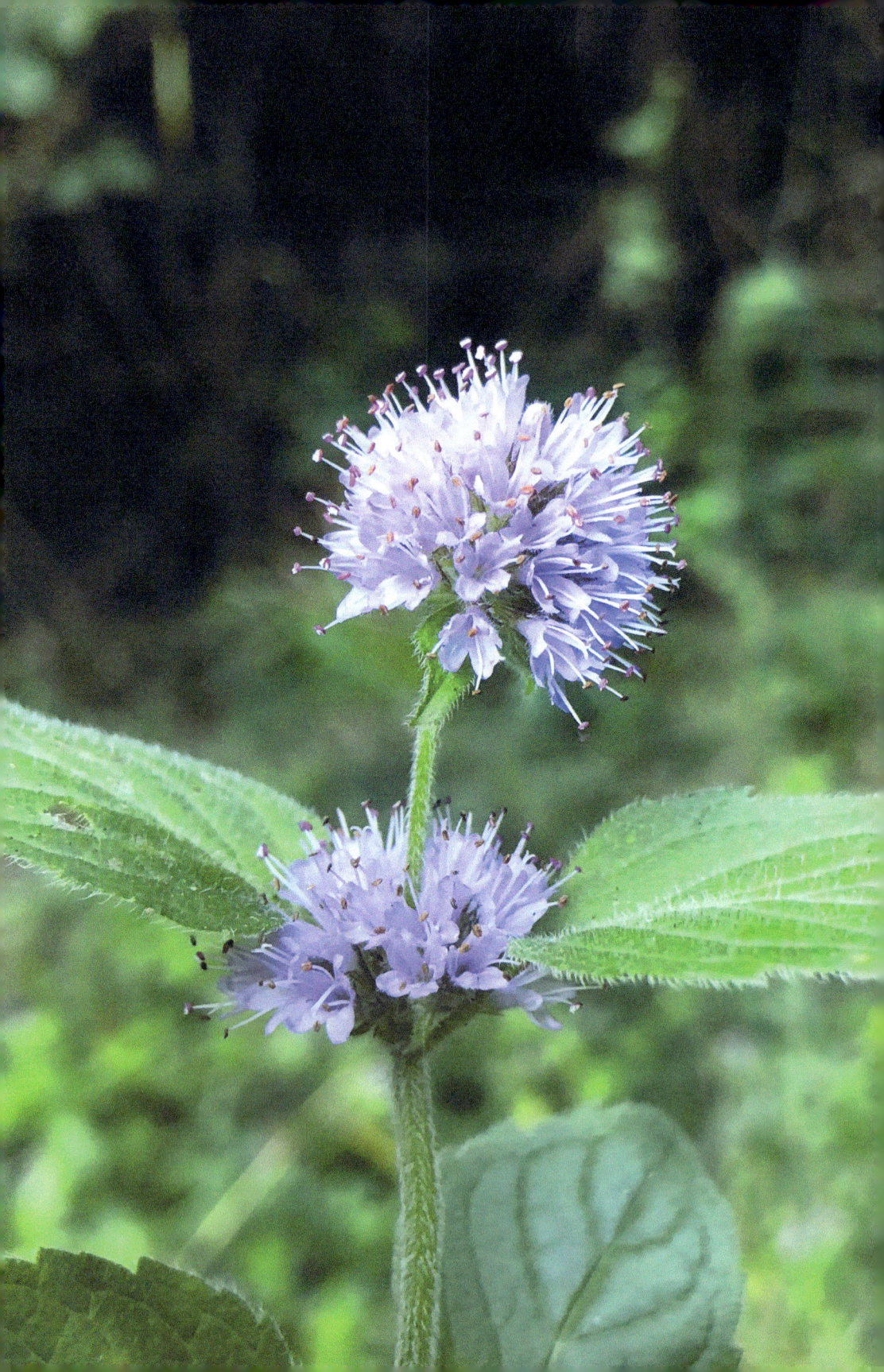

MINTS (WILD)
Mentha spp.

There are a number of Mint species that are native of naturalised in the UK. Water mint (*Mentha aquatica*), as the name suggests is found in damp habitats such as marshes, riverbanks and ponds. Wild mint (*Mentha arvensis*), also known as Corn mint, is found in grasslands, woodlands and disturbed habitats. Spearmint (*Mentha spicata*) is widely cultivated and naturalised in the UK, and Peppermint (*Mentha piperita*) is a cultivated hybrid between Water mint and Spearmint. The medical use of Mint plants, particularly for gastrointestinal issues, is presented in the works of most philosophers and physicians from Classical Antiquity to present-day medicine.

HISTORICAL USES

The oldest written records of Mint are attributed to King Hammurabi of ancient Babylon (1800BC), who prescribed them for gastrointestinal purposes. Similarly, the Greek physician Dioscorides mentioned Mint in his famous work *De Materia Medica*, written in the 1st century AD, as a remedy for the stomach and the relief of nausea.

The Greek philosopher Aristotle also wrote about the medicinal benefits of Mint, while the Roman naturalist Pliny the Elder discussed its therapeutic uses

ETYMOLOGY OF COMMON NAME
From Minthe, a nymph who was beloved by Hades and was transformed into the plant by either Persephone or Demeter.

PLANT LORE
In Greek mythology, the Minthe myth imbues the plant with themes of transformation and renewal.

USE
The leaves.

EDIBILITY
Used as a flavouring in salads or cooked foods.

HARVEST
In summer.

MEDICINAL PROPERTIES
Digestive, antibacterial, anti-inflammatory, analgesic, apoptotic and refrigerant.

ACTIVE CONSTITUENTS
Menthol, menthone, limonene cineole, rosmarinic acid, flavonoids, tannins.

LEFT: WILD MINT

in his encyclopaedic work *Naturalis Historia*.

John Gerard said of it in his *Herball*, 'Mint is marvellous for the stomacke. It is good against watering eies. It is poured into the eares with honied water.'

Nicholas Culpeper confirmed the virtues of Mint, calling it 'Wild or Horse Mint', '*It is good for wind and colic in the stomach, to procure the menses, and expel the birth and secundiues* [afterbirth]. *The juice dropped into the ears eases the pains of them and destroys the worms that breed therein. The juice laid on warm, helps the king's-evil, or kernels in the throat. The decoction or distilled water helps a stinking breath, proceeding from corruption of the teeth; and snuffed up the nose, purges the head. It helps the scurf or dandruff of the head used with vinegar.*'

MODERN RESEARCH

As previously mentioned, several species of mint grow wild in the UK, and all contain the compound menthol, which is believed to have the following properties:

Digestive

Menthol is what is thought to alleviate the gastrointestinal issues mentioned above and throughout history. It does so through its relaxing effects on the muscles of the digestive tract. A 2007 study showed that food passes through the stomach quicker when people take peppermint oil with meals, which relieves symptoms of indigestion.

Antibacterial

Menthol is also believed to have antibacterial properties that have been found to inhibit the spread of pathogens such as *Helicobacter pylori*, *Salmonella enteritidis*, *Escherichia coli* and *Staphylococcus aureus*. In one 2005 study, while inhibitory actions varied among the bacterial species tested, they were almost the same against antibiotic-resistant and antibiotic-sensitive strains of *Helicobacter pylori*, the cause of ulcers, and *Staphylococcus aureus*, the cause of soft tissue infections.

Anti-inflammatory

Peppermint is well-known for its anti-inflammatory effects, which are often attributed to its menthol, menthone and various flavonoid contents. The usefulness of Wild mint was justified in a study that revealed its anti-inflammatory properties exhibited a 68.30% reduction in swelling compared with diclofenac, which caused 77.87% inhibition.

Analgesic

The 2003 book *Clinical Botanical Medicine* by Yarnell et al. recommends application of a Wild mint leaf decoction for toothache treatments. This pain-relieving effect was further investigated in a 2019 study of the effects of peppermint oil compared with lidocaine drops for migraine attacks. The findings were that nasal application of Peppermint, as Culpeper rightly prescribed, caused considerable reduction in the intensity and frequency of headache and relieved the majority of patients' pain, similar to lidocaine. The study concluded that this nasal menthol can be used to relieve migraine headaches.

Contraceptive

It is also possible that Wild mint could have contraceptive effects. In animal studies the extract showed a reduction in the number of mice offspring, while body weight and libido of the treated animals remained unaffected. A significant decrease in the weight of the testis, epididymis, sperm count, motility, viability and normal morphology of the spermatozoa was however observed.

Anticancerogenic

Finally, a new way of formulating a solution of the essential oil has allowed the potential anticancer and antibacterial agents of Wild mint to be re-evaluated. A nanoemulsion (a combination of surfactants, in this case Wild mint oil, water and polysorbate) clearly displayed anticancer activity by the induction of early apoptosis (cell death) in thyroid cancer lines. Also, the same nanoemulsion demonstrated antibacterial activity against *Staphylococcus aureus*, confirming the earlier 2005 results. The results of this research are expected to substantiate the potential for use of Wild mint oil in therapeutic studies, as well as in anticancer and antibacterial therapy.

TOPICAL USES

Wild mint's antimicrobial action against *Staphylococcus* means that it acts as a natural antiseptic agent as it aids in treating skin problems and healing wounds.

DOSAGE

(as for Peppermint)

Tisane – 1–2tsp/5–10g. Drink freely.
Tincture – 1:5 45%, 2–4ml, 3 times per day – 20 drops = 1ml/1tsp = 5ml.

PRECAUTIONS

Not suitable for those who are pregnant or lactating.

Mint recipes

Medicinal recipes

Mint tisane

Pour 250ml boiling water over 1tsp/5g of dried Mint leaf and flower, and allow to steep for 10–15 minutes. Use for heartburn, to relax the muscles involved in the digestive process and ease travel sickness and ulcerative colitis. Use a strong tisane or boil the leaves in the water for 10 minutes to use for tooth pain.

Mint infused tincture 1:5 45%

If you are using 40% alcohol, ie. vodka, make a simple tincture by covering 1 part herb to 5 parts fluid.

If you are using Everclear or other 100% proof, use the following method for a specific tincture:

- 100g dried Mint herb
- 225ml alcohol
- 275ml water

Take 100g of dried herb and split into two parts of 50g each. Place 50g in the alcohol and the other 50g part in the boiled water. Steep/infuse in the water for 10 minutes. Strain thoroughly and top up if the water is less than 275ml. Add the infusion to the alcohol mix and leave for 14 days before straining. Using for heartburn, indigestion or nausea, one dose is usually sufficient, though sometimes a second is needed.

Mint balm

- 100g dried Mint herb
- 2tbsp alcohol, such as Everclear
- 1l grapeseed oil

Place the herb in the bottom of a jar with the Everclear. Allow to steep for 10 minutes and then add the oil. Allow the mix to steep/infuse for 4 weeks. Make into a balm by using a 1:3 ratio of melted beeswax to oil, ie. 1 part wax to 3 parts oil. Melt the wax pellets in the oil in a double boiler or bain-marie. Remove from the heat and allow to cool and set completely before using to soothe dry, irritated skin, insect bites, minor burns or muscle soreness as needed. Can also be used on the temples or chest for headache relief.

MISTLETOE
Viscum album

Viscum album, known as European or Common mistletoe, is an evergreen hemiparasitic plant native to the UK and usually found growing on the branches of various deciduous trees, including apple, oak, hawthorn and poplar. NB: Parts of the plant, particularly the berries, are toxic if ingested in large amounts.

HISTORICAL USES

Mistletoe use can be found in Ancient Greece for the treatment of the spleen and ailments related to menstruation. The Druids used it to treat almost every illness, even as an antidote for poisons and for infertility, while later it was used as a remedy for neuralgia, sciatica, epilepsy, bronchial asthma, diabetes mellitus, cramps, stroke, stomach problems, as an antihypertensive and for hot flushes in menopause.

Nicholas Culpeper's *Herbal* explained that Mistletoe *'made into powder, and given to drink, ... is good for falling-sickness. The fresh wood bruised, and the juice dropped into the ears is effectual in curing the imposthumes in them. Misseltoe is a cephalic and nervine medicine, useful for convulsive fits, palsy, and vertigo.'*

Robert Thornton's *Family Herbal* of

ETYMOLOGY OF COMMON NAME
Of Anglo-Saxon origin, from *mistel*, 'different', + *tān*, 'twig', because it looks unlike the tree it is found in.

PLANT LORE
One of the sacred herbs of the Druids, Mistletoe was gathered only by Druids, who are said to have spread their white cloaks on the ground to protect its fall to earth.

USE
The leaves and twigs.

EDIBILITY
Not edible, and the berries are TOXIC.

HARVEST
The leaves in spring.

MEDICINAL PROPERTIES
Nervine, anticonvulsant, antiviral, antihypertensive and anticancerogenic.

ACTIVE CONSTITUENTS
Lectins, polysaccharides, alkaloids, flavonoids, triterpenes, amines.

1814 advised that, '*The viscum should be separated from the oak about Christmas, then gradually dried. It is afterwards to be ground into a fine powder, which ought to be confined in a bottle, and kept in a situation where both light and air are excluded, as the admission of either tends to deprive this vegetable of its natural efficacy.*' He goes on to say that instances of the efficacy of Mistletoe in epilepsy '*are published in the writings of Paracelsus, Lemnius, Loseke, Hannes, Koelderer, Cole, Pliny, Swieten, Pfindel, Borellus, Boyle, Colbach, Baier, Cartheuser, and Hartmann.*'

Thornton continued, '*We are also informed, that the late Dr Fothergill and Dr Gilbert Thomson employed this medicine with great success in the cure of epilepsy; and my learned friend Dr Willan has experienced the utility of this plant in the treatment of that disease. The learned Dr Frazer has had equal success with this plant and published his experience in an ingenious work entitled* On Epilepsy, and the Use of the Viscus Quercinus (Mistletoe of the Oak), in the Cure of that Disease.'

MODERN RESEARCH

In the UK, there are several species of Mistletoe, but the most studied is European mistletoe. Modern research has confirmed and revealed the following uses:

Anticonvulsant

Culpeper's mention of 'falling sickness' relates to epilepsy and is also mentioned by Thornton. Mistletoe was used for the treatment of epilepsy and seizures until the 18th century, thereafter being rejected by scientists as a folklore remedy. Scientific interest was revived in the 20th century, leading to proof that Mistletoe is indeed antiepileptic (Amabeoku et al., 1998; Geetha et al., 2010, 2018; Gupta et al., 2012; Tsyvunin et al., 2016). It is thought to have sedative and calming properties, which might help in reducing the frequency and intensity of seizures, and some studies suggest it can modulate the immune system, which might indirectly affect neurological health.

Antiviral

A 2003 study found that Mistletoe also inhibits influenza virus replication and suppresses production by 99% without any toxic effect on host cells.

Antihypertensive

A 2016 study verified the use of Mistletoe for cardiac disorders, especially hypertension, confirming that it possesses antispasmodic effects as stated by Culpeper and vasodilatory effects, verifying its use in colic, diarrhoea and hypertension. Its calming effect is again thought to exert itself, this time on the cardiovascular system, while helping to improve circulation and heart function by dilating blood vessels and reducing the strain on the heart.

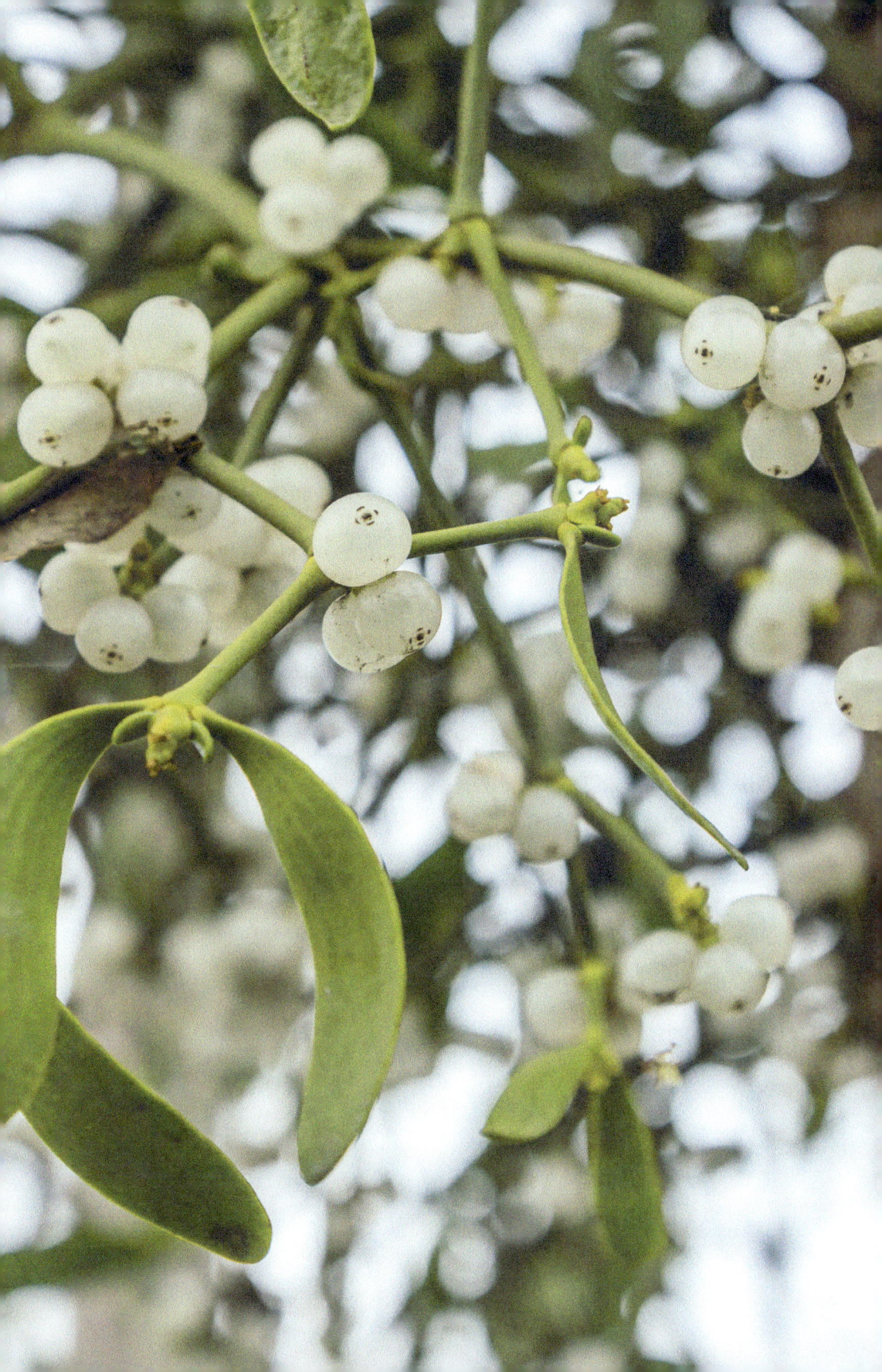

Anticancerogenic

For about the last 80 years, Mistletoe has been studied as a potential aid to cancer treatments. In a 2010 review, authors found 26 randomised controlled trials on the quality of life of cancer patients. Of those studies, 22 reported a benefit, 3 indicated no difference, and 1 did not report any result. Of those that did report a benefit, the improvements were mainly seen in the reduced side effects of conventional therapies such as chemotherapy or radiation. Fatigue, a particularly debilitating symptom of cancer, seems to improve.

In 2001, treatment with Iscador, a complimentary cancer product containing an extract of Mistletoe, was studied as part of a large study on 10,226 cancer patients. A total of 1668 patients were treated with Iscador and 8475 took neither Iscador nor any other Mistletoe product. Results showed that the survival time of patients treated with Iscador was longer for all types of cancer studied.

TOPICAL USES

A Mistletoe poultice was traditionally used for rheumatic, neuralgic and arthritic pains, and in 2008 a study of 30 patients found that in 25 cases with gonarthrosis (knee joint degeneration), there was an 80% decrease of pain symptoms, and a 75% increase of the mobility restricted mobility of the knee-joints was observed.

DOSAGE

Cold infusion – 1 heaped tsp. Dose: ½–1 cup, 3 times per day.
Tincture – (equivalent of) 1:5 45%. Dose – 3–5 drops, 3 times per day.

PRECAUTIONS

Mistletoe leaf is used widely and freely by European herbalists, with very little caution about toxicity, only a warning not to include the berries. As a precaution, children and pregnant or breastfeeding women should not use the plant.

Mistletoe recipes

Medicinal recipes

Mistletoe cold infusion

Use 1tsp/5g chopped or powdered Mistletoe leaf in 500ml water and let it stand overnight. Sweeten with honey and take the infusion first thing in the morning for arterial hypertension, insomnia, temporal arteritis and as a mild sedative.

Mistletoe decocted tincture, 1:5 45%

If you are using 40% alcohol, ie. vodka, make a simple tincture by covering 1 part herb to 5 parts fluid.

If you are using Everclear or other 100% proof, use the following method for a specific tincture:

- 100g dried Mistletoe leaf
- 225ml alcohol
- 175ml water

Divide your leaf into two equal 50g parts. Cover 50g with 225ml of alcohol such as vodka and place the other 50g in 175ml of water. Bring the water to a gentle boil, reduce heat and simmer for 20–40 minutes. Remove from heat and allow to cool a bit. Strain thoroughly and top up if the water is less than 175ml. Add the decoction to the alcohol mix and leave for 14 days before straining. Use for mild epilepsy, hypertension, headaches, arthritis and rheumatism.

Mistletoe compress

Soak a cloth in a decoction of the leaf and use as a compress for gout and sciatica, and rheumatic and neuralgic pains.

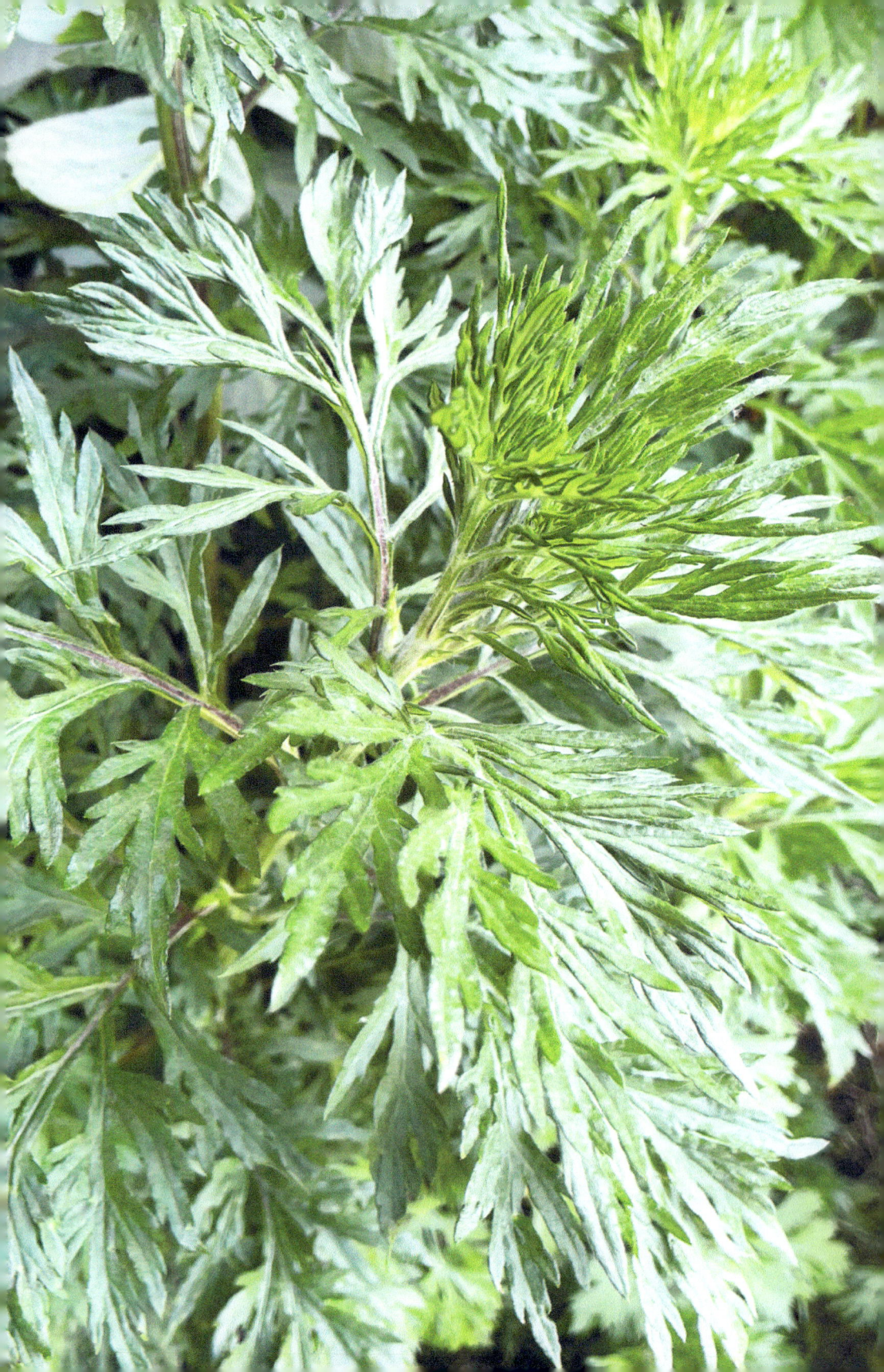

MUGWORT
Artemisia vulgaris

Commonly known as Mugwort, *Artemisia vulgaris* is native to the UK and found in waste areas, hedgerows and along roadsides. Mugwort has a long history of traditional use in herbal medicine and is also used in culinary dishes in some cultures.

HISTORICAL USES

Mugwort was well known in Ancient Egypt, Greece and Rome. Its name then, Artemisia, was believed to be derived from the name of the Greek goddess Artemis, the patron of pregnant women and new mothers. The properties of Mugwort were described in medical works in as early as the 1st century AD by Dioscorides in *De Materia Medica*, by Pliny the Elder in *Naturalis Historia*, followed in the next century by Galen in *De simplicium medicamentorum facultatibus* (Karl Gottlob Kühn).

Nicholas Culpeper's *Herbal* stated:

It is boiled among other herbs for drawing down the courses, by sitting over it, and for hastening the delivery, and helps to expel the afterbirth, and is good for the obstructions and inflammations of the mother [womb]. *It breaks the stone and provokes water. The herb itself being fresh is a special remedy upon the over-much taking of opium. Three drams of the powder of the dried*

ETYMOLOGY OF COMMON NAME
Germanic, probably corresponding to *midge* + *wort* for its use as an insect repellent.

PLANT LORE
In Coles' 1656 *Art of Simpling* it was noted that *'if a footman put Mugwort in his shoes, he may go forty miles and not be weary.'*

USE
The leaves.

EDIBILITY
The young fresh green leaves can be used in salads and smoothies.

HARVEST
In summer.

MEDICINAL PROPERTIES
Antioxidant, anti-inflammatory, digestive and antimicrobial.

ACTIVE CONSTITUENTS
Essential oils, flavonoids, coumarins, sesquiterpene lactones, phenolic acids, coumarins.

LEFT: MUGWORT

leaves taken in wine, is a speedy and certain help for the sciatica. A decoction made with camomile and agrimony, and the place bathed therewith while it is warm, takes away the pains of the sinews, and the cramp. The moxa, so famous in the eastern countries for curing the gout by burning the part affected, is the down which grows upon the underside of this.

MODERN RESEARCH

Modern research into Mugwort has found the following:

Digestive

The digestive benefits of Mugwort are primarily related to the sesquiterpene lactones, essential oils and flavonoids it contains. These stimulate digestive secretions, improve appetite and aid in the reduction of bloating and gas. The treatment of diseases related to the gastrointestinal tract was studied in 2011, and Mugwort was also found to have an antagonistic effect on the receptors while causing relaxation of smooth muscles, which further confirms its use as a relaxant for the gastrointestinal tract.

Antioxidant

In 2008, scientists from Cairo evaluated Mugwort and results showed that it exhibits antioxidant activity, which could help treat oxidative stress-related diseases. These results have since been confirmed in other studies, indicating that Mugwort could be used to combat signs of oxidative stress in the body, such as chronic fatigue and the previously mentioned digestive disorders.

Anti-dyslipidemic

In addition, animal studies have shown that Mugwort root may reduce the levels of cholesterol and triglycerides while increasing levels of HDL (good) cholesterol. In fact, the root was concluded to have the same lowering activity as rosuvastatin, a proprietary drug for lowering cholesterol.

Anticancerogenic

The aerial parts of Mugwort have been shown to demonstrate significant inhibitory effects against breast, cervical, aortic and kidney cell lines. Further studies then demonstrated that Mugwort essential oil induced apoptosis in leukemic cell lines, and in 2018 the plant was found to induce autophagy (death) in colon cancer cells. Based on these observations, it is suggested that Mugwort might be a promising source of new anticancer agents.

Antimicrobial

The essential oil from Mugwort has also exhibited inhibitory activity against *Escherichia coli*, *Salmonella enteritidis*, *Pseudomonas aeruginosa*, *Klebsiella pneumoniae* and *Staphylococcus aureus* as well as *Candida albicans* and *Aspergillus niger* fungi. This activity has been attributed to high levels of eucalyptol and thujone (Blagojević et al., 2006). A 2019 study confirmed the above and concluded that there is a potential for using this oil as a disinfectant and preservative against microorganisms.

Emmenagogue

Mugwort, as Culpeper pointed out, is known for hastening delivery and to expel the afterbirth, which it does by stimulating uterine contractions. In the same way, Mugwort is also used to stimulate menstrual flow, and is believed to do this via the essential oils it contains, particularly thujone and camphor (Lee et al., 1998).

TOPICAL USE AND MOXIBUSTION

Cosmetic products containing Mugwort have gained popularity in recent years owing to its soothing, anti-inflammatory properties, which mean it targets dry and irritated skin effectively.

One 2017 review found sufficient evidence to suggest that moxibustion, a traditional Chinese therapy that involves burning cones of moxa made from Mugwort on specific points of the body to promote the balance of the flow of Qi, is effective for pain reduction and symptom management in people with osteoarthritis in the knee. A separate 2018 review proposed that moxibustion may help reduce the haematological and gastrointestinal toxicities of chemotherapy or radiotherapy, improving quality of life in people with cancer.

In his 1814 *Family Herbal* Robert Thornton described the use of Mugwort as moxa as follows '*Moxa is a substance prepared in Japan from the dried tops and leaves of mugwort, by beating and rubbing them betwixt the hands till only the fine internal lanuginous fibres remain, which are then combed and formed into little cones. These, used as cauteries, are greatly celebrated in eastern countries for preventing and curing many disorders; but chronic rheumatisms, gouty, and some other painful affections of the joints, seem to be the chief complaints for which they can be rationally employed. The manner of applying the moxa is very simple: the part affected being previously moistened, a cone of the moxa is laid, which being set on fire at the apex, gradually burns down to the skin, where it produces a dark-coloured spot: by repeating the process several times, an eschar is formed of any desired extent, and this on separation leaves an ulcer, which is kept open or healed up as circumstances may require.*'

These days, practitioners generally hold a burning moxa stick close to, but not touching, the surface of the skin. In this method, the moxa material is compressed into a stick or pole, looking not unlike an oversized cigar that can be lit and allowed to smoulder, producing a unique form of very penetrating heat with the intention to warm and invigorate the flow of Qi in the body and dispel certain pathogenic influences.

DOSAGE

Tisane – 1–2tsp/5-10g. Drink ½ cup, 3 times per day.

PRECAUTIONS

When consumed in large doses, Mugwort may cause miscarriage, nausea, vomiting and nervous system damage. Furthermore, cases of hypertension have been reported. Mugwort should not be used for more than one week continuously. Continued, habitual use of mugwort can cause nervous problems, liver damage and convulsions. Not suitable for children or those who are pregnant or lactating.

Mugwort recipes

It is said that chewing fresh Mugwort leaves will help relieve fatigue and clear the mind.

Medicinal recipes

Mugwort tisane

Pour 250ml boiling water over 1–2tsp/5–10g of dried leaf and flower, and allow to steep for 10–15 minutes. Use to aid digestion, relieve menstrual cramps and promote relaxation, and to stimulate delayed menstruation.

Mugwort root decoction

Boil 1tsp/5g of the dried grated root for 10–15 minutes in 250ml of water. Use half a cup twice a day for high cholesterol and to regulate menstruation.

Mugwort infused oil

- 100g dried Mugwort herb
- 2tbsp alcohol, such as Everclear
- 1l grapeseed oil

Place the herb in the bottom of a jar with the Everclear. Allow to steep for 10 minutes and then add the oil. Allow the mix to steep/infuse for 4 weeks. Use a few drops of the oil on the face each day or add to your usual moisturiser to rejuvenate the skin.

Mugwort bath

- Handful of fresh Mugwort leaves (or 1–2 tablespoons dried)

Place the fresh or dried leaves in a heatproof bowl and pour over hot water to cover. Let the leaves steep for 15–20 minutes. Strain and add to a warm bath for relaxation, relief from muscle tension, and to promote overall well-being.

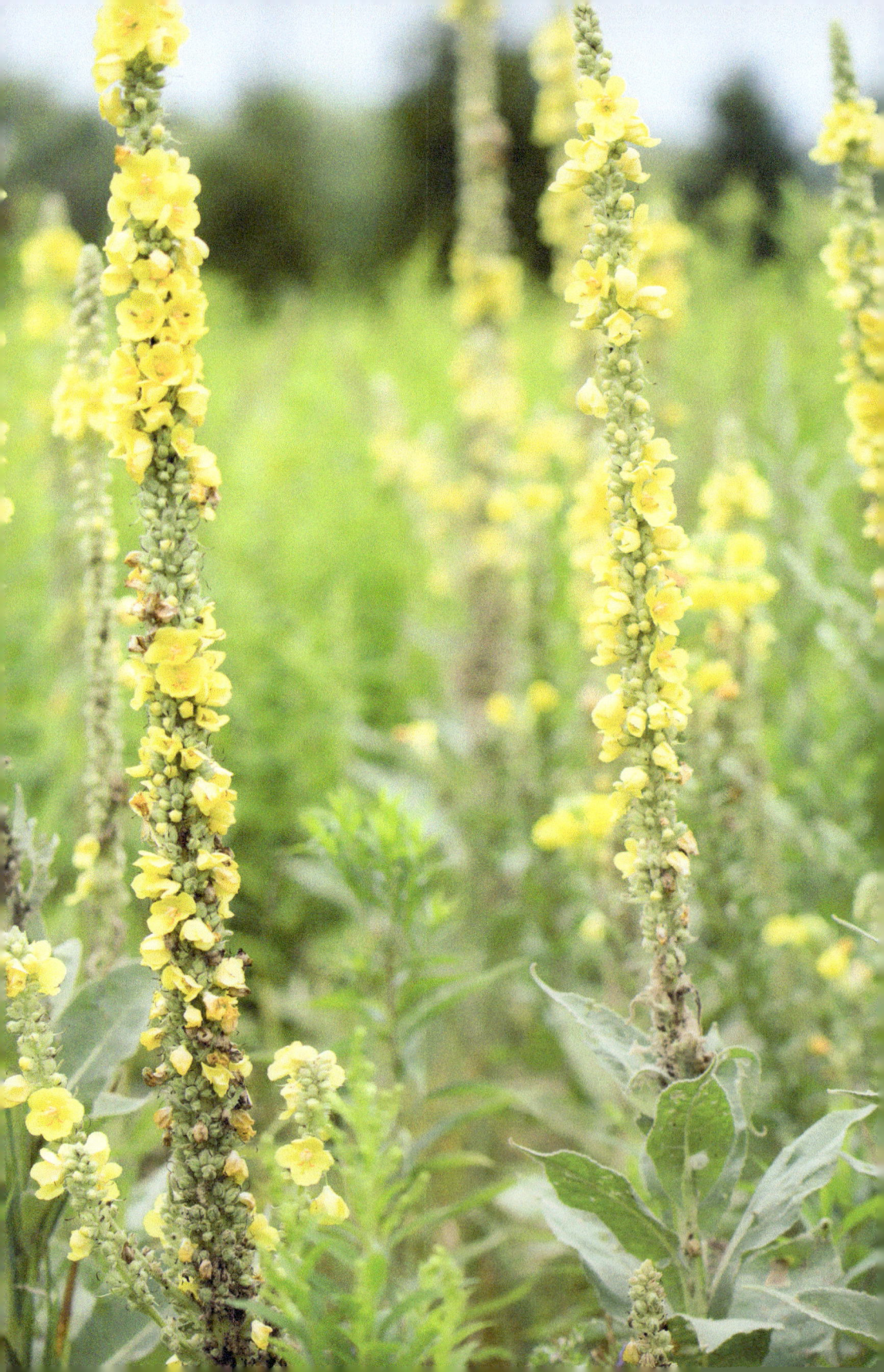

MULLEIN
Verbascum thapsus

The UK's native *Verbascum* species, Mullein, sometimes called Great or Common mullein, is known for its woolly leaves and tall spikes of yellow flowers. Mullein often grows in disturbed habitats, making it a common sight along roadsides, field margins and waste areas. It has a long history of traditional uses in herbal medicine and has also been used for dyeing and as torches (the dried stalks were historically dipped in wax and lit).

HISTORICAL USES

John Gerard mentioned in his *Herball* that '*The country people, especially the husbandmen in Kent, do give their cattel the leaves to drink against the cough of the lungs, being an excellent approved medicine for the same, whereupon they call it Bullocks Lungwort.*'

Nicholas Culpeper's *Herbal* stated, '*The decoction hereof drank, is profitable for those that are bursten, and for cramps and convulsions, and for those that are troubled with an old cough. The decoction gargled, eases tooth-ache, and the oil made by infusion of the flowers, is of good effect for the piles. The decoction of the root in red wine or water, is good for ague. Three ounces of the distilled water of the flowers drank morning and evening is a remedy for the gout. The juice of*

ETYMOLOGY OF COMMON NAME
Derived from Proto-Celtic *melinos*, 'yellow', or from Latin *mollis*, 'soft', referencing the plant's fluffy, downy leaves.

PLANT LORE
In certain traditions, Mullein was known as 'witch's candle'. It was believed that witches would use the stalks in their rituals, either as wands or as candles for their ceremonies.

USE
The flowers and leaves.

EDIBILITY
The leaves and flowers can be used in a salad.

HARVEST
Leaves just before flowering in the summer.

MEDICINAL PROPERTIES
Antispasmodic, antiparasitic, antitussive, demulcent, and antimicrobial.

ACTIVE CONSTITUENTS
Mucilage, volatile oil, saponins, flavonoids, iridoid glycosides, triterpenoids, phenolic acids, tannins.

the leaves and flowers laid on rough warts, as also the powder of the dried roots rubbed on, takes them away. The powder of the dried flowers is a remedy for bowel complaint, or the pains of the colic. The decoction of the root and the leaves, is of great effect to dissolve the tumours, swellings, or inflammations of the throat. The seed and leaves boiled in wine, draw forth thorns or splinters from the flesh, eases the pains, and heals them.'

In his 1897 *Herbal Simples*, William Fernie recommended what he described as the old Irish method of administering Mullein for coughs, *'put an ounce of the dried leaves, or a corresponding quantity of the fresh ones, in a pint of milk, which is boiled for ten minutes, and then strained. This is afterwards given warm to the patient twice a day, with or without sugar.'*

In her 1921 book *A Garden of Herbs*, Eleanour Sinclair Rohde explained that *'The Romans valued mullein highly for chest troubles, and they are supposed to have taught the English the use of it.'*

The Native Americans utilised Mullein both in tisanes and smoked to relieve respiratory disorders while tribes in the Malakand region of Pakistan are reported to still use Mullein for management of abdominal pain and also parasitic worms.

MODERN RESEARCH

This very recognisable plant has been the subject of much research, which has confirmed and found the following properties:

Antispasmodic

Culpeper's uses of Mullein for cramps have been confirmed in various studies showing that its combination of soothing and astringent properties is useful in treating cramps through intestinal relaxation, which also thus supports the traditional use of the tribes in tribes in the Malakand region.

Antiparasitic

Further to the above, Mullein's use for the management of parasites has also been confirmed. Test samples of the extract of Mullein proved comparable to albendazole against roundworms (*Ascaridia galli*) and tapeworms (*Raillietina spiralis*).

Antitussive

With regard to respiratory disorders and coughs, mentioned throughout the historic writings, this use has also been confirmed in many studies as far back as 1883, when an 'in-house' study was conducted at St Vincent's Hospital, in Dublin, Ireland on 7 patients with tuberculosis. Treatment consisted of placing Mullein leaves in a pint of milk (as per Dr Fernie's later recommendation) and boiling for 10 minutes; the mixture was strained and immediately given warm to drink, twice daily. Coughs improved considerably with each patient, but, one died owing to the severity of the tuberculosis.

Anti-inflammatory

Mullein contains various bioactive compounds, including flavonoids and saponins, which have demonstrated anti-inflammatory and antioxidant properties in laboratory studies. A 2021 study showed that Mullein can also be a possible treatment for inflammatory joint disease such as osteoarthritis. Study results showed that after 24 hours and then 6 days of treatment, a significant decrease was observed in pro-inflammatory enzymes, suggesting that the plant could be a potential candidate in the treatment of the early stages of osteoarthritis or mild joint inflammation.

Antiviral

A 2023 analysis reported that flavonoids found in Mullein flowers, phenyl-ethanoid glycoside, and iridoids demonstrated potent antiviral activity against Coronavirus, hepatitis B and *Herpes simplex* I. Meanwhile, the leaves had a higher antiviral impact against hepatitis C.

Antibacterial

The antibacterial activity of Mullein also comes from its phenyl-ethanoid glycosides, phenolic acids and terpenoids. In the same analysis as above, the methanol extract of leaves had slightly stronger antibacterial activity (50–62%) than that of the flowers (42–54%).

TOPICAL USES

Mullein flower oil is recommended for earache. Dr Fernie (*Herbal Simples*) stated that some of the most brilliant results had been obtained by a single application of Mullein oil, and that in acute or chronic cases, 2 or 3 drops of this oil should be put in the ear twice or thrice in the day. The antibacterial and anti-inflammatory properties of Mullein are likely be responsible for this action.

DOSAGE

Tisane – 1–2tsp/5–10g, 3 times per day.
Flower oil – 1–2g, 1:4 in olive oil for ears, 2–3 drops twice a day.

PRECAUTIONS

Not suitable for children or those who are pregnant or lactating.

Mullein recipes

Medicinal recipes

Mullein tisane

Pour 250ml boiling water over 1–2tsp/5–10g of the dried leaf and flower, and allow to steep for 10–15 minutes. Strain through a fine cloth or filter to remove the tiny hairs, which can be irritating to the throat. Use for respiratory issues such as asthma and coughs, digestive problems or as a general health tonic.

Mullein steam inhalation

- 1tbsp/15g of dried Mullein leaves and flowers
- 500ml boiling water

Add the flowers to a bowl and cover with the water. Cover the head with a towel and inhale the vapour.

Inhale deeply for 5–10 minutes to help relieve nasal congestion and respiratory discomfort.

Garlic and Mullein earache oil

- 100g fresh chopped Garlic leaves
- 50g Mullein flowers
- 500ml olive oil

Place the herbs in the bottom of a jar with the oil. Put the oven on its lowest setting and leave the door open. Allow the mix to steep/infuse for an hour. Strain and allow to cool before using a couple of drops placed in the ear canal. Store in the fridge.

Mullein poultice

- 1tsp fresh leaf (if using dried you will need to moisten with water first)
- 2tsp coconut oil
- cheesecloth or cotton bandage

Finely chop the herb into a pulp and add the coconut oil to make a paste. Spread the paste evenly over the desired area and wrap with the cloth or bandage. Use as a soothing anti-inflammatory for joints.

NETTLE (STINGING)
Urtica dioica

A very well-known and seriously underrated plant, Stinging nettle (*Urtica dioica*) has a long history of traditional uses in the UK and other parts of the world. It has been relied on as a food source, herbal medicine and fibre material used to make textiles, ropes and paper.

HISTORICAL USES

The use of Nettle goes as far back as the Romans where texts and medical writings mention it for therapeutic purposes. Notable figures such as Pliny the Elder, the Roman author and naturalist, documented various uses of Nettle in his encyclopaedia *Naturalis Historia*, including for warming and stimulating the skin, a process we now call urtication.

Nicholas Culpeper in his *Herbal* had a lot to say about this plant, including, '*The roots or leaves boiled … is a safe and sure medicine to open the pipes and passages of the lungs, which is the cause of wheezing and shortness of breath and helps to expectorate tough phlegm. The seed provokes urine and expels the gravel and stone in the reins or bladder. The seed or leaves bruised, and put into the nostrils, stays the bleeding of them and takes away the flesh growing in them called polypus. The juice of the leaves, or the decoction of them, or of the*

ETYMOLOGY OF COMMON NAME
Possibly from Anglo-Saxon *netel*, 'needle', for the stings, or from *net*, meaning something spun or sewn, for its use in making thread and cord.

PLANT LORE
In Celtic lore, thick stands of nettles indicate that there are fairy dwellings close by, and the sting of the nettle protects against fairy mischief.

USE
The whole herb.

EDIBILITY
Prepare young Nettle leaves as you would spinach.

HARVEST
Leaves in spring, seed in summer.

MEDICINAL PROPERTIES
Antispasmodic, antiparasitic, Antihistamine, anti-inflammatory, antioxidant, diuretic, antibacterial, antidiabetic and haemostatic.

ACTIVE CONSTITUENTS
Nutrients, flavonoids, phenolic acids, tannins, lignans, histamine.

root, is singularly good to wash either old, rotten, or stinking sores or fistulous, and gangrenes, and such as fretting, eating, or corroding scabs, manginess, and itch, in any part of the body …'

Robert Thornton's *Family Herbal* of 1814 recommended that '*Nettle broth is good against the scurvy. The expressed juice given a tablespoonful four times a day stops haemoptysis* [coughing up blood], *and lint dipped in it, and forced up the nostrils, has stopt bleeding of the nose, when every other remedy has failed. Cancers have been said to have yielded to the juice of nettles, as much being taken as four ounces a day. Paralytic parts being stung with this herb, have been found to regain vigour, as well as limbs lost from rheumatism. The seeds produce a fine oil, and taken inwardly in moderate quantity excite the system, especially* les plaisirs de l'amour, *and are very forcing, therefore should be cautiously employed. Excessive corpulency may be reduced by taking a few of these seeds daily.*'

In her 1894 *Occult Family Physician and Botanic Guide to Health*, Antonette Matteson advised that Nettle '*is a good blood remedy, and removes the phlegmatic superfluities left in the body by winter. Nettle is anti-asthmatic; the juice of the roots or leaves made into an electuary with honey and sugar opens the bronchial tubes of the lungs, the stoppage of which causes wheezing, shortness of breath, etc. It stimulates expectoration of phlegm very freely.*'

Fray's 1897 *Golden Recipes for the Use of All Ages* also provided an interesting remedy for weight loss using the seeds, '*simply from 20 to 30 crushed nettle seeds, taken night and morning daily, is the best remedy for stout people, which will prevent burdensome fat surrounding the kidneys and stopping the heart. Tried with good results.*'

MODERN RESEARCH

Nettles are one of the UK's most nutritious native plants, being high in amino acids, protein, flavonoids and minerals, including iron, calcium, magnesium, potassium and zinc. Nettles also contain the highest plant source of iron, making them excellent for combating anaemia and fatigue. The seeds are used as an adaptogen and will give an energy boost and uplift the mood, as Thornton points out. Modern research has also confirmed and found the following properties of Nettle:

Antihistamine

Nettle leaves contain histamine, which is why Culpeper and Matteson found them useful for treating wheezing and shortness of breath. They are still used to treat allergy symptoms such as hayfever, nasal congestion, sneezing or itching because they affect numerous receptors and/or enzymes involved in allergic reactions.

In 2017, in a clinical trial of 74 patients with symptoms of allergic rhinitis, subjects were randomly divided into two groups who were then given 150mg Urtidin®, a tablet containing

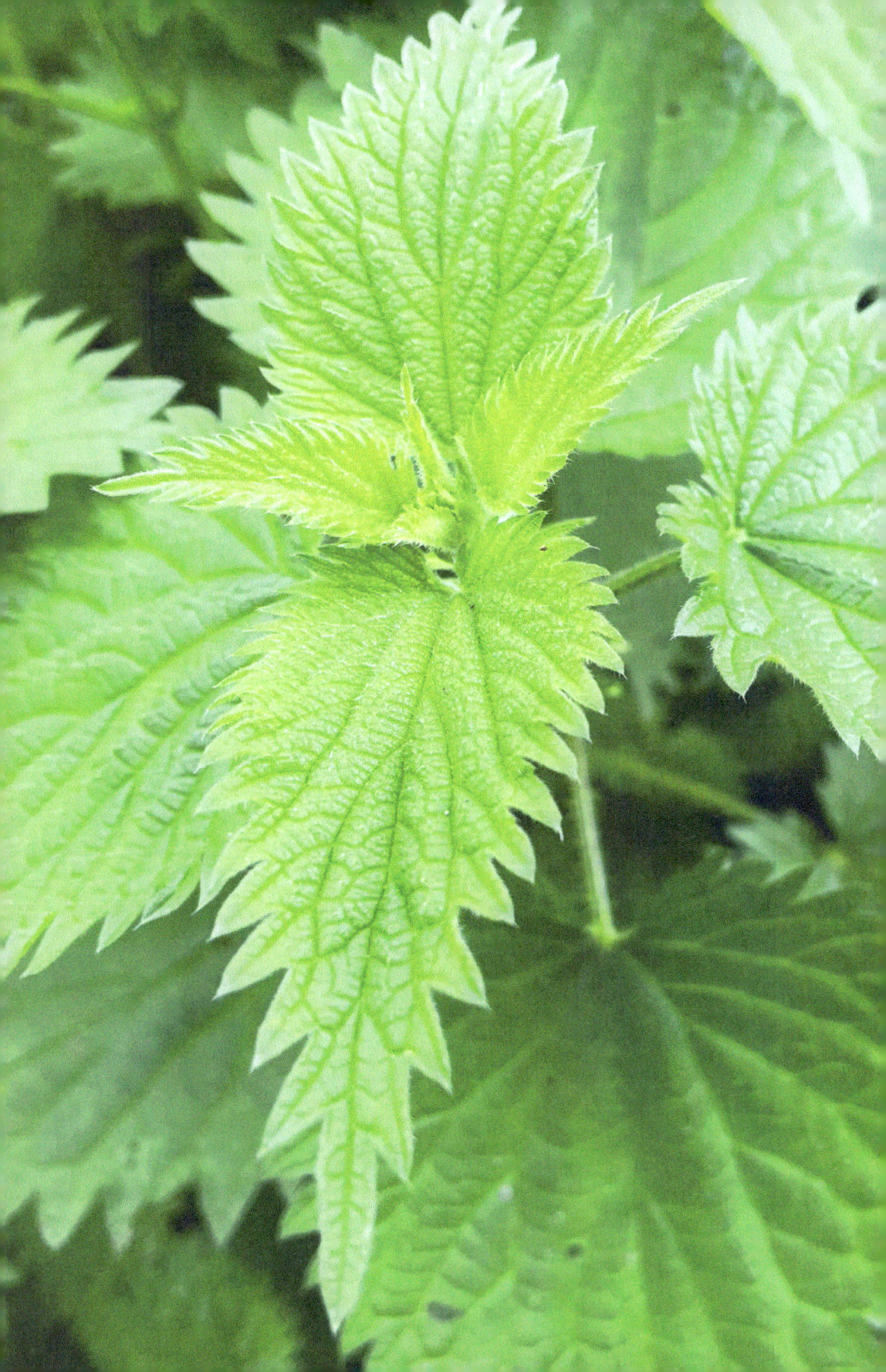

extract of Nettle, or a placebo for one month. A total of 40 patients completed the trial, and while a significant improvement in symptom severity was observed in both groups, a statistically significant reduction in mean nasal smear eosinophil (a type of white blood cell) count was observed after treatment with Nettle, suggesting a reduction in allergic response.

Haemostatic

Interestingly, the information by both Culpeper and Thornton regarding nasal bleeding also holds weight. Ankaferd Blood Stopper (ABS) is a haemostatic agent that contains a mixture of Thyme, Liquorice, Grape, Galangal and Nettle, and has been approved for the management of bleeding. It was found to be effective within 10 to 20 minutes in controlling bleeding in most patients after dental surgery.

Diuretic

Culpeper was also correct that Nettle is a natural diuretic and has been shown in studies to produce both diuretic and natriuretic effects (ie excreting excess sodium in the urine) without significant effect on potassium levels. A 2013 study showed that an intravenous infusion of Nettle extract produced a significant rise in urine volume, similar to furosemide (a diuretic medication). The diuretic and urinary disinfectant activity of Nettle is believed to be thanks to its glycolic and glyceric acid content, which leads to an increase in diuresis (De Vico et al., 2018).

Anti-inflammatory

Some of the anti-inflammatory compounds in Nettle include kaempferol, quinic acid and choline. Kaempferol has been described as a potent anti-inflammatory while quinic acid is effective in treating atherosclerosis owing to its ability to lower inflammation in the blood vessels (Seon-A Jang et al., 2017).

In human studies, applying a Nettle cream or consuming Nettle products appears to relieve inflammatory conditions, such as arthritis, and in a clinical trial of 37 people with acute arthritis, 50g of stewed Nettle leaves consumed daily, combined with 50mg of diclofenac, were shown to be as effective as the full 200mg dose of diclofenac over a two-week period.

In a further study by Christensen and Bliddal (2010), it was found that a combination of Nettle, fish oil and vitamin E reduced the need for analgesic and other drugs for the symptoms of osteoarthritis. It has also been shown that Nettle's anti-inflammatory activity lends itself to the treatment of rheumatoid arthritis as it inhibits pro-inflammatory cytokines in synovial fluid (Riehemann et al., 1999). Several studies have confirmed the inhibition of these pro-inflammatory cytokines and therefore inflammation in rheumatoid arthritis, the most recent being Dhouibi et al. in 2020.

Antiandrogenic

Another important use of Nettle has been in treating benign prostatic hyperplasia, also known as enlarged prostate. Clinical studies suggest that Nettle may have effects on sex hormone-binding globulin (SHBG) levels. SHBG is involved in regulating levels of hormones, including testosterone, which plays a role in prostate health. In addition, Nettle root extract shows activity against prostate cancer cells.

Antiestrogenic

Nettle root can also block oestrogen production throughout the body by inhibiting the enzyme aromatase, which may make it useful for the treatment of polycystic ovary syndrome. Because we also know that Nettle is an antihistamine, it can help balance histamine levels, which can go a long way towards also balancing out oestrogen levels.

Antidiabetic

Nettle root may also help improve insulin resistance. In an animal study, it increased both blood sugar balance and insulin resistance by increasing skeletal muscle insulin sensitivity (making the muscle cells more responsive to insulin). In 2017, a quasi-experimental study was conducted with type-2 diabetic patients who were given a decoction of Nettle per day for 8 weeks. At the end of the trial, blood glucose and body weight decreased significantly in the Nettle group. The findings of this study concluded that consumption of Nettle herbal tea could improve cardiovascular function and control blood glucose in diabetic patients.

Antibacterial

Culpeper's observation regarding the use of Nettle for 'old stinking sores' was confirmed when results from experiments showed that wounds treated with an ointment of Nettle extract healed in 9 days, while wounds not treated healed in 13 days. Histopathological examination also revealed that inflammation was significantly reduced, making the extract a novel drug candidate for wound-healing.

In addition, Nettle extracts showed significant antibacterial effect against some clinically important pathogenic bacteria, including *Staphylococcus epidermidis*, which lives on the skin and causes sepsis.

Anti-obesity

Finally, in a partial confirmation of Fray's findings, a recent study confirmed that Nettle seeds may indeed prevent obesity and its associated effects. In a 2024 study, rats were divided into four groups, comprising a control group, one group that received a high fat diet, another that received Nettle extracts and a final group that received a high fat diet as well as Nettle extracts. Results showed that the high fat diet led to weight gain that was partially moderated by the Nettle extract, but cholesterol levels were discovered to be highest in this group. It was concluded that the Nettle extract did not completely protect the rats from the effects of weight gain.

TOPICAL USE

Nettle's natural antihistamines also provide topical benefits in instances of insect bites, allergies, rashes and eczema, etc. Also, as seen from the above, Nettles are an anti-inflammatory, and in one 27-person study in 2000, applying a Stinging nettle cream on to arthritis-affected areas significantly reduced pain, compared to a placebo treatment.

DOSAGE

Tisane – 1tsp/5g, 3–4 times per day.
Root tincture – 1:5 45% – 2–6ml in water – 20 drops = 1ml/1tsp = 5ml.

PRECAUTIONS

Do not use Nettle in cases of reduced cardiac or renal function or with blood-thinners and medication for high blood pressure or diabetes. It is advisable to eat the young shoots and leaves, since as the plant flowers and bears fruits, it may contain higher amounts of cystolyths with maturity, which can irritate the kidneys (Gregory, 1997). Not suitable for children or those who are pregnant or lactating.

Nettle recipes

Medicinal recipes

Nettle tisane

Pour 250ml boiling water over 1tsp/5g of dried leaf and flower, and allow to steep for 10–15 minutes. Use for arthritis, asthma, allergic rhinitis, urinary infections, bronchitis, gingivitis, gout, kidney stones, laryngitis, sciatica and tendinitis. Nettle tea is also a very good tonic after taking antibiotics owing to its high vitamin and mineral content.

Nettle prostate tincture 1:5 45%

If you are using 40% alcohol, ie. vodka, make a simple tincture by covering 1 part herb to 5 parts fluid.

If you are using Everclear or other 100% proof, use the following method for a specific tincture:

- 50g dried Nettle root
- 25g dried Nettle leaves
- 25g Nettle seeds
- 225ml alcohol
- 275ml water

Split the dried root into two equal 25g parts. Cover 25g dried root, plus the leaves and the seeds, with the alcohol. Place the other 25g root in the water. Bring the water to a gentle boil, reduce heat and simmer for 20 minutes. Remove from heat and allow to cool a bit. Strain thoroughly and top up if the water is less than 200ml. Take ½–1tsp 2 or 3 times daily for 3 months. Discontinue use for 2 to 3 weeks, then repeat the cycle.

Nettle infused oil

- 100g dried Nettle herb
- 2tbsp alcohol, such as Everclear
- 1l grapeseed oil

Place the herb in the bottom of a jar with the Everclear. Allow to steep for 10 minutes and then add the oil. Allow the mix to steep/infuse for 4 weeks. Use as an anti-inflammatory for painful joints and as a topical antihistamine.

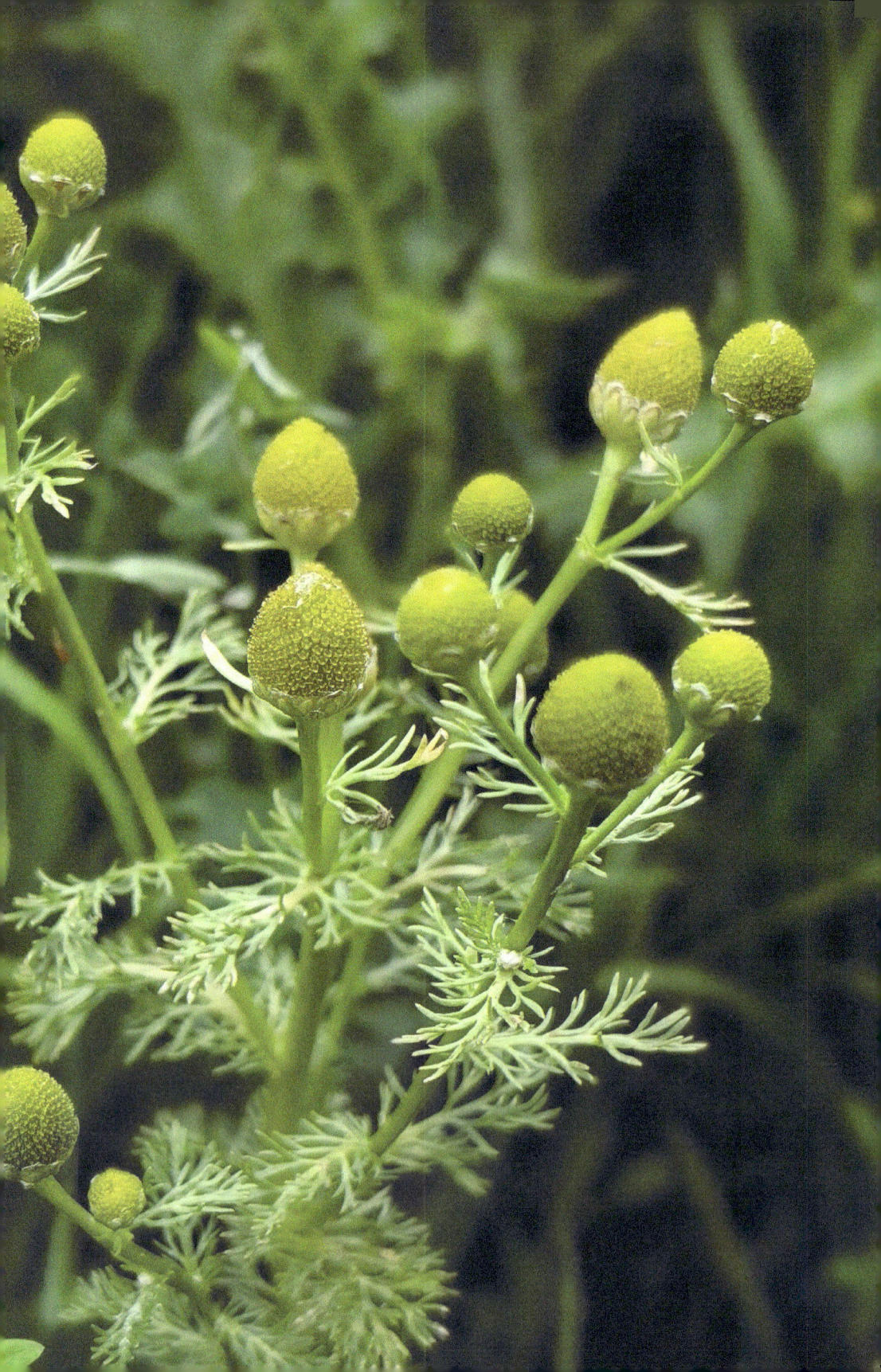

PINEAPPLEWEED
Matricaria discoidea

Matricaria discoidea, commonly known as Wild chamomile or Pineappleweed, belongs to the Daisy family, *Asteraceae*. Like its cousin, German chamomile, it is not native to the UK but was introduced by the Romans. However, unlike its cousin, it can be commonly found in various habitats, including grasslands, meadows, roadsides, waste grounds and disturbed areas.

HISTORICAL USES

Pineappleweed was used as a medicinal and aromatic plant by Native American tribes (Moerman, 1998). In particular it has documented use as an insect repellent by Blackfoot Indians and other indigenous groups of North America.

Nicholas Culpeper provides a list of actions for Chamomile, but it is likely that he is talking here about Roman chamomile, which belongs to a different taxonomic group within the *Asteraceae* family, though it possesses some similar properties.

Pineappleweed has an ethnomedical background in the UK dating back to the 19th century, with the plant having been mainly used in the form of tea or tincture for its anti-inflammatory and spasmolytic properties.

The tenth *State Pharmacopoeia of the USSR* (1968) allowed the use of the

ETYMOLOGY OF COMMON NAME
This refers to the fruit and the plant's crushed leaves that emit a fragrance reminiscent of Pineapple.

PLANT LORE
Pineappleweed is often seen as a symbol of simplicity and humility. Its ability to thrive in poor soil and harsh conditions reflects the idea that even in difficult circumstances one can find strength and flourish.

USE
The flower.

EDIBILITY
Eat raw in salads but you also the dried flowerheads for an energetic burst; they are great in a homemade trail mix.

HARVEST
In summer.

MEDICINAL PROPERTIES
Soporific, analgesic, anti-inflammatory, antimicrobial, anthelmintic.

ACTIVE CONSTITUENTS
Volatile oil, coumarins, flavonoids, phenolic acids, polyacetylenes.

LEFT: PINEAPPLEWEED

flowering parts of the Pineappleweed as a substitute for that of German chamomile, but only for external use, owing to its anti-inflammatory and spasmolytic activities.

MODERN RESEARCH

Most of the available modern research for the Chamomile family is on German chamomile, which is recommended by the German Commission E as a mild tranquilliser and sleep-inducer, but a 2004 study showed that the chemical constituents of Pineapple Weed are very similar to those of German Chamomile. Pineappleweed is used in the same manner, and is every bit as enjoyable. It also has the following properties:

Soporific

Chamomile tea and essential oils are widely used for their sedative effect. A 2024 study, undertaken to evaluate the effect of Pineappleweed extracts, showed that administration of the plant induced a prolonged sleep effect in rats, extending sleeping time 2.8 times compared to that found with the group administered a barbiturate.

The sedative effects, like those of German chamomile, are believed to be related to the flavonoid apigenin, which binds to benzodiazepine receptors in the brain.

Analgesic and anti-inflammatory

The same 2024 study that assessed the soporific effects of Pineappleweed above also found that the extracts had an analgesic effect in mice, prolonging the latent time of discomfort (by 72%) in a hot plate test compared to the control group that received acetaminophen.

As mentioned above, Pineappleweed contains apigenin, which has been studied for its anti-inflammatory, antioxidant, anticancer and neuroprotective properties. Another constituent is matricin, a sesquiterpene lactone that, when heated, degrades into chamazulene, which is particularly renowned for its anti-inflammatory effects. It inhibits the production of inflammatory cytokines, helping to reduce inflammation and alleviate symptoms of arthritis, skin irritation and gastrointestinal disorders, all conditions that German chamomile is also known for treating.

Antimicrobial

Pineappleweed's constituents coumarin and herniarin have shown a range of biological activities, including haemostatic and antiparasitic properties, as well as antimicrobial activity, with extracts causing inhibition of *Escherichia coli* cells *in vitro*.

The antimicrobial constituents of Pineappleweed, as with German chamomile, are thought to be α-bisabolol, luteolin, quercetin and apigenin and several studies have demonstrated these antibacterial activities against a wide range of pathogenic bacteria, such as *Staphylococcus aureus*, *Escherichia coli*, *Salmonella typhimurium* and *Helicobacter pylori* as well as fungal pathogens, including *Candida albicans*, *Aspergillus flavus* and *Cryptococcus neoformans*. These effects are attributed to the ability to disrupt cell membranes, interfere with bacterial enzyme activity and inhibit bacterial DNA replication.

Luteolin in particular has received widespread attention in recent years as a viable alternative for treating viral infections and related diseases. Structural fitting analysis has shown that luteolin can inhibit the replication of influenza virus, enterovirus, rotavirus, herpes virus, respiratory virus, coronavirus, and other viruses. In addition, luteolin protects cells against inflammatory damage and further promotes the repair of cells, tissues, and organs caused by virus infection and inhibits the activation of inflammatory factors.

Quercetin has also been studied for its potential antiviral activity against various viruses, including influenza and coronaviruses. It may inhibit viral replication and entry into host cells, as well as modulate host immune responses (Agrawal et al., 2020).

TOPICAL USES

A 2018 study confirmed the use of Pineappleweed as an insect deterrent against *Aedes aegypti*, a mosquito species that is a known vector of several important viruses, including yellow fever, dengue, chikungunya and zika. An essential oil from the plant was found to provide a 'proportion not biting' (PNB) value of 0.76, which was statistically equivalent to DEET, the main ingredient in most commercial insect repellents.

DOSAGE

Tisane – 1tsp/5g, 3 times per day.
Tincture – 1:5 45%, 5–10ml, 3 times per day – 20 drops = 1ml/1tsp = 5ml.

PRECAUTIONS

Pineappleweed contains coumarin, so care should be taken to avoid use with blood thinners. Not suitable for children or those who are pregnant or lactating.

Pineappleweed recipes

Medicinal recipes

Pineappleweed tisane

Pour 250ml boiling water over 1tsp/5g of the dried herb and allow to steep for 10–15 minutes. Use to calm down inflammation of respiratory and gastrointestinal tracts and to aid sleep.

Pineappleweed infused tincture 1:5 45%

If you are using 40% alcohol, ie. vodka, make a simple tincture by covering 1 part herb to 5 parts fluid.

If you are using Everclear or other 100% proof, use the following method for a specific tincture:

- 100g dried Pineappleweed
- 225ml alcohol
- 275ml water

Take 100g of dried herb and split into two parts of 50g each. Place 50g in 225ml alcohol and 50g in 275ml of boiled water. Steep/infuse in the water for 10 minutes. Strain thoroughly and top up if the water is less than 275ml. Add the infusion to the alcohol mix and leave for 14 days before straining. Use for insomnia and to relieve digestive discomfort, tension and anxiety.

Pineappleweed infused oil

- 100g dried Pineappleweed
- 2tbsp alcohol, such as Everclear
- 1l grapeseed oil

Place the herb in a jar with the alcohol and allow to steep for 10 minutes before adding the oil. Leave for 4 weeks and then strain. Use for all skin types to heal the skin, relax the nervous system and calm the mind. Using it to massage the muscles of the neck can relieve tension headaches, and it is also soothing for the feet at the end of the day to bring on a good night's sleep. The 'Chamomiles' also help skin regenerate and so it is perfect for use on scabs and scars.

Pineappleweed trail mix

- Cashews
- Chamomile/Pineappleweed buds
- Coconut flakes
- Chopped Dates
- Nettle seeds

Simply mix together and enjoy.

PLANTAIN
Plantago lanceolata/major

In the UK, several species of the genus *Plantago*, commonly known as Plantains, are native or naturalised. The two most well-known are Greater plantain (*Plantago major*), with its broad, oval-shaped leaves, and Ribwort plantain (*Plantago lanceolata*), which is characterised by narrow, lance-shaped leaves. Both have a long history of use in herbal medicine and folk remedies.

HISTORICAL USES

In her *Physica*, Hildegard of Bingen (1098–1179) recommended Plantain juice to treat insect bites and stings, saying '*Plantain is hot and dry. Take plantain and express the juice. Give it, strained through a cloth and mixed with wine or honey, as a drink to a person tormented by gicht (gout), and the gicht will cease. But one who has swollen glands, should dry the root over the fire, place it warm on the glands. He should tie a cloth over it and he will be better. Do not however, place it over scrofula, which would be harmed by it. One who is bothered by a stitch should cook plantain leaves in water. Having squeezed out the water, he should place them warm over the place where it hurts, and the stitch will cease. If a spider or any other insect touches or bites you, rub the bites with plantain juice, and it will relieve you.*'

ETYMOLOGY OF COMMON NAME
From Latin *planta* meaning 'sole of the foot', for the broad, flat leaves lying close on the ground.

PLANT LORE
In Celtic traditions, Plantain was considered a sacred herb. It was associated with the goddess Brigid, who was a deity of healing and protection. Plantain was often used in rituals and offerings to invoke her blessings.

USE
The leaves. Plantain is wild in two forms (*P. lanceolata* and *P. major*).

EDIBILITY
The young leaves are edible raw or cooked; seeds can be eaten.

HARVEST
In summer.

MEDICINAL PROPERTIES
Anti-inflammatory, antimicrobial, expectorant, vulnerary and cytotoxic.

ACTIVE CONSTITUENTS
Polysaccharides, iridoid glycosides, flavonoids, tannins, saponins.

In his *Herball*, John Gerard (1545–1612) wrote of Plantain, '*The juice dropped in the eies cooles the heate and inflammation thereof.*'

Nicholas Culpeper's *Herbal* recommended it as '*good to stay spitting of blood and other bleedings at the mouth and the too free bleeding of wounds. It is held an especial remedy for those that are troubled with the phthisic, or consumption of the lungs, or ulcers of the lungs, or coughs that come of heat. It is also good to be applied where any bone is out of joint, to hinder inflammations, swellings, and pains that presently rise thereupon. Briefly, the Plantains are singularly good wound herbs, to heal fresh or old wounds or sores, either inward or outward.*'

Robert Thornton wrote of it in his 1814 *Family Herbal*, '*It appears to be the great vulnerary of the ancients, and the leaves are now outwardly used by the common people to all fresh wounds.* He went on to describe many of the above and finished with, '*In short, there is too much reported of the medicinal virtues of this herb to have it as yet discarded from our Pharmacopoeias; but I have not had myself any experience of them.*'

MODERN RESEARCH

The two Plantain species, Ribwort and Greater, are used interchangeably. Research has confirmed the following:

Vulnerary

As the above all recognise, both Plantains are 'singularly good wound herbs'. An antibiotic effect was reported for *Plantago* species in 1988 (Grigorescu et al., 1973; Ravn and Brimer, 1988), which could explain the plant's topical use in difficult-to-heal skin wounds (Aliev, 1950; Quer, 1985).

A 1997 study by Guillen then presented data that indicated that upon oral administration, the aqueous extract of Greater plantain shows analgesic activities in addition to anti-inflammatory ones related to an inhibition of prostaglandins synthesis.

A 2000 study by Samuelsen found that more than a single compound is responsible for the healing effect of the plant. Thus glycosides, such as plantamajoside and acteoside, have antibacterial activities; flavonoids and caffeic acid contents have antioxidative activities; and pectic polysaccharides in the plant have been reported to be effective against ulcers. Finally, the saturated primary alcohols that are present in the leaf wax aid the healing of wounds and also contain compounds with anti-inflammatory activity.

Antitussive

In 2013, a study by Farkhi also confirmed the use that Culpeper recommended for Plantain in the respiratory system. Bulgarian clinical trials had suggested it may be effective in the treatment of chronic bronchitis (Tilford, 1997), and sedative and anti-cough effects in guinea pigs were also demonstrated (Boskabady et al., 2006). The allantoin constituent enabled cells in bronchioles to recover and

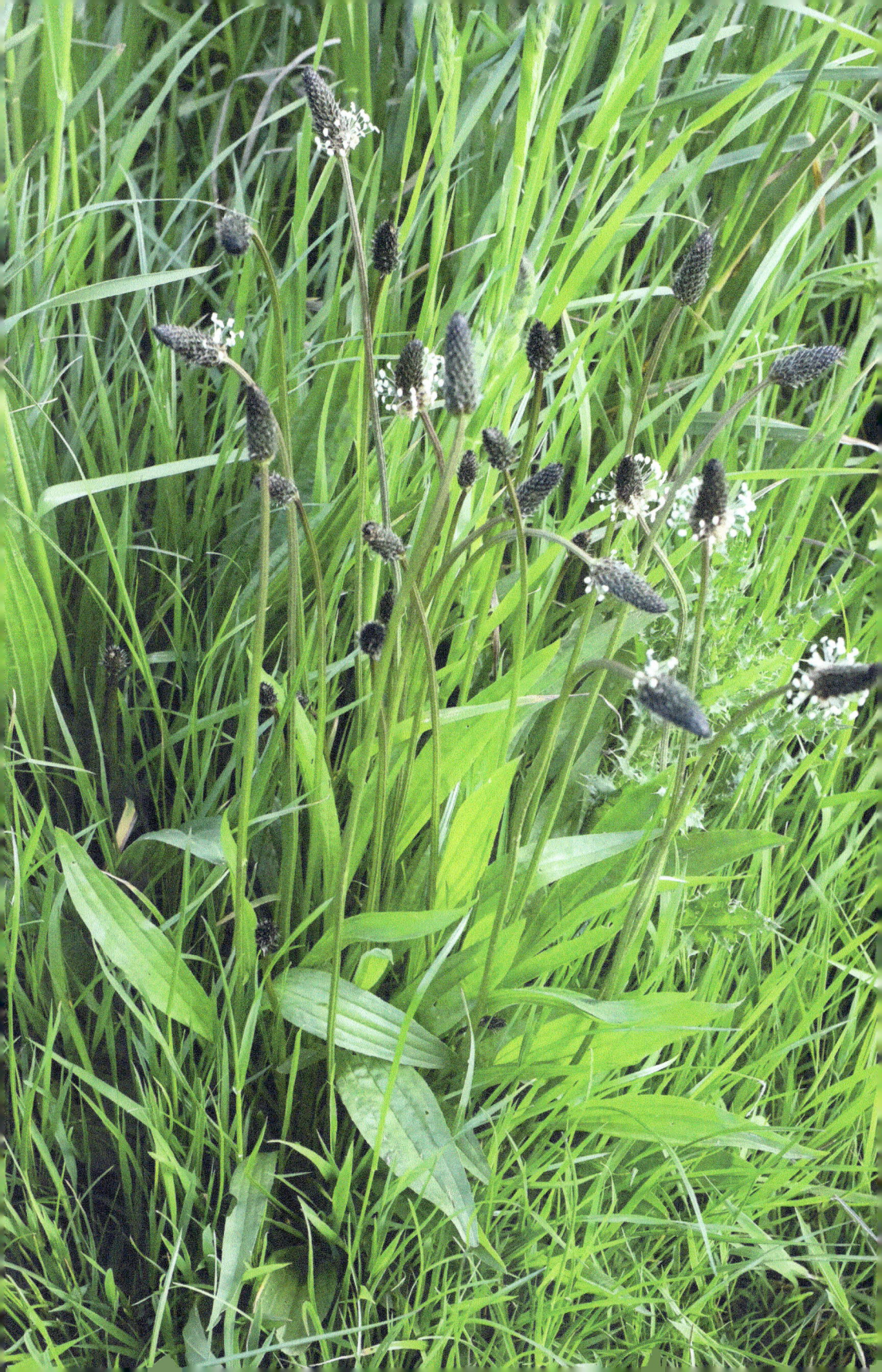

regenerate and the mucilagic compounds decreased lymphoid cell and nodule formation.

Anticancerogenic

Plantain extracts have shown cytotoxic activity against human renal adenocarcinoma, human melanoma and human breast adenocarcinoma cells (Gálvez et al., 2003; Beara et al., 2012). Then, in 2019, a study showed that Ribwort plantain leaf extract selectively inhibited the proliferation of triple-negative breast cancer cells. This was followed by a 2021 study by Rahamouz-Haghighi et al. that compared the two *Plantago* species and found that a methanolic extract of Greater plantain roots were more effective than that of Ribwort plantain roots on colon carcinoma cells.

Anti-obesity

The seed husks of the related *Plantago ovata* are known as Psyllium. They are rich in mucilaginous substances such as arabinose, xylose, galacturonic acid and trace amounts of other sugars. The effect of these substances on the human body includes a cholesterol-lowering effect and laxative and glycaemic index reduction from the seeds' high-water absorption capacity. When Psyllium is mixed with water it forms a gel-like mucilage, the viscosity of which may affect the absorption of glucose, fat and cholesterol.

TOPICAL USES

Plantain can draw out splinters, stings, poisons and infections from wounds. It can also treat ringworm. The leaves can be mashed or a cloth soaked in the tisane is placed directly over the area.

DOSAGE

Tisane – 1tsp/5g. Drink ½ cup, 3–4 times per day.
Tincture – 1:5 25% tincture, 1–2ml per day – 20 drops = 1ml/1tsp = 5ml.

PRECAUTIONS

Plantain can decrease the absorption of warfarin and iron, and is not suitable for anyone suffering from intestinal obstruction. Not suitable for children or those who are pregnant or lactating.

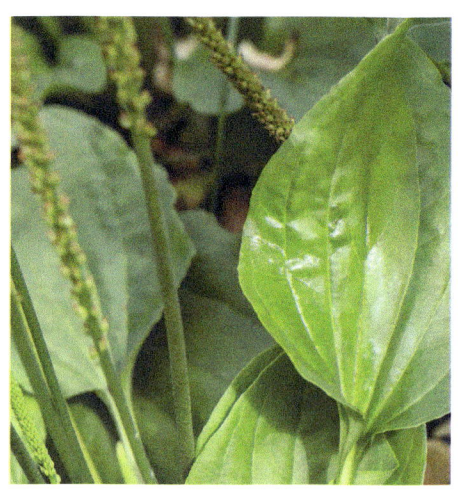

ABOVE: *PLANTAGO MAJOR*

Plantain recipes

Medicinal recipes
Plantain tisane
Pour 250ml boiling water over 1tsp/5g of the dried leaf and allow to steep for 10–15 minutes. Use for the treatment of diarrhoea, as well for haemorrhoids, cystitis, kidney stones and gallstones. Also, the plant is recommended against runny nose, bronchitis, sinusitis and asthma.

Plantain infused tincture – 1:5 25%
If you are using 40% alcohol, ie. vodka, you will need to dilute this at the ratio of 60ml water to every 100ml of Vodka to make a 25% medium and then cover 1 part herb to 5 parts fluid.

If you are using Everclear or other 100% proof, use the following method for a specific tincture:
- 100g dried Plantain herb
- 125ml alcohol
- 375ml water

Take 100g of dried herb and split into two parts of 50g each. Place 50g in 125ml alcohol and 50g in 375ml of boiled water. Steep/infuse in the water for 10 minutes. Strain thoroughly and top up if the water is less than 375ml. Add the infusion to the alcohol mix and leave for 14 days before straining. Use as an anti-inflammatory internally and externally as an analgesic (pain-relieving) for shingles.

Plantain compress
Soak cotton pads in a tisane of Plantain and use as a compress for itching, burning and pain.

Plantain salve
- 100g dried and powdered plant (Greater plantain is recommended for external use)
- 2 tbsp alcohol, such as Everclear
- 1l grapeseed oil

Place the herbs in a jar with the alcohol and allow to steep for 10 minutes before adding the oil. Leave for 4 weeks and then strain. Make into a salve by using a 1:4 ratio of melted beeswax to your oil mix, ie. 1 part wax to 4 parts liquid. Melt the wax pellets in the oil in a double boiler or bain-marie. Remove from the heat and allow to cool and set completely before using on wounds that refuse to heal.

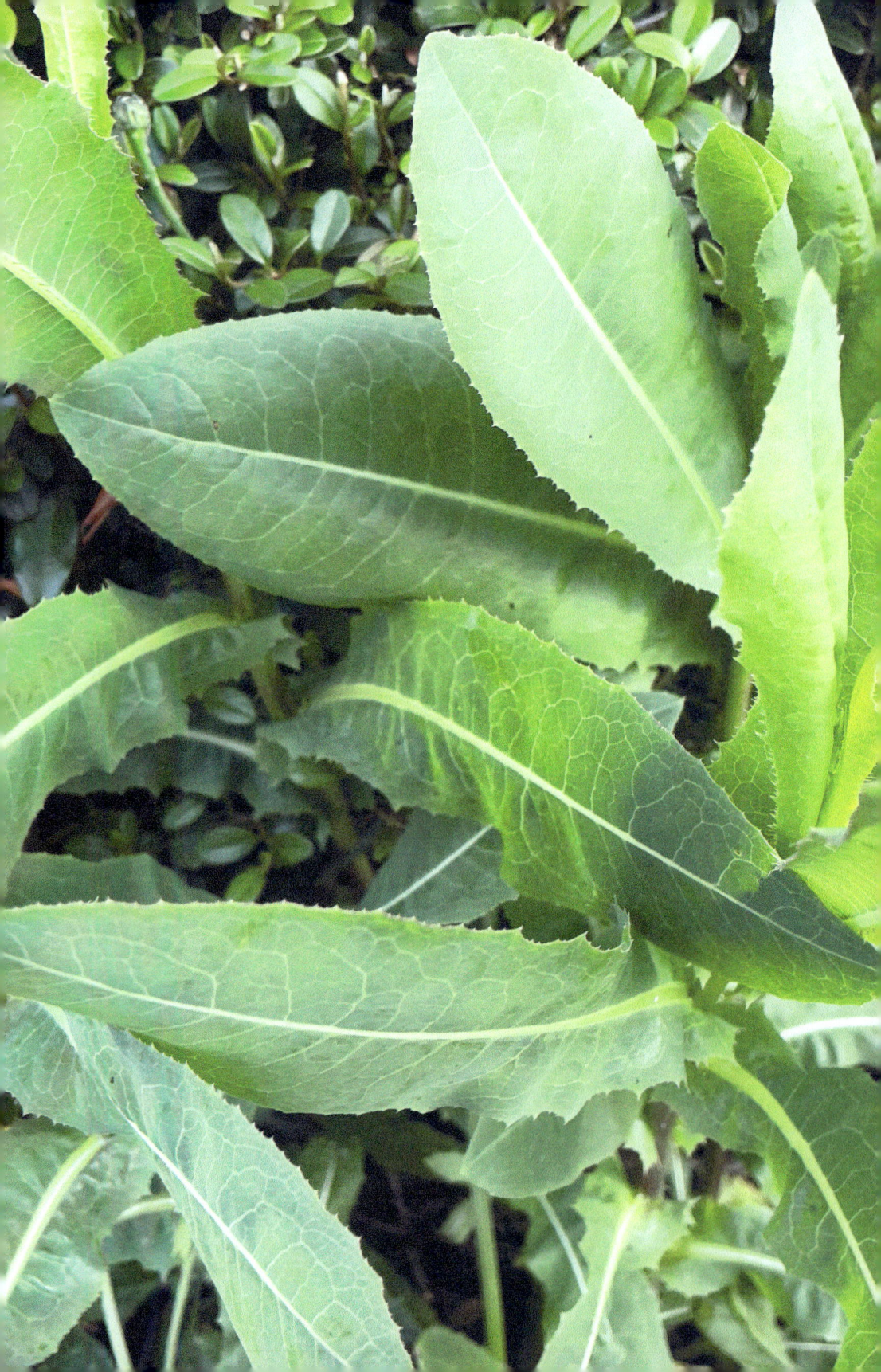

PRICKLY LETTUCE
Lactuca serriola

The wild lettuces are the ancestors of the garden lettuce. There are two species of Wild lettuce in the UK, and both are considered naturalised plants, meaning they have become established and reproduce in the wild without human intervention. Both are commonly found in various habitats, including roadsides, waste areas, disturbed sites and agricultural fields. Wild lettuce (*Lactuca virosa*), also called Opium lettuce, is known for its potential analgesic and sedative effects, while Prickly lettuce (*Lactuca serriola*) is more common but has a milder sedative and analgesic effect.

HISTORICAL USES

John Gerard (1545–1612) referred only to the cultivated garden lettuce variety in his *Herball*, saying of it, '*Lettuce cooleth the heat of the stomacke, called the heart-burning; and helpeth it when it is troubled with choler: it quencheth thirst, and causeth sleepe.*'

Nicholas Culpeper's *Herbal* said of the 'Great Wild Lettuce' (*Lactuca virosa*), '*A syrup made from a strong infusion of the plant makes an excellent anodyne, it eases the most violent pains of the colic, and other disorders and gently disposes the patient to sleep … The best way of giving it is to dry the juice which runs from the roots by*

ETYMOLOGY OF COMMON NAME
'Prickly' refers to the edges of the leaves while 'lettuce' is from the Latin word *lactūca*, which refers to the 'milk' or sap that is secreted from the stems.

PLANT LORE
Prickly lettuce is sometimes associated with endurance and resilience owing to its ability to thrive in challenging environments.

USE
The leaves and sap.

EDIBILITY
This is a wild lettuce and so can be used raw or cooked.

HARVEST
In summer, when in flower.

MEDICINAL PROPERTIES
Analgesic, anxiolytic, antibacterial, antihyperglycaemic.

ACTIVE CONSTITUENTS
Lactucarium, flavonoids, coumarins, triterpenes, alkaloids, phenolic acids.

LEFT: PRICKLY LETTUCE

incision; if one ounce be put in a gallon of wine there is produced and excellent quieting medicine, a teaspoonful of which is a dose in a glass of water.'

While Culpeper is referring to Wild lettuce, the usual source of the latex sap called lactucarium, this can be hard to find. It is recognised that lactuarium from the much more obtainable Prickly lettuce is still of superior quality. A single plant of Wild lettuce has been found to give 56 grains whereas Prickly lettuce yields 25 grains.

'The sap is obtained by cutting the stem of the lettuce at the time of flowering and collecting the milky juice that flows out into a vessel containing a little water. It is then left in a dry place until it concretes into a solid mass,' according to Thompson's *Organic Chemistry*. The juice, in drying, loses about half its weight of water. By making another cut a short distance below the first, and so proceeding several times daily, the whole of the juice contained in the plant may be collected.

MODERN RESEARCH

As it is more easily obtained, I have chosen to include those modern studies that refer to Prickly lettuce, *Lactuca serriola*. These studies have found the following properties:

Analgesic

Prickly lettuce has exhibited potent analgesic activity in studies carried out in 1992 by Fayyaz et al. In 2006, Wesołowska et al. evaluated the analgesic properties and found that the component lactucopicrin, a sesquiterpene lactone, is responsible for both the sedative and analgesic effect of Prickly lettuce as it acts on the central nervous system.

Anxiolytic

In a 2009 clinical trial of seeds on mixed anxiety depressive disorder, results showed that Prickly lettuce had a significant effect in reducing anxiety and depressive symptoms.

Antihyperglycaemic

A 2019 study to investigate the hypoglycaemic action of Prickly lettuce in male rats indicated that it restored cell function and insulin secretion. Furthermore, the extract improved glucose tolerance significantly, which suggests that it could be applied as a therapy for chronic hyperglycaemia.

Antibacterial

A triterpenoid saponin isolated from the stem possesses antibacterial activity, and in 2022 a study was initiated to investigate the effect of Prickly lettuce against *Porphyromonas gingivalis* and *Prevotella intermedia*, the causes of periodontitis. Results showed strong antibacterial and anti-biofilm activity against both, revealing that Prickly lettuce could be used in the treatment of periodontal disease in respect of its favourable bioactivity, easy availability and simple extraction process.

TOPICAL USES

The milky latex given out by Wild lettuce leaves and stem is traditionally applied topically to cure warts.

DOSAGE

Tisane – ½tsp/2.5g, 3 times per day.
Seed decoction – 3-5gm (Ansari, 1888; Kabir, 1951).

PRECAUTIONS

The Physicians Desk Reference (PDR) for Herbal Medicines 2000 provides a warning about Wild Lettuce that should be equally applied to Prickly lettuce, '*The following signs of poisoning can occur through overdosage or following intake of the fresh leaves, as in salads: outbreaks of sweating, acceleration of breathing, tachycardia, pupil dilation, dizziness, ringing in the ears, vision disorders, pressure in the head, somnolence, on occasion also excitatory states. The toxicity is, however, relatively low. Following gastrointestinal emptying as well as instillation of activated charcoal, the treatment of poisonings should proceed*'.

Avoid if you have enlarged prostate or glaucoma. Members of this plant family can cause allergic reaction. Not suitable for children or those who are pregnant or breastfeeding.

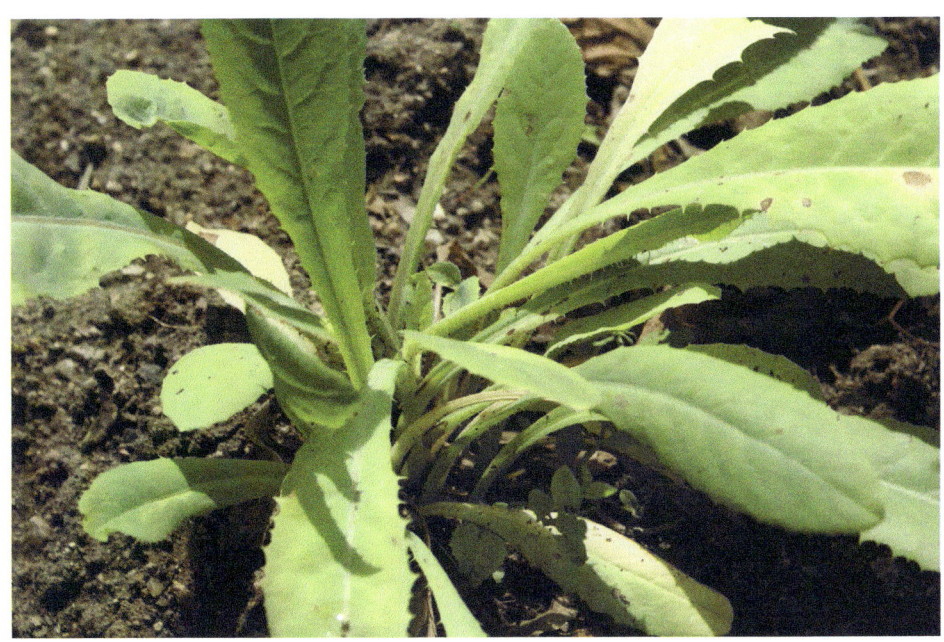

Prickly lettuce recipes

Medicinal recipes

Prickly lettuce tisane

Pour 250ml boiling water over ½tsp /2.5g of the dried leaf and allow to steep for 10-15 minutes, before straining. Use for anxiety, pain relief and as a sedative.

Prickly lettuce seed decoction

Boil 1tsp/5g of the seed in 250ml of water for 15 minutes. Use for headache, insomnia, nervousness, hypertension, etc.

Prickly lettuce infused oil

- 100g dried Prickly lettuce leaves
- 2tbsp alcohol, such as Everclear
- 1l grapeseed oil

Fill a glass jar with the dried Prickly lettuce leaves. Pour the carrier oil over the leaves until they are fully covered. Seal the jar and place it in a sunny spot for 2-3 weeks, shaking it occasionally. Strain the oil through a fine mesh strainer or cheesecloth. Apply the oil to the affected area for pain relief and to reduce inflammation.

Prickly lettuce poultice

- Fresh leaves
- A clean cloth or gauze

Crush or chop fresh Prickly lettuce leaves to release their juices. Apply the crushed leaves directly to the affected area. Cover with a clean cloth or gauze to keep the leaves in place. Leave the poultice on for 20-30 minutes. Remove the poultice and rinse the area with warm water. Use for bruises, insect bites or joint pain.

SCARLET PIMPERNEL
Anagallis arvensis

Scarlet pimpernel is a member of the Primrose family and is commonly found in grasslands, meadows, cultivated fields and disturbed areas. It has a long history of use in traditional medicine and folklore.

HISTORICAL USES

In his *Naturalis Historia*, Pliny wrote that Scarlet pimpernel was good for liver complaints, while in his *De Materia Medica* Dioscorides claimed that it dispelled the depression that followed liver complaints. The Greeks used its juice to cure eye problems, including cataracts.

Early herbalists termed the Scarlet pimpernel (*Anagallis arvensis*) the male, and the blue variety (*A. ccerulea*) the female. Gerard said of 'Pimpernell' in his *Herball* '*Both the sorts of Pimpernell are of a drying faculty without biting, and somewhat hot, with a certaine drawing quality, insomuch that it doth draw forth splinters and things fixed in the flesh. The juyce cures the toothach being snift up into the nosethrils, especially into the contrary nosethril.*'

Nicholas Culpeper mentioned Pimpernel but only in relation to an aquatic species, *Anagallis aquatica*, which we now know as a variety of Speedwell.

In India, the whole plant is used as a

ETYMOLOGY OF COMMON NAME
The flower serves as the emblem of the fictional hero, the Scarlet Pimpernel.

PLANT LORE
In England, the Scarlet pimpernel plant is sometimes called 'shepherd's weatherglass', because the flowers only open in the sunshine, and so can be used to predict the weather.

USE
All parts.

EDIBILITY
Not edible. Has shown some toxicity in grazing mammals.

HARVEST
In summer.

MEDICINAL PROPERTIES
Vulnerary, antimicrobial, anti-inflammatory, spermicidal, uroprotective and hepatoprotective.

ACTIVE CONSTITUENTS
Triterpenoid saponins, flavonoids, alkaloids, coumarins, essential oil.

sedative, stimulant and anti-asthmatic, and an anti-flatulent for cattle. In Navarra, a poultice, decoction, ointment or infusion is used as an antihaemorrhagic and antiseptic. In Taiwan, the whole herb of *Anagallis arvensis* is used for liver complications, and in Italy, *Anagallis arvensis* was used in veterinary practices for curing mastitis, because of its powerful anti-inflammatory and emollient (moisturising) properties.

MODERN RESEARCH

This little plant has some promising properties according to modern research:

Vulnerary and antimicrobial

The traditional use of Pimpernel as a wound-healing remedy was examined in research in 2011 that confirmed the presence of both antimicrobial and anti-inflammatory effects. The methanolic extract was antibacterial against *Escherichia coli* and *Bacillus subtilis* but also produced inhibition in *Candida albicans* and COX-1 and COX-2 enzymes (the measure for anti-inflammatory responses).

The alcoholic extract of herb has been found to be effective for anti-leishmania (ie antiparasitic) activity. Saponins seem to have a role as the antimicrobial constituent, as they can cause damage to cells, and significant activity was recorded for the ethanolic extract of Pimpernel against *Proteus vulgaris*, which is a gram-negative bacillus that can cause urinary tract infections.

Antiviral activity has also been found, but in extracts made with ethanol, for poliovirus as well as for HSV-1. The saponins present in Pimpernel are responsible for its antimicrobial and antiviral properties and have broad spectra that not only inhibit the cytopathogenesis in the host cell but also minimise the production of new viruses.

Spermicidal

Interestingly, the plant has been noted for its semen-coagulating and spermicidal activities. Anagalligenone, the sapogenin isolated from the plant, revealed spermicidal activity in human semen at a concentration of 0.008% and caused the instantaneous immobilisation of spermatozoa in one minute. These findings might help to decrease the incidence of pregnancy without using female contraceptives.

Uroprotective and hepatoprotective

The traditional use of Pimpernel for liver and kidney diseases was evaluated in 2022, and also confirmed. It was found to significantly reduce bladder weight, vesical vascular permeability, oedema and haemorrhage. It was concluded that Pimpernel might act as uroprotective and hepatoprotective owing to the presence of antioxidants.

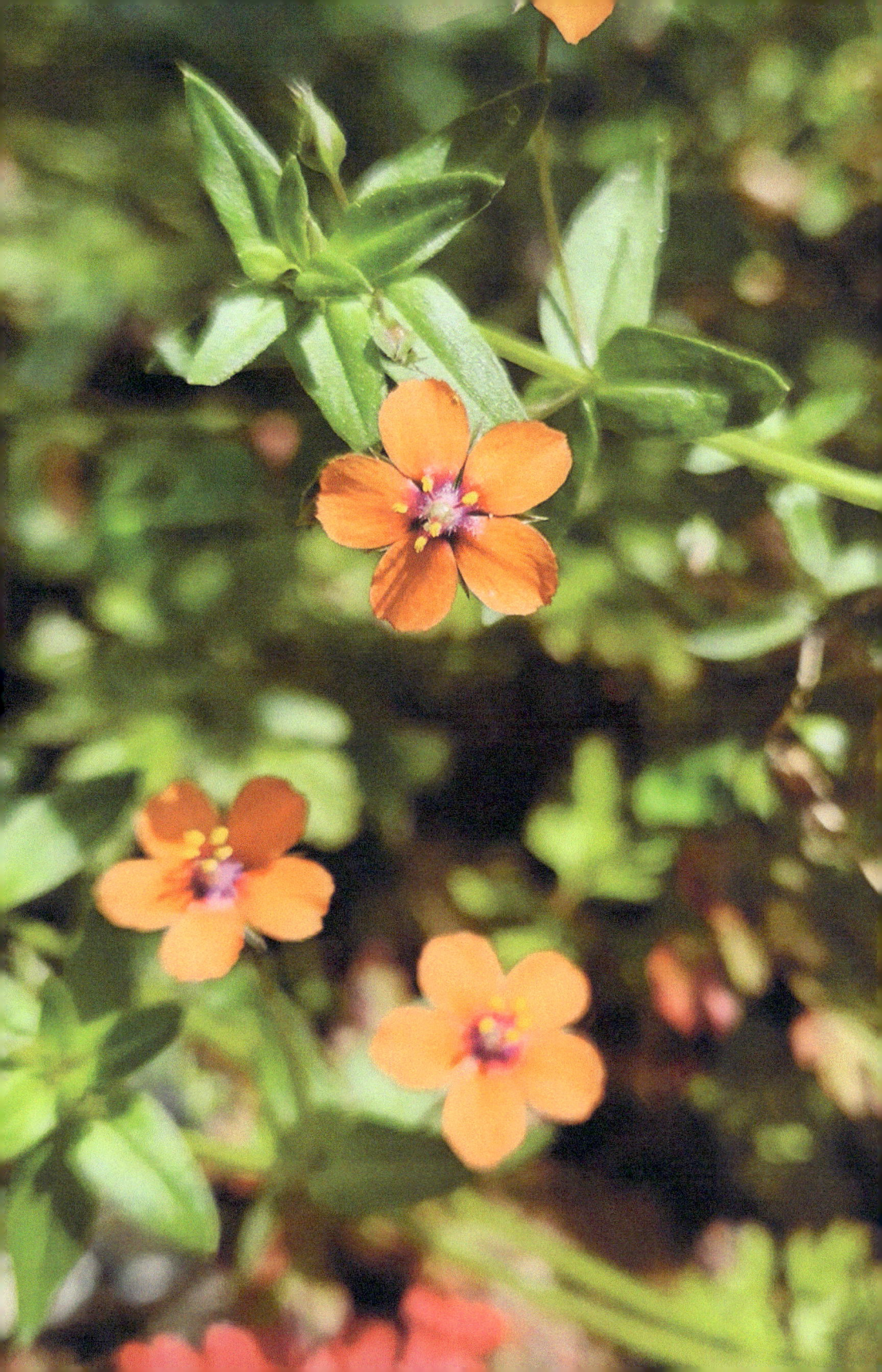

Anticancerogenic

A 2022 study aimed at the effect of Pimpernel on the growth of breast cancer cells showed that it reduced both cell cycle progression and cell growth. Additionally, the oestrogen receptors that develop the cancer were decreased, while the protein that regulates cell survival and the histone γ-H2AX (a tumour suppressor) was increased. Pimpernel therefore has an anticancer effect and is recommended for breast cancer treatment.

TOPICAL USES

The plant is used topically for healing both in humans and animals where it is administered against pruritus, warts and skin inflammations. Pimpernel was the most effective antimycotic agent among 22 tested plant extracts, in the aqueous extract, against *Trichophyton mentagrophytes* (ringworm), *Trichophyton violaceum* (*Tinea capitis*) and *Microsporum canis* (Canine/Feline ringworm).

DOSAGE

Tisane – ½tsp /2.5g, 3 times per day.

PRECAUTIONS

Large doses or long-term administration could lead to gastroenteritis and nephritis, owing to cucurbitacins present in the plant. Not suitable for children or those who are pregnant or lactating.

Scarlet pimpernel recipes

Medicinal recipes

Scarlet pimpernel tisane

Pour 250ml boiling water over ½tsp/2.5g of the dried herb and allow to steep for 10–15 minutes. Sip hourly, for the treatment of liver and kidney disorders, oedema and water retention.

Scarlet pimpernel skin compress

Soak a cloth in a tisane of the dried herb and apply it to the affected areas 2–3 times a day. Use to treat fungal infections such as ringworm.

Scarlet pimpernel poultice

- 1tsp fresh Scarlet pimpernel leaf (if using dried you will need to moisten with water first)
- 2tsp coconut oil
- cheesecloth or cotton bandage

Finely chop the herb into a pulp and add the coconut oil to make a paste. Spread the paste evenly over the desired area and wrap with the cloth or bandage. Use against warts, fungal infections and other skin inflammations.

SELF-HEAL
Prunella vulgaris

Self-heal is native to the UK and is widespread in various habitats, including grasslands, meadows, woodlands and disturbed areas. It is actually part of the Mint family, characterised by its square stems, opposite leaves and spikes of tiny purple flowers. Self-heal has a long history of medicinal use and is valued for its wound-healing and anti-inflammatory properties.

HISTORICAL USES

In his *Herball*, John Gerard recommended Self-heal as follows, '*a decoction made with wine or water, doth join together and make whole and sound all wounds, both inward and outward, even as Bugle doth. Prunel* [Self-heal] *bruised with oil of Roses and vinegar, and laid to the forepart of the head, assuageth and helpeth the pain and aching thereof. To be short, it serveth for the same that Bugle doth, and in the world there are not two better wound herbs, as hath been often proved.*'

Nicholas Culpeper's *Herbal* stated, '*it is an especial herb for inward or outward wounds. Take it inwardly in syrups for inward wounds, outwardly in unguents and plasters for outward. Where the sharp humours of sores, ulcers, inflammations or swellings need to be repressed, this compound will be effectual; it will also*

ETYMOLOGY OF COMMON NAME
Inherited from Middle English *selfhele*, *selfehale* and *sylfhele*, from 'self' and 'heal'.

PLANT LORE
Self-heal was gathered at night, during the dark of the moon by the head Druid with his sacred sickle.

USE
All parts.

EDIBILITY
The leaves and flowers are used in salads.

HARVEST
In summer, when in flower.

MEDICINAL PROPERTIES
Anti-inflammatory, anticancerogenic, antiviral, anti-osteoporosis, haemostatic and tonic.

ACTIVE CONSTITUENTS
Triterpenoid saponins, favonoids, phenolic acids, tannins.

stay the flux of blood from wounds, and solder up their lips, and cleanse the foulness of sores, and speedily heal them. It is a remedy for green wounds.'

In his 1936 book *Herbal Manual*, Harold Ward wrote, *'The 1 ounce to 1 pint infusion is taken in wineglass doses for internal bleeding, used blood-warm as an injection in leucorrhea, and may be used to gargle sore and relaxed throats.'*

MODERN RESEARCH

Culpeper was correct that this plant is an 'especial' herb for inward or outward wounds. Research has so far shown the following:

Anti-inflammatory

The ability of Self-heal, as described by the historical writers, derives from its many active components such as rosmarinic acid and ursolic acid, which have significant anti-inflammatory and immunosuppressive effects. The water extracts of stems and leaves markedly inhibited rat paw swelling and mouse auricular swelling in a 2017 study. It can be applied as a salve to speed the healing of injuries and taken internally to improve healing from surgery and to speed the healing of internal injuries.

The flavonoid extract of the plant shows an anti-osteoperosis effect, increasing bone formation and decreasing trabecular bone loss and bone mass loss. A 2022 study found that when combined with Gentian, the expression of catabolic factors and inflammatory levels was reduced. Administration of the combination in mice with cartilage destruction was shown to inhibit the inflammatory processes, suggesting that the combination could be used as an alternative herbal medicine to treat patients with Osteoarthritis.

Anticancerogenic

Anti-tumour activities of extracts from Self-heal have been investigated and found to inhibit metastasis and promote the apoptosis (programmed cell death) of many kinds of tumour cells through different pathways, significantly inhibiting breast cancer, liver cancer, thyroid cancer cells and lymphoma. A 2021 study into the effects of Self-heal on thyroid cancer cell lines found that it inhibits the proliferation and migration of cells, both *in vitro* and *in vivo*, and suggested that Self-heal has the potential to be developed into a new anticancer drug for the treatment of thyroid cancer.

Antiviral

A number of antiviral studies have identified compounds in Self-Heal that are active against both HIV and *Herpes simplex* virus and were found to decrease HSV-1 and HSV-2 virus lesions in guinea pigs.

An August 2020 study has provided evidence that Self-heal has anti-SARS-CoV-2 activity and may be developed as a novel antiviral approach against COVID-19 infection. To

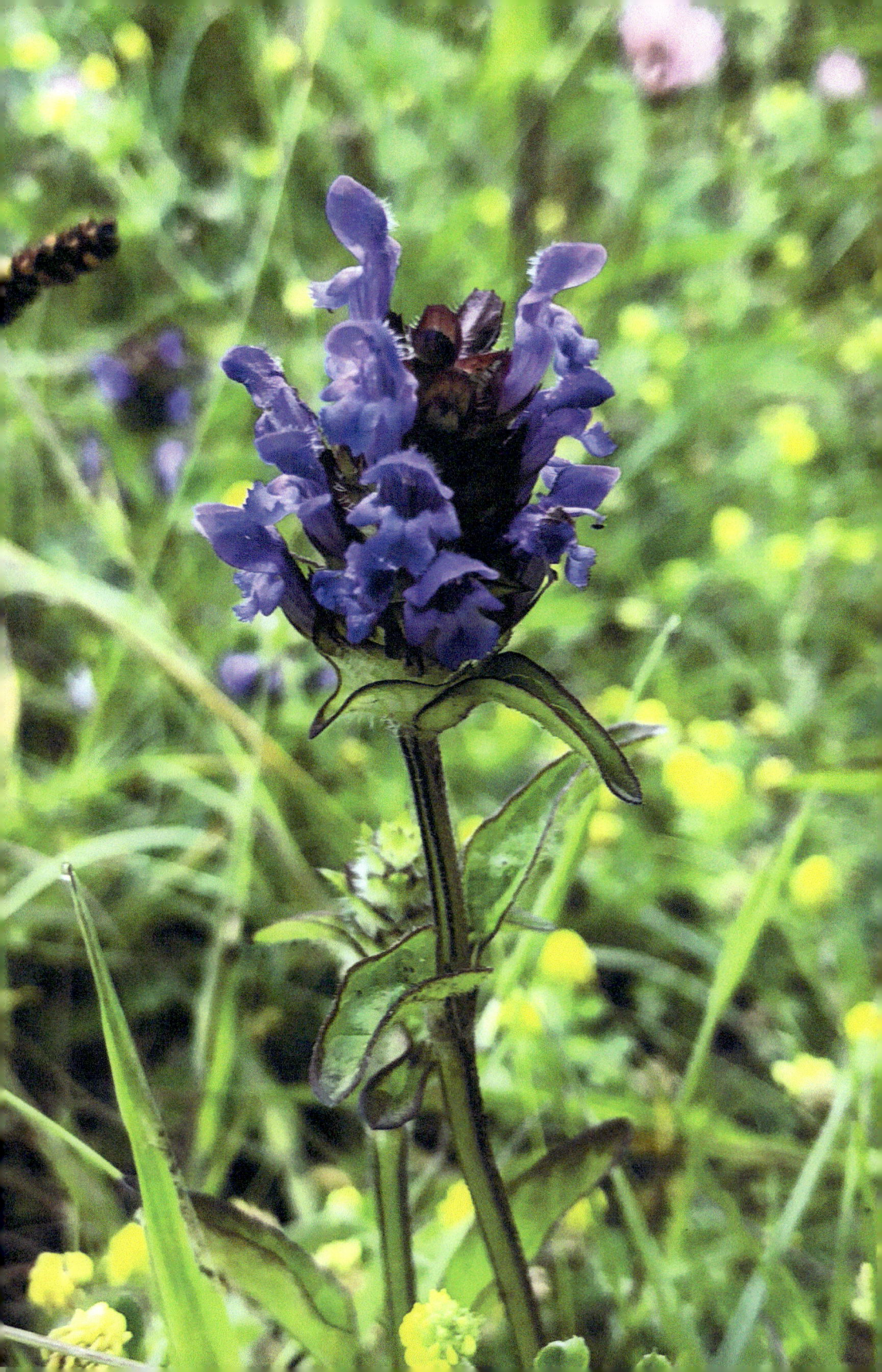

define the mechanisms of the actions, the study demonstrated that Self-heal is able to directly interrupt the virus from binding to its receptor and therefore blocking the virus' entry. The results demonstrated that a combination of Self-heal and the antiparasitic drug suramin increased the blocking effect against SARS-CoV-2.

TOPICAL USES

Self-heal should be part of any topical application for cold sores. It can also be used to clean wounds, and a strong infusion made from the leaves can be used as a mouthwash to promote overall oral health. It can also be used as a sitz bath formula for promoting a faster clearance of *Herpes* outbreaks and tissue repair around the sores.

DOSAGE

Tisane – 1tsp/5g, 2–3 times per day.

PRECAUTIONS

Not suitable for children or those who are pregnant or lactating.

Self-heal recipes

Medicinal recipes

Self-heal tisane

Pour 250ml boiling water over 1tsp/5g of the dried herb and allow to steep for 10–15 minutes. Use after surgery to aid internal healing and as an aid to healing from flu and COVID. It can also be used as a gargle against oral inflammation and sore throat.

Self-heal compress

Soak a cloth in a tisane of the dried herb and apply it to the affected areas 2–3 times a day. Use to treat cuts and wounds, insect bites, or skin irritations and also for haemorrhoids.

Self-heal bath

- 50g Self-heal herb
- 1l of water

Steep the herb in the water for 15 minutes, then strain and add to the bathwater to soothe and heal *Herpes* outbreaks.

Self-heal balm

- 100g dried flowers and leaves
- 2tbsp alcohol, such as Everclear
- 1l grapeseed oil

Place the herbs in a jar with the alcohol and allow to steep for 10 minutes before adding the oil. Leave for 4 weeks and then strain. Make into a salve by using a 1:3 ratio of melted beeswax to oil. Alternatively, make into a balm by using a 1:3 ratio of melted beeswax to your oil mix, ie 1 part wax to 3 parts liquid. Melt the wax pellets in the oil in a double boiler or bain-marie. Remove from the heat and allow to cool and set completely before using as a topical anti-inflammatory treatment for the healing of injuries and cold sores.

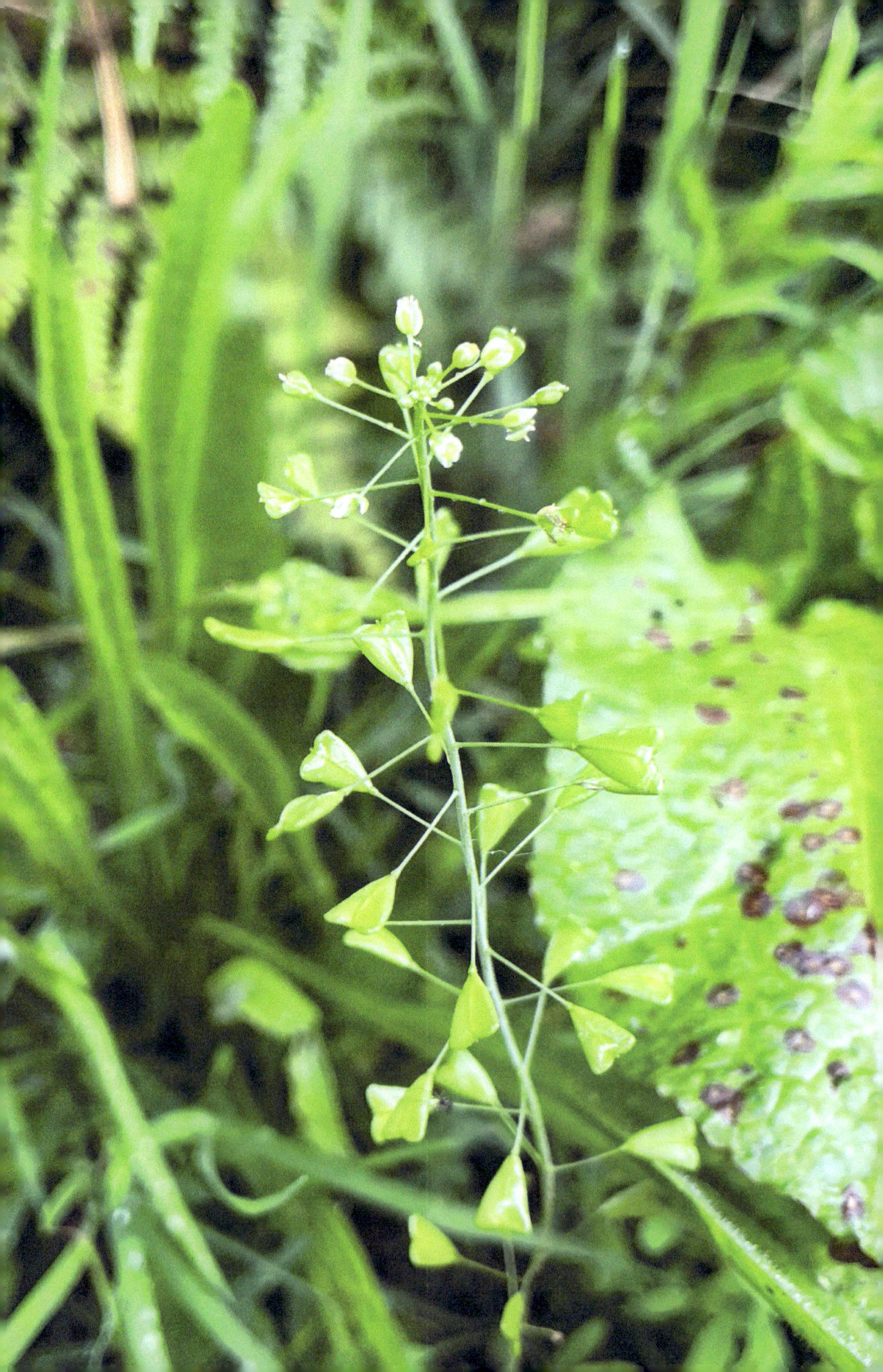

SHEPHERD'S PURSE
Capsella bursa-pastoris

Shepherd's purse is not thought to be native to the UK but has been in the country for so long that it is considered an 'archaeophyte'. It is a member of the Brassicae family and is commonly found in disturbed areas, such as fields, gardens and roadsides. It is characterised by distinctive heart-shaped seed pods. Shepherd's purse has a long history of use in traditional medicine and culinary applications.

HISTORICAL USES

Nicholas Culpeper's *Herbal* said, '*It helps all fluxes of blood, either caused by inward or outward wounds; as also flux of the belly, and bloody flux, spitting blood, and bloody urine, stops the terms in women; being bound to the wrists of the hands, and the soles of the feet, it helps the yellow jaundice. The herb being made into a poultice, helps inflammations and St Anthony's fire* [ergot poisoning]. *The juice being dropped into the ears, heals the pains, noise, and mutterings thereof. A good ointment may be made of it for all wounds, especially wounds in the head.*'

Harold Ward's 1936 book *Herbal Manual* stated, '*The infusion of 1 ounce to 1 pint is administered in wineglass doses for kidney complaints and dropsy. Often combined with Pellitory-of-the-Wall and Juniper berries.*'

ETYMOLOGY OF COMMON NAME
Named from its heart-shaped seed pods, which resemble little pouches that were worn by medieval peasants.

PLANT LORE
Eating the seeds of the first three Shepherd's purse plants one sees is said to protect against all manner of diseases for the rest of the year.

USE
All aerial parts, fresh.

EDIBILITY
As a substitute for cress. The fresh or dried root is a ginger substitute.

HARVEST
In summer.

MEDICINAL PROPERTIES
Astringent, diuretic, emmenagogue, haemostatic/styptic.

ACTIVE CONSTITUENTS
Flavonoids, alkaloids, fatty acids, coumarins.

LEFT: SHEPHERD'S PURSE

MODERN RESEARCH

Shepherd's purse contains various phytochemicals that contribute to its potential medicinal properties as follows:

Diuretic

According to Mills and Bone (2000), Shepherd's purse is a soothing, mildly stimulating diuretic, most indicated in cases of haematuria (blood in the urine) and urinary sediment. These properties may be attributed to its content of flavonoids, potassium and some tannins, and confirms Harold Ward's findings.

Antihaemorrhagic/Styptic

Culpeper was correct to say that Shepherd's purse is excellent to stop bleeding, both internally and externally. It is believed that this is due to its flavonoids and tannins, which help constrict blood vessels, promote blood clotting and reduce bleeding time. In fact it is now approved by the German Commission E for:
- Nosebleeds
- Premenstrual syndrome (PMS)
- Wounds and burns

Shepherd's purse has also been studied in relation to gynaecological conditions and been found to be a uterine antihaemorrhagic. It is utilised in the treatment of uterine myomas, one of the most common causes of menorrhagia (heavy menstrual bleeding). Intravenous and intramuscular injections have been found effective in menorrhagia owing to function abnormalities and fibroids (Weiss, 1988).

In a 2015 clinical trial of 100 women with postpartum haemorrhage the experimental group were given 10 sublingual drops of Shepherd's purse extract plus an infusion of oxytocin, and the control group 10 sublingual drops of the placebo plus an infusion of oxytocin. Results showed a significant decrease in the amount of postpartum bleeding in both groups, but the mean decrease in the amount of bleeding was significantly more in the Shepherd's purse group.

Another clinical study in 2018 took place in patients affected with heavy menstrual bleeding. The experimental group received mefenamic acid every 8 hours and two Shepherd's purse capsules every 12 hours. In the control group, the patients received mefenamic acid and placebo. Compared with the control group, extracts of Shepherd's purse capsule appeared to be more effective in reducing menstrual bleeding.

Anti-inflammatory

In 2019, the anti-inflammation potential of Shepherd's purse was investigated using an *in vivo* mouse paw oedema model and found that inflammatory development process was significantly inhibited by the plant. This again appears to be due to the flavonoid content of Shepherd's purse.

A 2022 study has further found that

the flavonoids in Shepherd's purse can prevent development of cataracts. It is believed that it does so by reducing oxidative stress damage and inhibiting apoptosis (cell death) of lens cells.

Anticancerogenic

Shepherd's purse also contains Fumaric acid and this was shown to have an inhibitory effect on tumours in mice in 1979. In fact, the extract caused 50 to 80% inhibition of the solid growth of Ehrlich tumour cells of the animals. The Chemoprevention Branch (National Cancer Institute, National Institutes of Health) has tested dozens of chemopreventive compounds in rats and found that significant chemopreventive (i.e., anticancer) effects have been produced with fumaric acid (Boone et al., 1992).

In 2019, cancer cells were exposed to hot water extracts of both Broccoli and Shepherd's purse for a 72-hour period, and results showed that while Broccoli inhibited the growth of cancer by only 13%, Shepherd's purse showed an inhibitory rate of 67%.

TOPICAL USES

Shepherd's purse is sometimes applied directly to the skin as an infusion of 3–5g drug to 150ml water for nosebleeds, superficial burns and bleeding skin injuries.

DOSAGE

Tisane – 1tsp/5g, 3 times per day.
Tincture – 1:5 45%, 1–2tsp in water – 20 drops = 1ml/1tsp = 5ml.

PRECAUTIONS

It is recommended that this herb be avoided in cases of cortisone treatments, birth control pill treatments, insomnia, psychic or neurological diseases showing hyperactivity, depressive states, hyperthyroid, epilepsy, Parkinson's disease, paralysis, leukaemia or allergies. Not suitable for children or those who are pregnant or lactating.

Shepherd's purse recipes

NB: The dried herb quickly loses its effectiveness and should not be stored for more than a year.

Medicinal recipes

Shepherd's purse tisane

Pour 250ml boiling water over 1tsp/5g of the fresh herb and allow to steep for 10-15 minutes. Use for the treatment of internal bleeding, heavy periods, etc. Can also be used externally to soothe the skin and stop bleeding.

Shepherd's purse infused tincture – 1:5 45%

If you are using 40% alcohol, ie. vodka, make a simple tincture by covering 1 part herb to 5 parts fluid.

If you are using Everclear or other 100% proof, use the following method for a specific tincture:

- 100g fresh Sheperd's purse herb
- 225ml alcohol
- 200ml water

Cover 50g fresh herb with 225ml alcohol. Then steep/infuse another 50g of fresh herb in 200ml of water (adjusted to take into account the latent water content of the fresh herb) for 15 minutes. Strain thoroughly and top up if the water is less than 200ml. Add the infusion to the herb and alcohol mix and leave for 14 days before straining. Use for the treatment of nephrolithiasis (kidney stones).

Shepherd's purse poultice

- 1tsp fresh leaf (if using dried you will need to moisten with water first)
- 2tsp coconut oil
- cheesecloth or cotton bandage

Finely chop the herb into a pulp and add the coconut oil to make a paste. Spread the paste evenly over the desired area and wrap with the cloth or bandage. Use to heal bleeding wounds, as well against rheumatic and muscular pain.

SOLOMON'S SEAL
Polygonatum spp.

In the UK, there are several species of *Polygonatum*, commonly known as Solomon's seal, that are native or have become naturalised over time. I am concentrating on two native species, Fragrant Solomon's seal (*Polygonatum odoratum*) and Common Solomon's seal (*Polygonatum multiflorum*).

HISTORICAL USES
In his *Herball*, John Gerard noted that, '*As touching the knitting of bones and that truly which might be written, there is not another herb to be found comparable to it for the purposes aforesaid; and therefore in briefe, if it be for bruises inward, the roots muſt be ſtamped, some ale or wine put thereto and ſtrained and given to drinke … as well unto themselves as to their cattle, it being applied 'outwardly in the manner of a pultis' for external bruises.*'

Nicholas Culpeper's *Herbal* added that: '*The root of Solomon's Seal is found by experience to be available in wounds, hurts, and outward sores, to heal and close up the lips of those that are green, and to dry up and reſtrain the flux of humours to those that are old. It is singularly good to ſtay vomitings and bleeding wheresoever, as also all fluxes in man or woman; also, to knit any joint, which by weakness uses to be often out of place, or will not ſtay in long*

ETYMOLOGY OF COMMON NAME
From the root depressions that supposedly look like the marks of a wax seal of King Solomon.

PLANT LORE
The biblical King Solomon is said to have placed his seal upon this plant when he recognised its great medicinal value.

USE
The root.

EDIBILITY
The young shoots of the plants may be boiled and served like asparagus.

HARVEST
In autumn.

MEDICINAL PROPERTIES
Antidiabetic, vulnerary, anti-inflammatory, demulcent and tonic.

ACTIVE CONSTITUENTS
Saponins, phenolics, steroidal saponins, polysaccharides and lectins.

when it is set; also to knit and join broken bones in any part of the body, the roots being bruised and applied to the places; yea, it hath been found by experience ... It is no less effectual to help ruptures and burstings, the decoction in wine, or the powder in broth or drink, being inwardly taken, and outwardly applied to the place. The same is also available for inward or outward bruises, falls or blows, both to dispel the congealed blood, and to take away both the pains and the black and blue marks that abide after the hurt.'

The rhizome of both species is famous in Traditional Chinese Medicine and used as a nutritious tonic for removing dryness, promoting secretion of fluid and quenching thirst. It is also a remedy in TCM to treat lung disease and upset stomachs, improve insulin resistance and diabetes (*P. odoratum*) aid liver injury, cancer, diabetes, alopecia, atherosclerosis and neurodegenerative diseases (*P. multiflorum*).

MODERN RESEARCH

Like its relative, Lily-of-the-valley, Solomon's seal contains convallarin, a poisonous glycoside, though in small enough amounts to be therapeutic rather than toxic and have a mildly regulating effect on the heart. Modern research has so far discovered the following other properties for this plant:

Antidiabetic

In the traditional treatment of diabetes mentioned above, administration is via a decoction of Fragrant Solomon's seal root and was confirmed in a 2009 study. A 9-day treatment significantly reduced blood glucose levels in type-1 diabetic mice and showed that the blood glucose levels in treated groups were steadily lowered during the whole experiment. In another experiment, a 30-day administration with extracts was shown to prevent and reduce hyperglycaemia in type-2 diabetic rats.

Vulnerary

As John Gerard pointed out, this plant is wonderful as a vulnerary. The root is astringent as well as demulcent, both qualities that speed up the healing process; in addition, the roots also contain allantoin, a substance also contained in Comfrey, which led to that plant being called knitbone. It also contains polysaccharides that are particularly useful in the joints, tendons and ligaments to improve flexibility and range of motion. A 2014 study using rats showed that their wounds dressed with Fragrant Solomon's seal root showed considerable signs of faster healing compared with those who received the placebo control treatment.

Cognitive support

One of Common Solomon's seal's main uses is in the prevention of neurodegenerative diseases and cognitive decline. The main constituents relevant for this are anthraquinones, particularly emodin, which has been shown to have a protective effect against brain

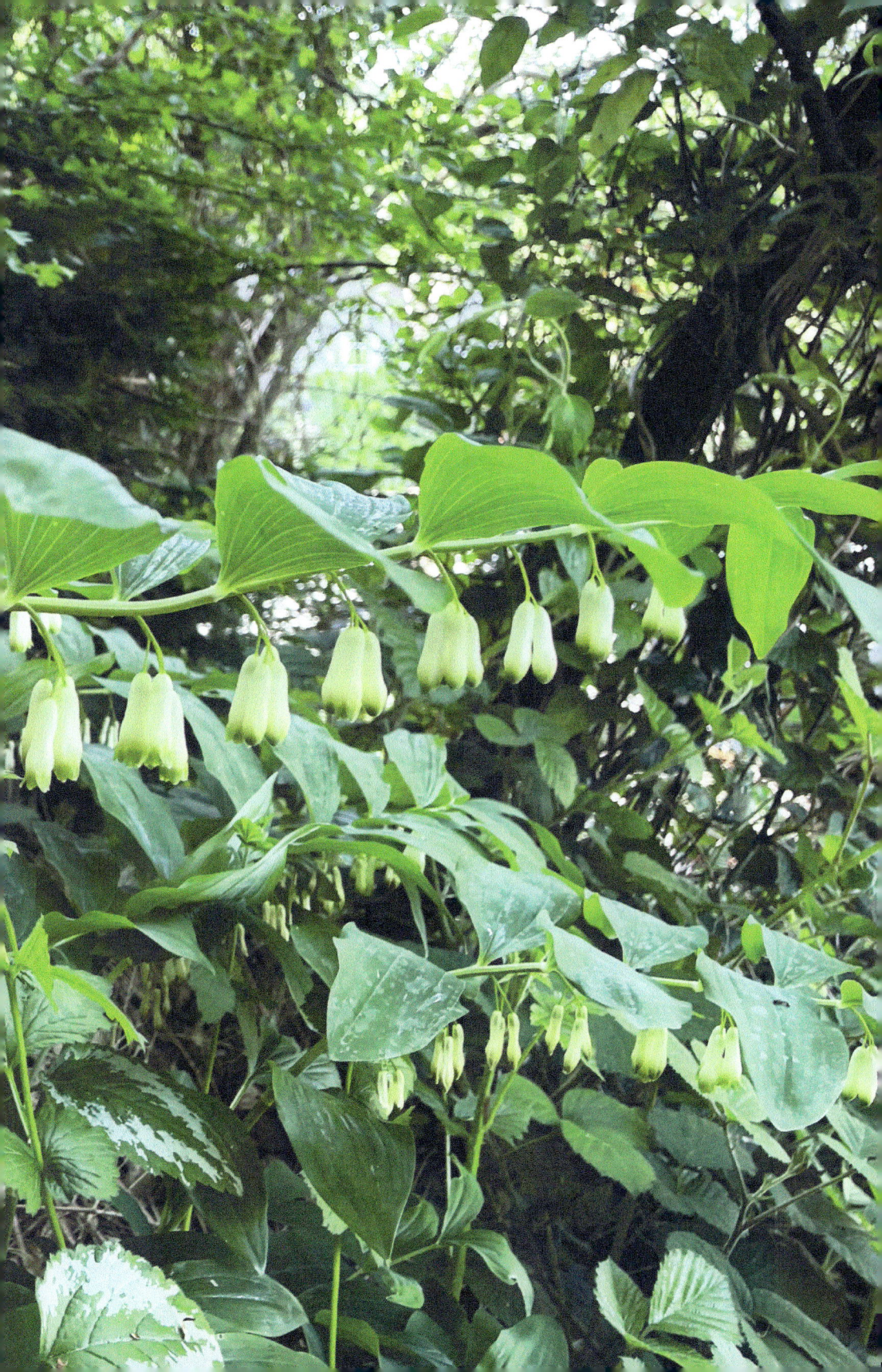

disturbances induced by severe cerebral injury (Gu et al., 2003), and also to inhibit lipid peroxidation in rat brain cells (Sato et al., 1992).

Anti-inflammatory

People have traditionally used Solomon's seal (both varieties) to ease heartburn, ulceration and indigestion caused by inflammation, and a 2016 study confirmed that this activity is attritutable to the quercitrin and scutellarein-7-glucoside in the plant.

Expectorant

Choong (2004) reported that Solomon's seal is used for the treatment of respiratory diseases in Eastern medicine, and Lee et al. (also in 2004) found that it is the kaempferol derived from the plant that was responsible for this efficacy. A 2015 study then demonstrated that the plant acted by increasing airway mucin-secreting cells and suggested its possible use as a mild expectorant during the treatment of chronic airway diseases.

Antiosteoporotic

In a 2014 study a combined extract of *Morus alba* (Mulberry) and Solomon's seal leaves increased the density of cells that form bone tissue. The increased cortical thickness and density of bone-forming cells in the tibia were also observed. This effect is probably related to the calcium, potassium and phosphorus, in the root, which are essential for bone strength and density.

Antimicrobial

Solomon's seal contains saponins, which are phytochemicals known for their antimicrobial properties, including effectivess against bacteria, fungi and viruses. A 2018 study on Solomon's seal leaf and stem extracts found that it possessed high antibacterial effects against *Staphylococcus epidermidis*, *Enterococcus faecium*, *Enterococcus faecalis* and *Staphylococcus aureus*.

TOPICAL USES

As mentioned, Solomon's seal is astringent as well as demulcent, both qualities that speed up healing, and it is known for external use in the treatment of bruises, ulcers or boils, redness of the skin and for bruises.

DOSAGE

Up to 250mg daily, but also see below.

PRECAUTIONS

Overdosage of Solomon's seal can lead to nausea, diarrhoea, gastric complaints and queasiness. In recent years, there have been increasing reports of hepatotoxicity that have affected the clinical efficacy and safety of Common Solomon's seal in particular. It is not suitable for children or those who are pregnant or lactating.

Solomon's seal recipes

Medicinal recipes

Solomon's seal cold infusion

Steep 2tsp of the root in 1 litre of cold water overnight and drink a cup up to 3 times per day as a mild expectorant, to soothe heartburn, ulceration and indigestion, and promote overall well-being.

A herbal healing salve

- 1 part Solomon's seal
- 1 part Calendula
- 1 part Comfrey
- 1 part Horsetail
- 1 part Daisy
- 1 part St John's wort
- 2tbsp alcohol, such as Everclear
- 1l grapeseed oil

Place the herbs in a jar with the alcohol and allow to steep for 10 minutes before adding the oil. Leave for 4 weeks and then strain. Make into a salve by using a 1:4 ratio of melted beeswax to oil. Weigh or measure out the wax pellets and place them with the herbal infused oil in a double boiler or bain-marie. Heat over a low heat until the wax is fully melted and then stir well. Remove from the heat and allow to cool slightly. Use for the relief of muscular-skeletal discomfort associated with sprains, muscle strain, joint flexibility, etc.

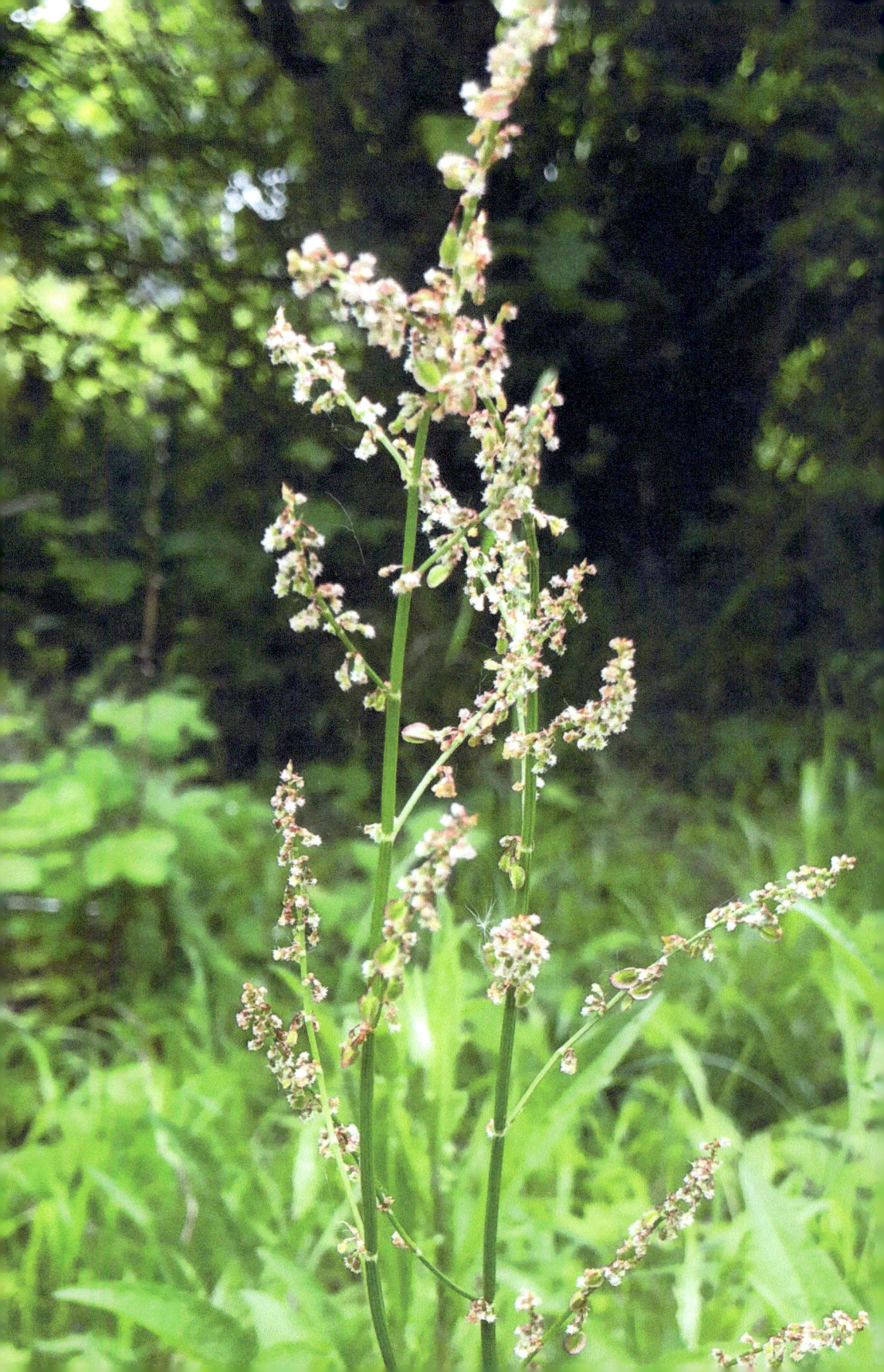

SORRELS
Rumex spp.

Common sorrel is probably the best known of the Sorrels. It belongs to the *Rumex* family, which includes the Docks and approximately 200 other species in the Buckwheat family. It is commonly used as a culinary herb, adding a tangy flavour to salads, soups, sauces and other dishes. It is also used as a traditional medicinal herb.

HISTORICAL USES

In his *Herball*, John Gerard counted eight different kinds of Sorrel: Garden, Bunched or Knobbed, Sheep's, Roman or Round-leaved, Curled, Barren, Dwarf sheep's and Great broad-leaved Sorrel, and said of them, '*The Sorrells are moderately cold and dry. Sorrell doth undoubtedly cool and mightily dry, but because it is sour, it likewise cutteth tough humours. The juice hereof in summertime is a profitable sauce in many meats and pleasant to the taſte. It cooleth a hot ſtomach ... The leaves are with good success added to decoctions which are used in agues. The leaves taken in good quantity, ſtamped and ſtrained into some ale ... cooleth the sick body. The leaves are eaten in manner of a spinach tart ... The seed of Sorrell drunk in wine ſtoppeth the lask and bloody flux.*'

Nicholas Culpeper's *Herbal* explained, '*The decoction of the roots is*

ETYMOLOGY OF COMMON NAME
Late Middle English *sorele*, of Germanic origin; related to 'sour' after the taste of the leaves.

PLANT LORE
It was believed that the cuckoo eats sorrel leaves to strengthen its voice.

USE
The leaves, seed and root.

EDIBILITY
Yes in moderation; the leaves have a tangy, sour-lemon flavour.

HARVEST
From April to November.

MEDICINAL PROPERTIES
Diuretic, laxative, antioxidant, cytotoxic, antimicrobial, anti-inflammatory, antihypertensive and antihyperglyceemic.

ACTIVE CONSTITUENTS
Oxalic acid, flavonoids, anthraquinones, tannins.

LEFT: COMMON SORREL

taken to help the jaundice, and to expel the gravel and the stone in the reins or kidneys. The decoction of the flowers made with wine and drank, helps the black jaundice, as also the inward ulcers of the body and bowels. A syrup made with the juice of Sorrel and fumitory, is a sovereign help to kill those sharp humours that cause the itch. The juice thereof, with a little vinegar, serves well to be used outwardly for the same cause, and is also profitable for tetters, ringworms, etc. It helps also to discuss [soften] *the kernels in the throat; and the juice gargled in the mouth, helps the sores therein.'*

MODERN RESEARCH

Sorrel has been used in folk remedies from ancient times to treat various health disorders, and modern research has so far confirmed the following:

Diuretic

Sorrel stimulates the flow of urine, thereby ensuring detoxification of the kidneys. This explains Culpeper's use of it 'to expel the gravel and the stone in the reins or kidneys'.

Antimicrobial

Gescher et al. in 2011 reported the antiviral nature of the extract from the aerial parts of Sorrel. Their results showed high amounts of oligomeric and polymeric proanthocyanins and flavonoids, which displayed significant antiviral activity against *Herpes simplex* virus type 1 (HSV-1).

Beckert and Hensel, in 2013, then reported antibacterial activity of Sorrel against the gram-negative bacterium *Porphyromonas gingivalis,* which is regarded as one of the main agents of periodontitis and often known as 'gum disease'. The seed of the plant is also used to manage haemorrhages owing to its astringent property (Felter and Lloyd, 2016; Hussain et al., 2015; Vasas et al., 2015). Both of these findings may explain Culpeper's use of the juice, which when 'gargled in the mouth, helps the sores therein'.

Anti-inflammatory

Anti-inflammatory activity of several Sorrel species was evaluated and the authors discovered that the rhizome extracts of Common sorrel and Sheep's sorrel both showed significant inhibitory action against COX-1 (inhibitors of COX enzymes are used in medications that treat chronic pain syndromes. They are in the anti-inflammatory class of drug) (Mimica-Dukić, 2016).

Antioxidant and anticancerogenic

The antioxidant capacity of Sorrel is reported to be approximately the same as that in Japanese green tea (Alzoreky and Nakahara 2001). Antioxidants can inhibit the growth and proliferation of cancer cells, and strong cytotoxic properties from Sorrel have been shown against five human tumour cell lines including lung, ovarian, central nervous system, intestines and melanoma.

The high levels of antioxidants in Sheep's sorrel have also been

RIGHT: WOOD SORREL

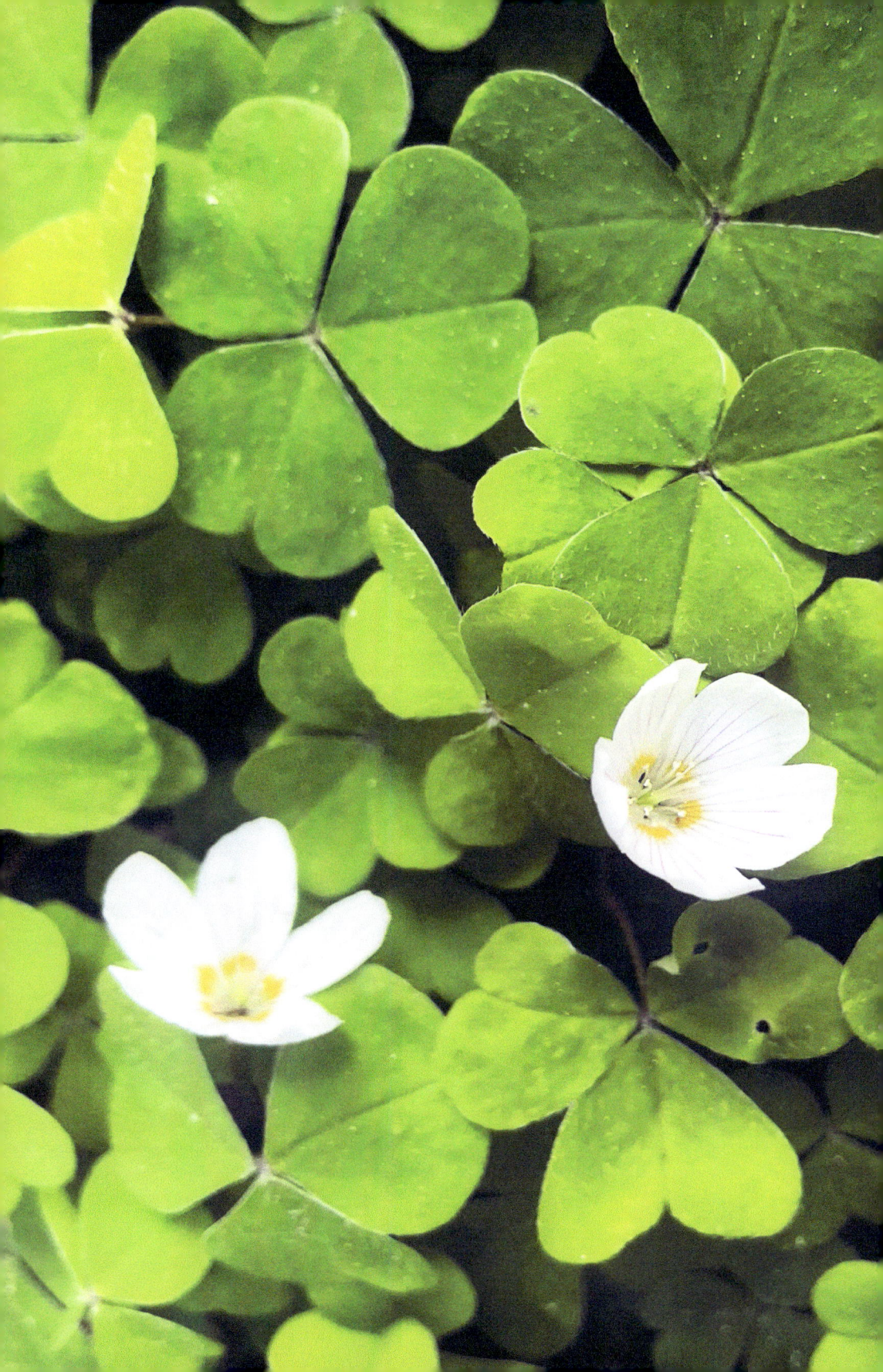

demonstrated by *in vitro* studies. This level of antioxidant activity may be the reason for the inclusion of this herb in the alternative cancer remedy Essiac (made together with Burdock, Slippery elm and Turkey rhubarb). This remedy was originally a herbal formulation from the Ojibwe Indians in Canada and was discovered in 1922 by Rene Caisse, a Canadian nurse whose aunt, after using the remedy for two years, fully recovered from an inoperable stomach cancer with liver involvement. Other terminal patients taking the remedy began to improve, and Caisse eventually handed over the recipe to the Resperin Corporation in 1977, for the sum of one dollar, so that cancer patients might obtain the mixture. Essiac has been shown to inhibit cell proliferation and induce differentiation in human prostate cancer cell lines (Ottenweller et al., 2004; Tai et al., 2004).

I have not been able to find any published human clinical studies of the Essiac formula. However, a laboratory study revealed that, among mice injected with human cancer cells, those given oral and intravenous Essiac showed more tumour necrosis and cell degradation than the control mice.

Essiac has been found to exhibit significant antioxidant activity with immunomodulating effects. It also exhibited significant cell-specific cytotoxicity towards ovarian carcinoma cells, and in another *in vitro* study indicating inhibition of tumour growth in prostate cells.

In 2018, rats with leukaemia were treated with a water extract of the same four herbs above and the animals successfully recovered weight loss and restored normal total white blood cell, lymphocyte and neutrophil counts. Results showed that S1PR1 (a receptor that promotes cancer proliferation) decreased by 14.6-fold in the leukemic rats after using this plant mixture.

Antihypertensive

Finally, a 2018 study showed that Common sorrel can reduce the risks of hypertension and even possibly stroke, as seen by preliminary data conducted in a rat model.

Antihyperglycaemic

2020 research into Sheep's sorrel for antihyperglycaemic potential found that nearly all the extracts exerted strong inhibition and, in particular, alcohol extracts showed outstanding inhibition of enzymes related to type-2 diabetes. These findings suggest that these alcohol extracts may provide alternative approaches for diabetes therapy as antihyperglycaemic agents.

TOPICAL USES

Traditionally, water from boiled Sorrel has been used to wash chicken pox sores, boils, shingles-afflicted skin, poison ivy rashes, blisters, acne and other skin sores. It is thought to ease pain, relieve itches and speed up the healing process.

DOSAGE

Sorrel can be eaten directly in salad or as a dressing when mixed with olive oil.

PRECAUTIONS

Oxalate poisonings are conceivable only with the consumption of very large quantities of the leaves as a salad. Bello et al. (2019) showed that cooking reduces the oxalic acid concentration of *Rumex acetosa* to a negligible amount. Not suitable for children or those who are pregnant or lactating.

Sorrel recipes

Medicinal recipes

Sorrel decoction

Pour 250ml boiling water over 1tsp/5g of the dried herb and lightly simmer for 5-10 minutes. Use for respiratory issues and as a gargle for gum disease. Use topically to wash chicken pox sores, boils, shingles-afflicted skin, rashes, blisters, acne and other skin sores. It is supposed to ease pain, relieve itches and speed up the healing process.

Sorrel infused tincture – 1:5 45%

If you are using 40% alcohol, ie. vodka, make a simple tincture by covering 1 part herb to 5 parts fluid.

If you are using Everclear or other 100% proof, use the following method for a specific tincture:

- 100g dried Sorrel herb
- 225ml alcohol
- 275ml water

Cover 50g dried herb with 225ml alcohol. Then steep/infuse another 50g of dried herb in 275ml of water for 15 minutes. Strain thoroughly and top up if the water is less than 275ml. Add the infusion to the dried herb and alcohol mix, and leave for 14 days before straining. Use for gastritis and gastric ulcers.

Lemon aid

- 120g Sheep's sorrel leaves (crushed)
- 600ml water
- 30ml/2tbsp honey
- a few Mint leaves

Mix all of the ingredients and serve after 15 minutes for its antioxidant effects.

SPEEDWELL
Veronica spp.

There are many species of Speedwells native and naturalised in the UK. All belong to the *Veronica* genus and are characterised by small blue flowers.

HISTORICAL USES

Nicholas Culpeper's *Herbal* described this as a '*small and very useful plant*'. He went on to say, '*it is also reckoned among the vulnerary plants, both used inwardly and outwardly: it is likewise pectoral, and good for coughs and consumptions; and is helpful against the stone and strangury, as also against pestilential fevers. An infusion of the leaves, drank constantly in the manner of tea, is greatly recommended as a provocative to venery, and a strengthener; it has been called a cure for barrenness, taken a long time in this manner.*'

In her 1894 *Occult Family Physician and Botanic Guide to Health*, Antonette Matteson recommended an infusion, which, '*taken freely, opens all obstructions in the kidneys and bladder, also the pores of the skin. It is an excellent cleanser of the blood. It removes blotches and cutaneous eruptions. It is one of the best medicines for children in the spring, combined with some one of the medicines recommended under that head.*'

In Romanian folk medicine, Common speedwell has been used for kidney

ETYMOLOGY OF COMMON NAME
From the propensity for most *Veronica* blooms to lose their petals after just a few days.

PLANT LORE
Associated with magical ointments allowing mortals to see faeries, and with healing afflictions of the eyes.

USE
All parts.

EDIBILITY
The raw flowers are edible and a decorative addition to salads.

HARVEST
When in flower.

MEDICINAL PROPERTIES
Antimicrobial, antitussive, expectorant and tonic.

ACTIVE CONSTITUENTS
Iridoid glycosides, flavonoids, triterpenoids, phenolic acids.

diseases, coughs and catarrh, and was known for its wound-healing properties and its indication in lung diseases and hypercholesterolemia.

MODERN RESEARCH

Most modern research pertains to *Veronica officinalis* (Common speedwell) and *Veronica persica* (Bird's eye speedwell), though there are many other varieties of Speedwell with varying degrees of medicinal properties as follows:

Antimicrobial

In a 2015 analysis of Common speedwell (and others) activity against gram-positive bacteria like *Listeria monocytogenes*, *Listeria ivanovii* and *Staphylococcus aureus* was attributed at least in part to the high β-sitosterol content, but also to the presence of campesterol and stigmasterol.

In 2018, Bird's eye speedwell was analysed for its antimicrobial, scolicidal (anti-tapeworm) and anti-inflammatory activities. The results presented *Bacillus subtilis* as the most susceptible to the extract, while *Pseudomonas aeruginosa* was the most resistant strain. The extracts demonstrated significant activity against *Echinococcus granulosus* (tapeworm) with dose-dependent inhibitions of the juvenile worms.

Bird's eye speedwell extract also demonstrated antiviral activity (against *Herpes simplex* viruses HSV-1 and HSV-2) and an antifungal effect against *Candida albicans* and *Aspergillus niger* (Sharifi-Rad et al., 2018).

Anti-inflammatory and expectorant

Bird's eye speedwell has also exhibited high anti-inflammatory activities and this, in addition to its antimicrobial activity, makes it promising as a treatment of infectious, neurodegenerative and inflammatory disorders.

A 2013, a study sought to confirm the traditional use of Common speedwell for the treatment of lung diseases, finding that it reduced inflammation in the lungs by suppressing white blood cell activation, which validates the observations by Culpeper of the plant as a respiratory healer.

A 2022 study aimed at comparing the effect of Bird's eye speedwell on the airways, showed that the plant significantly reduced inflammation in the lung tissue and showed for the first time that Bird's eye speedwell also effectively suppresses white blood cell activation, and inhibits eotaxin cells, making it a potential pharmacological agent to prevent inflammatory airway diseases related to allergies.

TOPICAL USES

Common speedwell is also administered externally in the form of an ointment or lotion as a healing agent with antimicrobial and anti-inflammatory effects. In 2015, a clinical study was conducted on a topical cream made from an extract of Common speedwell. Results showed that after 56 days of treatment, wrinkles decreased significantly, with dermatological scores 66% lower than

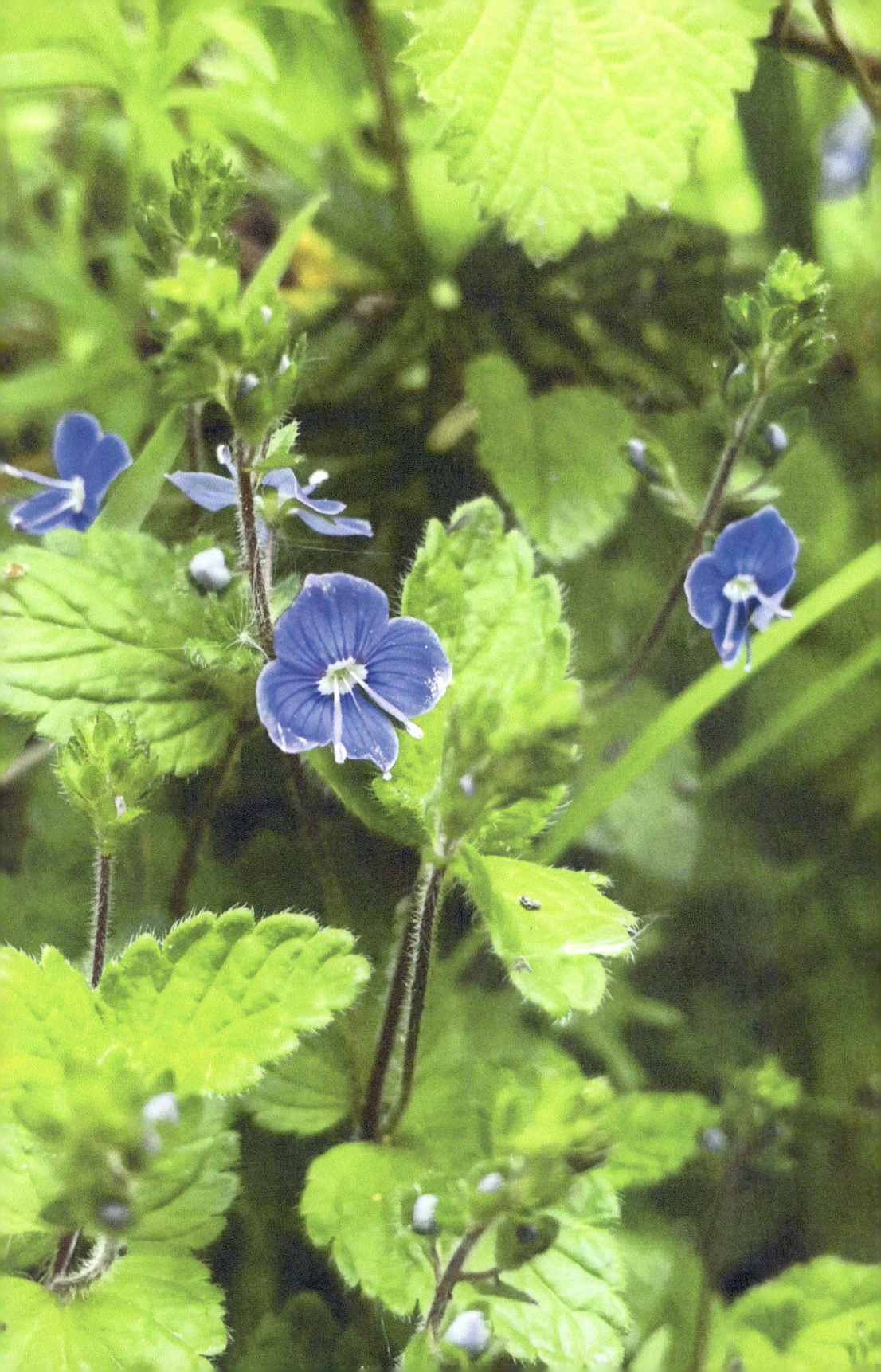

that of placebo treatment, demonstrating that Speedwell is a potent anti-wrinkle agent in human skin.

In 2018 a pharmaceutical formulation consisting of a microemulsion of Bird's eye speedwell was tested for anti-inflammatory effects on rat paw oedema and resulted in a total reduction of inflammation.

DOSAGE

Tisane – 1tsp/5g. Drink a half cup 3–4 times per day.

PRECAUTIONS

Not suitable for children or those who are pregnant or lactating.

Speedwell recipes

Medicinal recipes

Bird's eye speedwell tisane

Pour 250ml boiling water over 1–2tsp/5–10g of the dried leaf and flower and allow to steep for 10–15 minutes. Use to ease the discomfort of the respiratory, gastrointestinal and lower urinary tracts.

Speedwell compress

Soak a cloth in a tisane of the dried herb and apply it to the affected areas 2–3 times a day. Use for ulcers, wounds and eczema.

Common speedwell infused oil

- 100g Speedwell herb
- 2tbsp alcohol, such as Everclear
- 1l grapeseed oil

Place the herbs in a jar with the alcohol and allow to steep for 10 minutes before adding the oil. Leave for 4 weeks and then strain. Use as a topical healing treatment and anti-wrinkle balm.

Speedwell poultice

- fresh Speedwell leaves and/or flowers
- hot water
- clean cloth or gauze

Mix the chopped herbs with enough hot water to form a paste. Spread the paste onto a clean cloth or gauze. Apply the poultice directly to the affected area of the skin, such as wounds, bruises or insect bites. Leave the poultice on for 20–30 minutes before removing and rinsing the area with cool water.

SPURGES
Euphorbia spp.

There are many species of Spurge to be found in the UK. The focus here is on *Euphorbia peplus* (Petty spurge), characterised by small, inconspicuous green flowers, and *Euphorbia helioscopia* (Sun spurge), which is slightly larger and has yellow–green flowers. Both have a milky sap, which is toxic and can cause irritation to the skin and eyes in some individuals. Despite this toxicity, spurges have traditionally been used in herbal medicine.

HISTORICAL USES

John Gerard said of 'Sunne Spurge' in his *Herball*, '*First the milke and sap is in speciall use, then the fruit and leaves, but the root is of least strength.*' He also writes of tasting Spurge, '*Some write by report of others, that it enflameth exceedingly, but my selfe speak by experience; for walking along the sea coast at Lee in Essex, with a Gentleman called Mr. Rich, dwelling in the same towne, I tooke but one drop of it into my mouth; which neverthelesse did so inflame and swell in my throte that I hardly escaped with my life. And in like case was the Gentleman, which caused us to take our horses, and poste for our lives unto the next farme house to drinke some milke to quench the extremitie of our heat, which then ceased.*'

Nicholas Culpeper's *Herbal* stated,

ETYMOLOGY OF COMMON NAME
Spurge is from the Latin ex and *purgare* meaning to 'purge out', and refers to the purgative properties of these plants.

PLANT LORE
In European folklore, Petty spurge was believed to protect against evil spirits and was hung above doorways and windows to ward off evil.

USE
The caustic sap.

EDIBILITY
Not edible! TOXIC.

HARVEST
In summer.

MEDICINAL PROPERTIES
Anticancerogenic, anti-inflammatory, antimicrobial, antidiabetic.

ACTIVE CONSTITUENTS
Diterpenoids, latex, flavonoids, alkaloids, triterpenes.

'It is a strong cathartic, working violently by vomit and stool, but is very offensive to the stomach and bowels by reason of its sharp corrosive quality, and therefore ought to be used with caution.'

MODERN RESEARCH

As Culpeper said, Spurge should be used internally with caution. Its traditional use was to treat digestive problems as it has a purgative effect, but with many other safer alternatives, Spurge is no longer used internally. Externally, the plants have been used for centuries as traditional folk medicine for treating sunburns, corns and waxy growths. Much of the modern research is concentrated in this area as follows:

Anticancerogenic

In 2011, scientists in Australia carried out a clinical study of the sap of Petty spurge on 36 patients with non-melanoma skin cancer lesions. The patients were treated once a day for three consecutive days using a cotton bud to apply enough of the sap to cover the surface of each lesion. After one month 41 of the 48 cancers had completely gone. In all cases of successful treatment, the skin was left with a good cosmetic appearance.

Further studies have shown that both Petty and Sun spurge markedly inhibit the proliferation of cancer cell lines, such as breast, colorectal and lung cell lines, which means that they could be exploited as cancer treatments after further evaluation.

Anti-inflammatory

In 2013, the antimicrobial, pharmacological and cytotoxic activities of the different extracts were evaluated and found to have anti-inflammatory activity compared with indomethacin (an NSAID). All the extracts exhibited significant analgesic activity.

Antimicrobial

The above study also tested Petty spurge extracts against *Staphylococcus aureus*, *Bacillus subtilis*, *Salmonella typhi*, *Escherichia coli* and *Candida albicans*. The ethanol and methanolic extracts showed high antimicrobial activity against all strains, which the authors conclude was caused by the presence of phenolics, triterpenes and sterols.

Similarly, in 2020, Sun surge extracts were tested against six human pathogenic microorganisms: *Escherichia coli*, *Bacillus subtilis*, *Staphylococcus aureus*, *Klebsiella pneumoniae*, *Salmonella typhi* and *Pseudomonas aeruginosa*; and three fungal strains: *Trichoderma*, *Rhizopus nigricans* and *Aspergillus niger*. The results showed that extracts were active against all tested microbes, with *E. coli* being the most susceptible and *S. typhi* the most resistant bacteria.

Antidiabetic

The antioxidant effects of the Spurges led scientists to investigate their antidiabetic efficacy. In 2021, the results of a study of Sun spurge showed that extracts contained starch-blocking

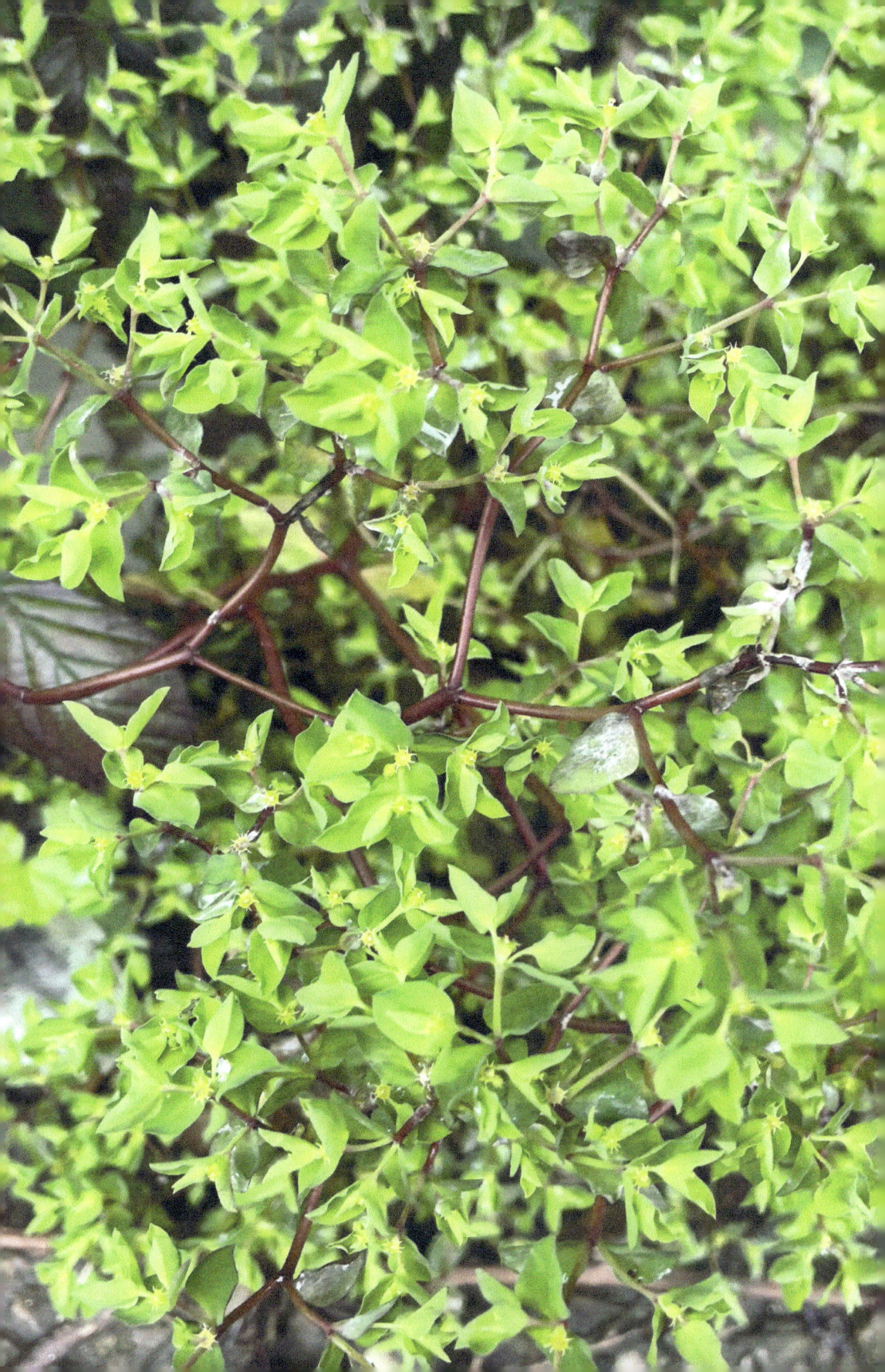

activity, with a methanol extract demonstrating the highest antidiabetic activity.

Petty spurge was studied in 2023 using rats with type-2 diabetes. The diabetic rats received treatment with the extract for 4 weeks, and results showed an enhanced insulin resistance, hyperglycaemia, dyslipidaemia, inflammation and redox imbalance, and upregulated adiponectin, meaning Petty spurge possesses potent radical-scavenging and anti-diabetic effects.

DOSAGE

Not for internal use.

PRECAUTIONS

The drug is severely irritating to mucous membranes and skin. Ingestion leads to salivation, burning pains in the stomach, colic, diarrhoea and nephritis. One case of death has been reported. Chronic application of the drug promotes tumour formation, so internal administration is no longer advised.

Spurge recipes

Medicinal recipes

First of all, if you are going to collect the sap of this plant, wear gloves! It will burn on contact with skin! Make an incision into the fleshy part of the stem or branch. The sap will exude easily and can be collected as with Prickly lettuce.

Spurge sap for warts and sunspots

You can use either Petty or Sun spurge for this application. Once you have obtained your sap, apply one drop carefully, using a cotton bud, to warts and non-melanoma lesions for 2–4 days. Initially, the skin will irritate and then scab, but you will soon see new skin appearing.

Spurge poultice

- 1tsp fresh leaf and stems of either Spurge
- 2tsp coconut oil
- cheesecloth or cotton bandage

Crush or grind the herb into a pulp and add the coconut oil to make a paste. Spread carefully over the affected area only and wrap with the cloth or bandage. Use against sunburns, corns and waxy growths.

STITCHWORT, GREATER
Stellaria holostea

The Stitchworts, Greater and Lesser, are native to the UK but I have not been able to find any mention of this plant by Culpeper either under this name or its pseudonyms such as Addersmeat or Startwort. However, it is a relative of Chickweed (*Stellaria media*) and has many of the same soothing properties. The Stitchwort species are found in woodlands, hedgerows, grasslands and on roadside verges.

HISTORICAL USES

In his 1897 edition of *Herbal Simples*, William Fernie tells us that Gerard said that folk, in his day, '*are wont to drink it in wine (with the powder of acorns) against the pain in the side, stitches, and such*'. Fernie went on to say that the apothecary John Parkinson (1567–1650) mentioned that '*in former days it was much commended by some to clear the eyes of dimness by dropping the fresh juice into them.*'

MODERN RESEARCH

This is not a plant that has received a lot of scientific attention, but phytochemical profiling has shown that phenolic acids, such as ferulic, chlorogenic and *p*-coumaric acid, flavonoids and flavonoid

ETYMOLOGY OF COMMON NAME
Derived from the fact that the plant was once used as a herbal remedy for a stitch.

PLANT LORE
Some say that if you pick Greater stitchwort, you will cause a thunderstorm.

USE
The leaves, stalks and flowers.

EDIBILITY
The leaves and shoots can be used in salads or lightly cooked as a vegetable.

HARVEST
In spring.

MEDICINAL PROPERTIES
Anti-inflammatory, antifungal and antibacterial.

ACTIVE CONSTITUENTS
Saponins, flavonoids, polysaccharides, essential oils.

glucosides, such as chrysoeriol, rutin and naringin, are the most abundant compounds in this plant and may have the following properties:

Antimicrobial
Scientific analysis undertaken in 2002 on the seeds of 21 Scottish plant species from 14 different families showed that Stitchwort displayed activity against one bacterial species, *Pseudomonas aeruginosa*, the cause of pneumonia, septicaemia and UTIs. Then, in 2023, potential activity was discovered against some fungi such as *Fusarium oxysporum*, which can cause a broad spectrum of infections, including keratitis and onychomycosis.

Anti-inflammatory
The same study found that Stitchwort also has anti-inflammatory activity when it was demonstrated to significantly inhibit both COX-1 and COX-2 pro-inflammatory enzymes by 71.24% and 72.83%, respectively. Molecular docking studies indicated that chlorogenic acid and chrysoeriol are the main contributors to such anti-inflammatory activity.

TOPICAL USES
Like Chickweed, Stitchwort leaves have cooling, anti-inflammatory and healing properties. An ointment made from the crushed leaves is very soothing for eczema, bites, heat rash and even psoriasis.

DOSAGE
As per Chickweed

PRECAUTIONS
Not suitable for children or those who are pregnant or lactating.

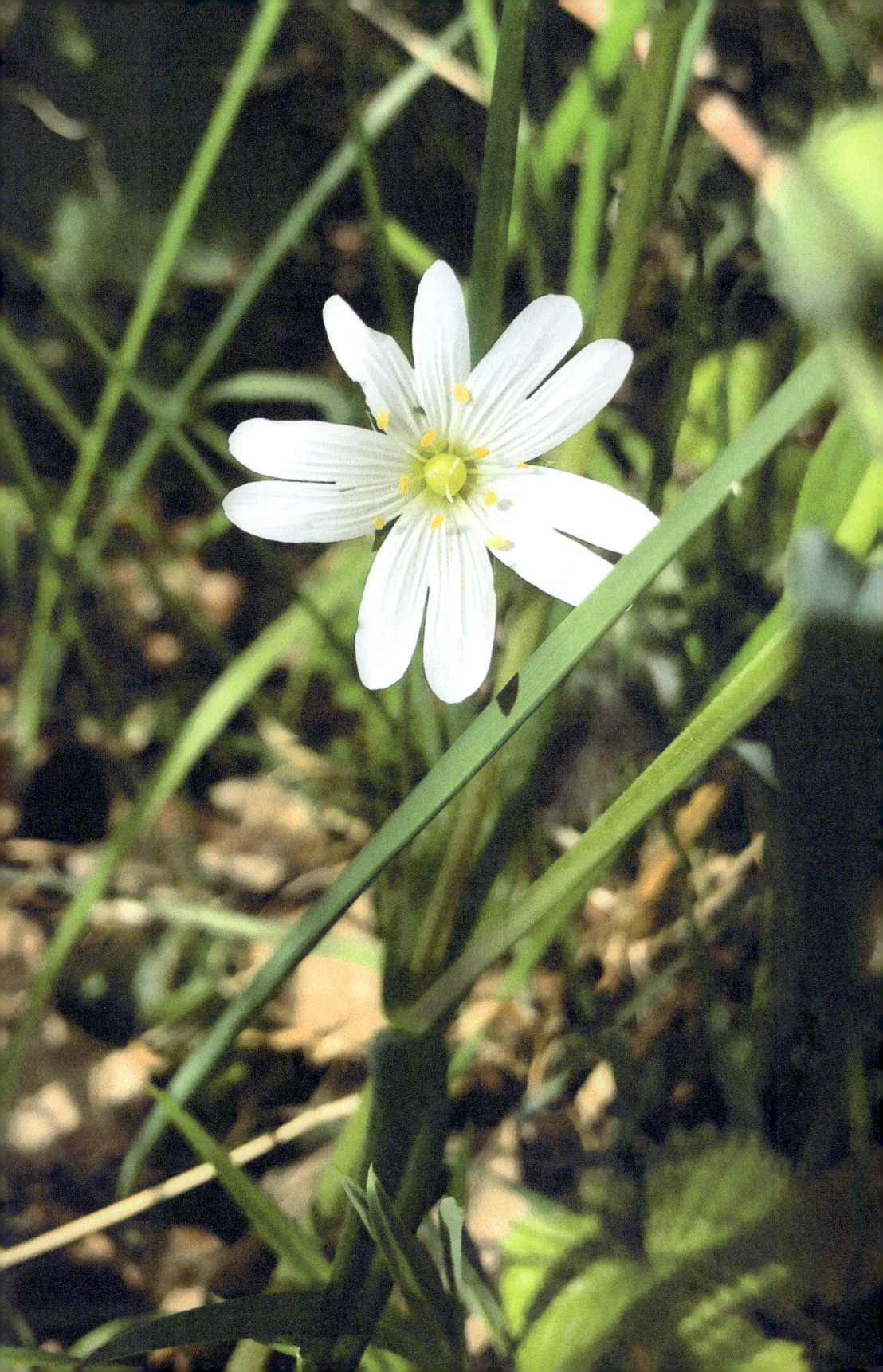

Stitchwort recipes

Medicinal recipes

Stitchwort infusion

Pour 250ml boiling water over 2tsp/10g of the dried leaf and allow to steep for 10–15 minutes. Use to relieve inflammation and soothe tension. Use 1–2 cups daily to aid digestion and reduce inflammation.

Stitchwort poultice

- 1tsp fresh Stitchwort leaf (if using dried you will need to moisten with water first)
- 2tsp coconut oil
- cheesecloth or cotton bandage

Finely chop the herb into a pulp and add the coconut oil to make a paste. Spread the paste evenly over the desired area and wrap with the cloth or bandage. Use as an astringent and antioxidant against various skin problems such as eczema and psoriasis.

Stitchwort salve

- 100g dried leaves and stems
- 2 tbsp alcohol, such as Everclear
- 1l grapeseed oil

Place the herbs in a jar with the alcohol and allow to steep for 10 minutes before adding the oil. Leave for 4 weeks and then strain. Make into a salve by using a 1:4 ratio of melted beeswax to oil mix, ie 1 part wax to 4 parts liquid. Melt the wax pellets in the oil in a double boiler or bain-marie. Remove from the heat and allow to cool and set completely before using to soothe irritations, rashes or minor wounds.

ST JOHN'S WORT
Hypericum spp.

There are several species of *Hypericum* native to the UK including Saint John's wort (*Hypericum perforatum*) and Hairy St John's wort (*Hypericum hirsutum*). Hairy St John's wort flowers just before St John's wort and is slightly larger leafed with the titular hairy stem. Both are native to the UK and typically grow in sunny locations, such as meadows, fields and roadsides. An easy way to distinguish between the two is that Hairy St John's wort buds will not stain your fingers red when crushed.

HISTORICAL USES

The classical physicians Galen, Dioscorides, Pliny and Hippocrates recommended St John's wort as a diuretic, wound-healing herb, which offered treatment for menstrual disorders and a cure for intestinal worms and snakebites (Foster, 2000; Castleman, 2001; Redvers et al., 2001).

In 1525, the Swiss physician Paracelsus recommended St John's wort for treating depression, melancholy and overexcitation (Clement et al., 2006).

John Gerard explained in his *Herball* that, 'The leaves, floures, and seeds stamped, and put into a glasse with oile olive, and set in the hot sun for certain weeks together, and then strained from

ETYMOLOGY OF COMMON NAME
Refers to John the Baptist, as the plant blooms around the time of the feast of the Saint in late June.

PLANT LORE
The Celts passed it through the smoke of the summer solstice fire, then wore it into battle for invincibility.

USE
The flowers and flower tops.

EDIBILITY
The flowers can be used for making mead.

HARVEST
In summer, when in flower.

MEDICINAL PROPERTIES
Analgesic, anti-Inflammatory, antiviral, vulnerary, antidepressant, antimicrobial, anxiolytic.

ACTIVE CONSTITUENTS
Hypericin, hyperforin, flavonoids, phenolic acids, essential oil.

those herbs, and the like quantitie of new put in and sunned in like manner, doth make an oile of the colour of bloud, which is a most pretious remedie for deep wounds and those that are thorow the body, for the sinues that are prickt, or any wound made with a venomed weapon.'

Nicholas Culpeper's *Herbal* commented, 'It is a singular wound herb; it heals inward hurts or bruises; made into an ointment, it open obstructions, dissolves swellings, and closes up the lips of wounds.'

Harold Ward's 1936 *Herbal Manual* suggested, 'Indicated in coughs, colds, and disorders of the urinary system. It was prescribed more often by the English herbal school of a hundred years ago than it is to-day and was noticed as far back as Culpeper for 'wounds, hurts and bruises'. Indeed, an infusion of the fresh flowers in Olive oil, to make the 'Oil of St. John's Wort', is still used as an application to wounds, swellings, and ulcers. Internally, the infusion of 1 ounce of the herb to 1 pint of boiling water is taken in wineglass doses.'

MODERN RESEARCH

St John's wort has been the subject of several pharmacopoeias and monographs, including the *British Herbal Pharmacopoeia* (1996) and the European Directorate for the Quality of Medicines (EDQM), 2000, among others (Parfitt, 1999; Beara et al., 2001).

A number of studies of the biological activities of *Hypericum* species have shown that while *H. perforatum* is richer in flavonoids and hyperforin (recognised as one of the most crucial components for the antidepressive activity) other *Hypericum* species including Hairy St John's wort nevertheless have important properties. Modern research has found and confirmed the following:

Antiviral

The constituents in St John's wort, particularly hypericin and pseudohypericin, have been found to inhibit viruses, including *Herpes simplex* 1 and 2, HIV-1, Cytomegalovirus (CMV, the cause of mononucleosis and pneumonia), HPIV, Indiana virus and equine infectious anaemia virus.

Because of this antiviral research and in response to the *in vitro* and animal studies, clinical trials were undertaken on HIV patients. In one study, 18 HIV patients were treated solely with standardised St John's wort extract (weekly intravenous injection and daily oral intake), providing a daily intake of 2mg of hypericin. The 16 patients showed stable or even

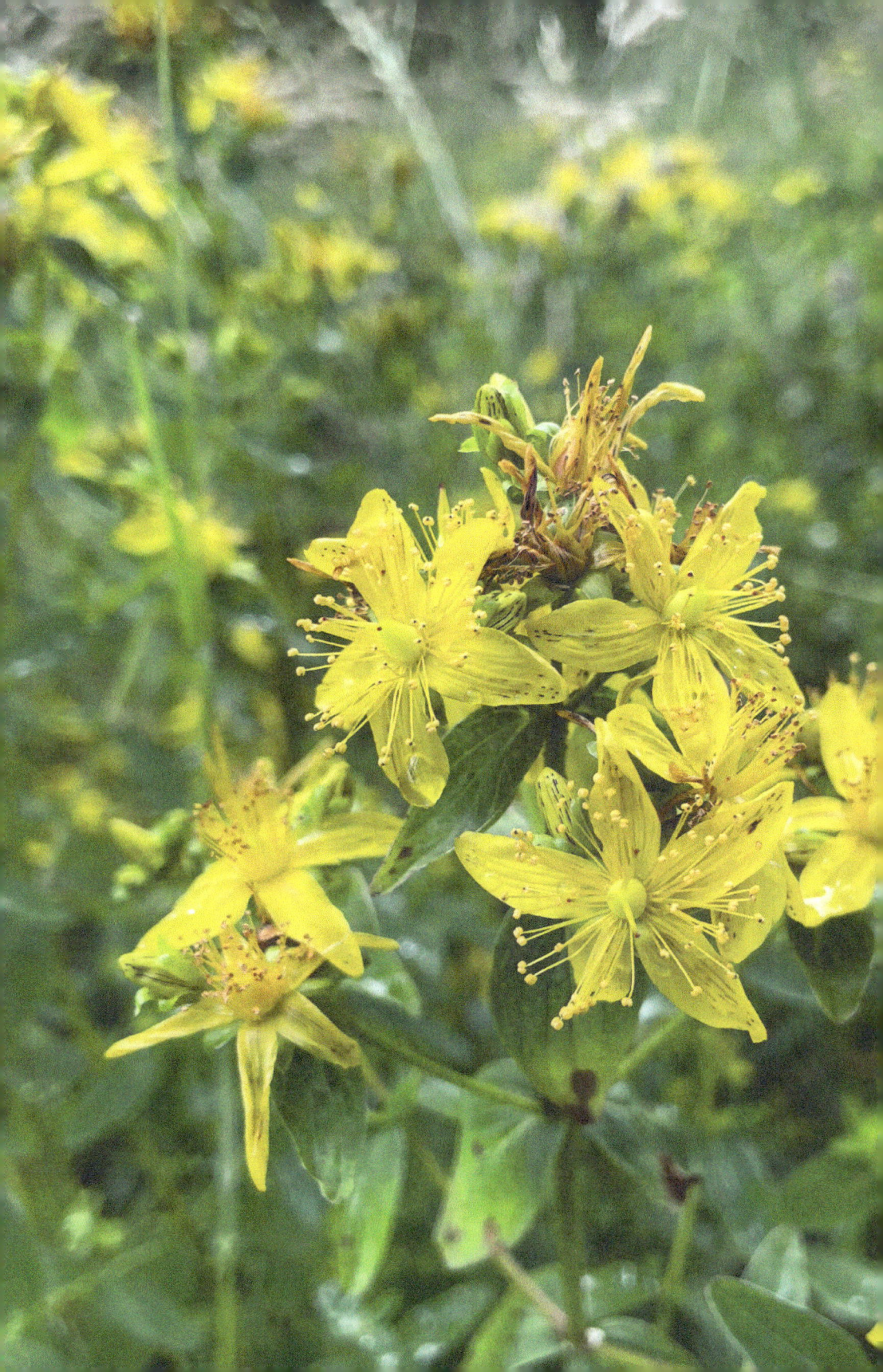

increasing counts of helper T-cells over the 40 months of observation. Furthermore, none of the otherwise known viral complications to CMV, *Herpes* or Epstein-Barr virus was encountered in these 16 patients.

A 2021 study into the use of St John's wort in the fight against COVID-19 concluded that it could be effective and that compounds may be screened using *in vitro* and *in vivo* analyses to indicate its inhibitory potency. Research on these effects of St John's wort is ongoing.

Hypericin and pseudohypericin have also been found to be present in Hairy St John's wort, though it appears that it is in less abundance than in St John's wort and may not therefore have the same antiviral effects.

Antidepressant and anxiolytic

With regard to its best-known use, depression, St John's wort has been tested in over 3,000 patients against placebo and various controls. A 1996 analysis of 23 randomised trials with a total of 1,757 outpatients with mild to moderate depression revealed that St John's wort was significantly superior to placebo and comparably effective to standard antidepressants while producing fewer side effects. The official German Commission E monograph for St John's wort lists psychovegetative disturbances, depressive states, fear and nervous disturbances as clinical indications for St John's wort.

The clinical evaluation of St John's wort began with an initial study of six depressed women, aged 55–65. The results demonstrated a significant improvement in symptoms of anxiety, apathy, hypersomnia and insomnia, anorexia, psychomotor retardation, depression and feelings of worthlessness. No side effects were observed. Since this initial study, a total of 1,592 patients have been studied in more than 25 double-blind controlled studies, and St John's wort extract has produced improvements in many psychological symptoms without producing significant side effects.

Furthermore, St John's wort did not interfere with REM sleep as other antidepressants did and was shown to increase the intensity of deep sleep during the total sleeping period as demonstrated by brain wave studies. While St John's wort improved sleep quality it did not act as a sedative (ie it did not reduce sleep onset) and nor did it change total sleep duration. It has also been shown to improve memory.

The above studies have also shown St John's wort to be effective in the treatments of seasonal affective disorder (SAD). Patients who fulfilled criteria for major depression with seasonal pattern were randomised in a 4-week treatment study with 900mg of St John's wort extract combined with either bright or dim light. The significant reduction in the

Hamilton Depression scale in both groups (72% and 60%, respectively) indicated that St John's wort extract may offer support to patients with SAD as a sole therapeutic agent as well as in combination with light therapy.

The antidepressive activity of St John's wort is due to the presence of Hyperforin, a phloroglucinol, and it is the only species which contains hyperforin in abundant amounts (Umek et al., 1999, Smelcerovic and Spiteller, 2006).

Analgesic and anti-inflammatory

In accordance with Gerard's and Culpeper's findings, St John's wort has also been shown to be analgesic and anti-inflammatory. In a 2017 animal study, low doses of St John's wort were shown to provide relief from acute and chronic pain sensitivity and to augment opioid analgesia. Clinical studies highlighted dental pain conditions as a promising St John's wort application and that St John's wort analgesia appears at low doses owing to its content of hyperforin and hypericin and minimising the risk of herbal–drug interactions produced by hyperforin.

In 2006, ethanol extracts of the aerial parts of six *Hypericum* species including Hairy St John's wort, were tested for anti-inflammatory activity in comparison with indomethacin (an NSAID). It was found that Hairy St John's wort in particular produced anti-inflammatory activity with no correlation between the amount of hypericin in the extracts and their anti-inflammatory activity.

In 2017, a comparative analysis of the phenolic compounds of 7 *Hypericum* species was conducted. The second best in flavonoid content was extract of Hairy St John's wort, with the largest share of orientin and its 2'-O-acetyl derivative. Orientin has been shown to have significant anti-inflammatory properties and may well be the reason that Hairy St John's wort showed such activity.

Anticancerogenic

In 2021, regular use of St John's wort was shown to reduce colorectal cancer risk in humans and prevent genotoxic effects of carcinogens in animal models. In established cancer, St John's wort and its hyperforin content have been shown to exert therapeutic effects by their ability to downregulate inflammatory mediators and inhibit pro-survival kinases, angiogenic factors and extracellular matrix proteases, thereby counteracting tumour growth and spread.

TOPICAL USES

Topical application of St John's wort extracts inhibits *Staphylococcus aureus* infection and speeds the healing time for wounds, including burns. Its anti-inflammatory properties are particularly indicated in the pain resulting from sciatica.

DOSAGE

Tisane – 1tsp/5g, 2–3 times per day.
Tincture – 1:5 45%, up to 2–4ml, 3 times per day – 20 drops = 1ml/1tsp = 5ml.

PRECAUTIONS

Extracts of St John's wort do appear to interact with other medications, especially drugs that impact liver and intestinal enzyme function. The fresh plant can be phototoxic, and it can break down contraceptives more quickly and therefore make them less effective. It may also cause a hypotensive episode that is poorly responsive to resuscitation under anaesthetic. Use alongside other antidepressants has resulted in serotonin syndrome. Not suitable for children or those who are pregnant or lactating. (EDQM 2000)

St John's wort recipes

Medicinal recipes

St John's wort tisane

Pour 250ml boiling water over 1tsp/5g of the dried herb and allow to steep for 10–15 minutes. Use to treat dyspepsia, liver diseases, rhinitis, neuralgia, anxiety and tension. This tisane is particularly good for treating the winter blues or SAD during winter months. The average time to notice the effect of the herb is between 2 and 6 weeks.

St John's wort infused tincture 1:5 45%

If using 40% alcohol, ie. vodka, cover 1 part herb to 5 parts fluid.

If using Everclear or other 100% proof, use the following method for a specific tincture:

- 100g fresh St John's wort
- 225ml alcohol
- 275ml water

Cover 50g fresh flowers with 225ml alcohol. Then steep/infuse another 50g of herb in 275ml water for 15 minutes. Strain thoroughly and top up if the water is less than 275ml. Add the infusion to the dried herb and alcohol mix, and leave for 14 days before straining. Use for the treatment of mild to moderate depression, SAD and anxiety.

St John's wort infused oil

- 100g flowers
- 2tbsp alcohol, such as Everclear
- 1l grapeseed oil

Place the herbs in a jar with the alcohol and allow to steep for 10 minutes before adding the oil. Leave for 4 weeks and then strain. Use as a topical treatment for nerve pain from shingles, neuralgia, etc.

HSJW anti-inflammatory salve

- 100g flowers and leaves
- 2tbsp alcohol, such as Everclear
- 1l grapeseed oil

Place the herbs in a jar with the alcohol and allow to steep for 10 minutes before adding the oil. Leave for 4 weeks and then strain. Make into a salve by using a 1:4 ratio of melted beeswax to your oil mix, ie 1 part wax to 4 parts liquid. Melt the wax pellets in the oil in a double boiler or bain-marie. Remove from the heat and allow to cool and set completely before using as a topical anti-inflammatory treatment for wounds and bruises, etc.

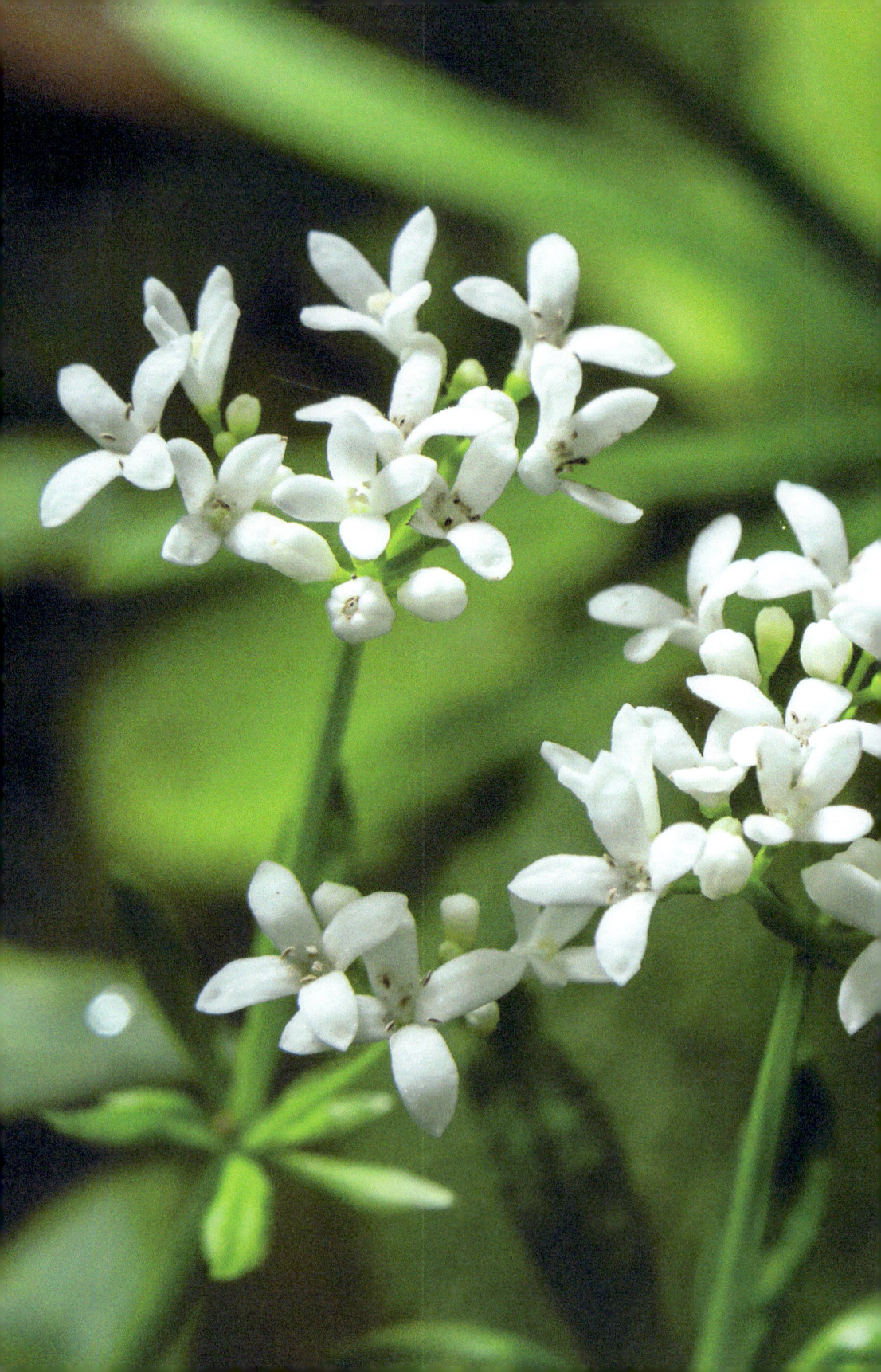

SWEET WOODRUFF
Galium odoratum

Sweet woodruff is native to the UK, where it can be found growing in woodlands, shady hedgerows and damp, shaded areas. It is related to Cleavers and the Bedstraws. In addition to its medicinal uses Woodruff has been traditionally used to infuse beverages and desserts, including cakes, custards and jellies.

HISTORICAL USES

Nicholas Culpeper's *Herbal* declared 'The Woodruffe is accounted nourishing and restorative, and good for weakly consumptive people; it opens obstructions of the liver and spleen and is said to be a provocative to venery.'

In her 1921 book *A Garden of Herbs*, Eleanour Sinclair Rohde said of Woodruff, 'Its bruised leaves were laid on cuts, and woodruff tea was esteemed an "excellent cordial drink".'

William Fernie's 1897 edition of *Herbal Simples* explained that 'fragrant and exhilarating tea may be made from the leaves and blossoms of the sweet Woodruffe, and this is found to be of service in correcting sluggishness of the liver.'

Harold Ward summarised in his 1936 *Herbal Manual*, 'In faulty biliary functioning and general liver sluggishness. Tonic properties particularly applicable to the digestive apparatus. Dose, two

ETYMOLOGY OF COMMON NAME
'Wood' for the location the plant prefers and 'ruff', derived from the Old English *rofe*, a wheel, which the leaf whorls resemble.

PLANT LORE
Medieval soldiers carried Woodruff in their helmets as it was believed to bring success in battle.

USE
Aerial parts.

EDIBILITY
Used to flavour wine, juice, punch, beer, jam, ice cream as well as jellies.

HARVEST
In summer, just as it flowers.

MEDICINAL PROPERTIES
Hepatoprotective, antimicrobial, anti-inflammatory, antihypoxic.

ACTIVE CONSTITUENTS
Coumarins, tannins, flavonoids, polysaccharides, essential oils.

LEFT: SWEET WOODRUFF

tablespoonfuls of the *1 ounce to 1 pint boiling water infusion*.'

MODERN RESEARCH

This plant has been found to contain coumarin, asperuloside, monotropein, tannins, iridoids, anthra-quinones, flavonoids and traces of nicotinic acid, which underlie the following medicinal properties:

Hepatoprotective

The claims of the historical writers of Woodruff as a treatment for the liver are substantiated by a study that found the hepatoprotective activity at a dose of 25mg/kg was not inferior to the reference drug silibor.

Antimicrobial and anti-inflammatory

Studies also suggest that this plant may have anti-inflammatory activity and an anthraquinone derivative in this plant showed an inhibitory effect against cell division in the *Herpes simplex* virus-1 (HSV-1).

An extensive study showed that the plant is effective against *Escherichia coli*, and actually changes the hydrophobicity (tendency to repel water) of the cellular surface and causes the bacterium to lose its haemagglutination (clumping) capacity (Vlase et al., 2014; Wojnicz et al., 2012). The plant has also shown strong antibacterial activity on *Staphylococcus aureus* and *Listeria* (Vlase et al., 2014).

Antihypoxic and sedative

A 2015 study was carried out on the sedative and antihypoxic activity of extract from Woodruff. Hypoxia prevents the utilisation of oxygen and plays a key role in diseases such as coronary heart disease, myocardial infarction, ischaemic stroke and other brain dysfunctions as well as lungs, liver, kidney and foetal pathology. This study found that a dose of 100mg/kg showed a high antihypoxic activity, which is almost double that for the reference drug bilobil, a medication that treats dementia. Furthermore, the extract revealed a dose-dependent sedative activity on the central nervous system but without an adverse effect on skeletal muscle tone and coordination. This means Woodruff could be a good treatment for insomnia and nervous tension, and is no doubt why it was traditionally used as a tonic or cordial for nervous agitation.

Antioxidant

A 2018 study compared the polyphenolic content of Woodruff with its cousins *Galium aparine* (Cleavers) and *Galium verum* (Lady's bedstraw). The results showed that all three had strong antioxidant capacity, with the highest antioxidant activity belonging to Woodruff.

TOPICAL USES

As Eleanour Sinclair Rohde said, traditionally the crushed leaves of Woodruff were used topically to reduce swelling and to accelerate wound-healing, and the water extract was found to have a significant healing effect in case of burns in a 2013 study. This inflammation reduction and control of infection reflects the effects of antioxidant, anti-inflammatory and antimicrobial components of this plant.

DOSAGE
Tisane – 1tsp/5g, morning and evening.

PRECAUTIONS
The usage of the plant for sweets was prohibited in Germany in 1974, owing to Woodruff's low level of toxicity, which increases upon drying, and is particularly problematic for children, owing to their lower body mass. The toxicity stems from the presence of coumarin, which can create sickness and headaches, and damage the liver when ingested in greater quantities. Do not use this remedy if you are taking conventional medicine for circulatory problems or if you are pregnant or lactating.

Sweet woodruff recipes

Medicinal recipes
Woodruff tisane
Pour 250ml boiling water over 1tsp/5g of the dried herb and allow to steep for 10–15 minutes. Use for insomnia and to help relaxation and digestion.

Woodruff poultice
- 1tsp fresh Woodruff leaf (if using dried you will need to moisten with water first)
- 2tsp coconut oil
- cheesecloth or cotton bandage

Finely chop the herb into a pulp and add the coconut oil to make a paste. Spread the paste evenly over the desired area and wrap with the cloth or bandage. Use as an anti-inflammatory and wound-healer. Also, for use against trigeminal neuralgia.

Woodruff syrup
- 500ml tisane
- 500g sugar
- 25ml tincture, optional (preservative)

Warm your tisane over a low heat and bring to a simmer. Then cover partially and reduce the liquid down to half its original volume, ie. 250ml. Add the sugar and stir constantly, but do not let the mix boil. Remove the syrup from the heat and add the tinctures at a ratio of 5%. Syrups keep for up to 2 years unopened. After opening, store in the refrigerator and use within 1 month. Add to sparkling water for a relaxing cordial.

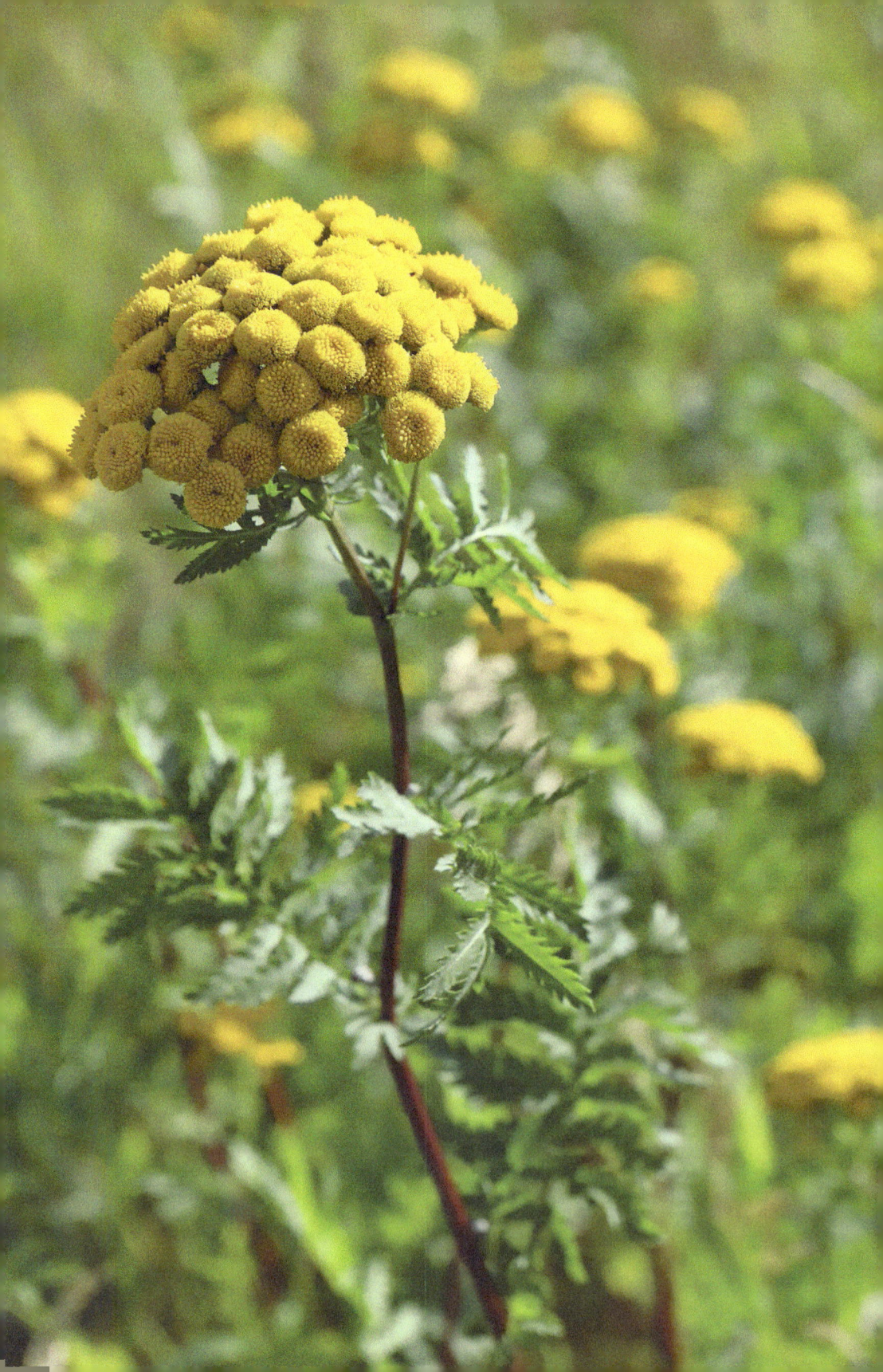

TANSY
Tanacetum vulgare

Tansy belongs to the *Asteraceae* family, commonly referred to as the Aster, Daisy or Sunflower family. It is naturalised but not native to the UK even though it has been present for several centuries. It is commonly found in waste areas, roadsides, fields and disturbed habitats.

HISTORICAL USES

During medieval times, Tansy was the go-to herb for ridding the body of worms. It was also used as a digestive aid. Additionally, meat was covered with Tansy leaves to repel insects.

Nicholas Culpeper's *Herbal* stated, 'It is an agreeable bitter, an anti-flatulent and a destroyer of worms, for which case a powder of the flowers should be given from six to twelve grains at night and mornings. Worms are often the cause of putrid fevers and epileptic fits, and sometimes bring on a consumption. The flowers are the part to be used, and they should be given in powder, but there requires care in the collecting of them, to obtain all their virtue. Clip off a quantity of Tansy flowers, before they are over blown, close to the stalk. It cleanses and heals ulcers in the mouth or secret parts, and is very good for inward wounds, and to close the tips of green wounds, and to heal old, moist, and corrupt running sores in the legs or elsewhere. Being bruised

ETYMOLOGY OF COMMON NAME
The word Tansy comes from the Greek word *athanatos*, which means 'immortal', and referred to the long life cycle of the plant.

PLANT LORE
In Greek mythology Zeus gave the shepherd Ganymede a drink of Tansy to make him immortal.

USE
The flowers and leaves.

EDIBILITY
Not edible, TOXIC.

HARVEST
When in bloom.

MEDICINAL PROPERTIES
Antimicrobial, anti-inflammatory, nootropic.

ACTIVE CONSTITUENTS
Alkaloids, flavonoids, triterpenoids, phenolic acids, essential oils.

LEFT: TANSY

and applied to the soles of the feet and handwrists, it wonderfully colls the hot fits of agues, be they never so violent.'

Robert Thornton's *Family Herbal* of 1814 related that, '*In the year 1771, the late Dr David Clarke, of Edinburgh, published, in the third volume of the Edinburgh Essays Physical and Literary, a paper on the gout, in which he recommends the use of an infusion of tansy in that disorder; and he mentions cases in which it was of use: eg A gentleman, under fifty years of age, who had been subject to the gout for about fifteen years, on finding his disorder increase, he about seven years ago had recourse to an infusion of tansy to remove it; he filled every morning a tea-pot, capable of holding an English pint of liquor, with the dried flowers, leaves, and stalks of tansy, and then poured as much boiling water over them as the pot would hold, and let it stand till night, when he drank, at going to bed, the whole of the cold infusion: by following constantly this method he has remained free of the gout for seven years, excepting a slight fit which he had after spraining his ancle. He was not sensible of its operating by stool, by perspiration, or by urine; though Dr Clarke thought that it acted on his bowels, as he had regularly two stools in the day. Another person, fifty-two years of age, had remained free from the gout for three years, by drinking near a pint of the infusion of tansy daily, and by eating some of the fresh tansy in the morning, while it was in season: before using this remedy he had regularly a fit of the gout, which confined him from one to four months in the winter.'*

Harold Ward gave the following recipe in his 1936 *Family Herbal*, '*Tansy herb is probably the best of all the media for getting rid of worms in children, and a dose according to age should be given night and morning fasting. The infusion of 1 ounce to 1 pint of boiling water is used.*'

MODERN RESEARCH

Culpeper is correct in that the plant expels worms, but we now know that the essential oil in the leaves contains thujone. This is toxic, and as little as 15g can kill an adult. Its use in herbal medicine is controversial, and caution is advised. Nevertheless, the following medicinal properties of Tansy have been discovered:

Antimicrobial and anti-inflammatory

In a 2017 study, essential oil from Tansy showed activity against *Bacillus subtilis*, *Escherichia coli* and *Staphylococcus aureus*, with camphor and caryophyllene oxide responsible for antibacterial activity.

It has also been shown to be as efficient as the antifungal drugs bifonazole and ketoconazole against aiborne fungal species such as *Aspergillus fumigatus*, *Aspergillus ochraceus*, *Aspergillus versicolor* and *Aspergillus niger*, as well as some plant pathogens.

Extracts of Tansy were found to have significant wound-healing and anti-inflammatory activities driven mainly by the α-humulene content.

Nootropic

In 2016, a study showed that extracts of Rose, Tansy and Nettle improved spatial learning in rats and that this herbal group could have anti-dementia properties and improve spatial learning and memory.

Neurotec® is a medication that contains the above extracts and is an Iran Food and Drug Administration (IFDA)-approved medication for treatment of peripheral neuropathies in diabetic patients. A clinical trial was carried out on patients with tinnitus, who attended otolaryngology clinic between 2015 and 2016, the trial concluding that a three-month treatment with Neurotec capsules accompanied by educational counselling was of benefit for managing symptoms in patients with chronic tinnitus.

TOPICAL USES

Externally, Tansy is used as a poultice on swellings and some eruptive skin diseases. It is also used externally to kill lice, fleas and scabies, though even external use of the plant also carries the risk of toxicity.

DOSAGE

Tisane – ½tsp/2.5g, once per day.

PRECAUTIONS

The plant is poisonous if large quantities are ingested. There have been cases of death in North America from drinking strong brews of the tisane, possibly as an abortifacient. Not suitable for children or those who are pregnant or lactating.

Tansy recipes

Medicinal recipes

Tansy insect repellent

I like to use a simple bunch of dried Tansy hanging from doorways to repel flies in the summer. You can also make a repellent spray as follows:

- fresh Tansy leaves and flowers
- 1 cup of water
- spray bottle

Boil the water and add the fresh Tansy leaves and flowers. Simmer for 10–15 minutes. Allow the mixture to cool, then strain it into a spray bottle. Spray the mixture around the house or on exposed skin to repel insects. Do NOT use near pets.

Tansy poultice

- 1tsp fresh Tansy leaf (if using dried you will need to moisten with water first)
- 2tsp coconut oil
- cheesecloth or cotton bandage

Finely chop the herb into a pulp and add the coconut oil to make a paste. Spread the paste evenly over the desired area and wrap with the cloth or bandage. Use to relieve rheumatism and external injuries such as sprains, but note precautions.

Tansy infused oil

- 100g Tansy leaves and flowers
- 2tbsp alcohol, such as Everclear
- 1l grapeseed oil

Place the herbs in a jar with the alcohol and allow to steep for 10 minutes before adding the oil. Leave for 4 weeks and then strain. Use as a topical treatment to relieve muscle aches, joint pain and minor skin irritations.

TOADFLAX
Linaria vulgaris

Yellow toadflax is the UK's native Toadflax and is also known as Butter-and-eggs. It can be found in a variety of habitats, including grasslands, meadows, roadsides, wastelands and disturbed areas. In addition to its medicinal use, Yellow toadflax was historically used to produce yellow and green dyes from the flowers and leaves.

HISTORICAL USES

John Gerard reported in his *Herball* that in his time Toadflax was called Linaria or Flaxweed, and that '*The decoction of Toad-Flax taketh away the yellowness and deformity of the skin, beeng washed and bathed therewith. The same drunken, openeth the stoppings of the liver and spleen, and is singular good against the jaundice which is of long continuance and the same decoction doth also provoke urine, in those that piss drop after drop, unstoppeth the kidneys and bladder.*'

Nicholas Culpeper's *Herbal* commented on the plant, '*This is frequently used to spend the abundance of those watery humours by urine which cause the dropsy. The decoction of the herb, both leaves and flowers, in wine, taken and drank, doth somewhat move the belly downwards, opens obstructions of the liver,*

ETYMOLOGY OF COMMON NAME
From the resemblance of the flower to the wide mouth of a toad and in early summer to a Flax plant.

PLANT LORE
In England, Toadflax seeds strung on a linen thread were said to ward off evil and break hexes.

USE
All aerial parts.

EDIBILITY
Not edible.

HARVEST
When in bloom.

MEDICINAL PROPERTIES
Astringent, anti-dyslipidemic, antihistamine, diuretic and antiviral.

ACTIVE CONSTITUENTS
Alkaloids, flavonoids, triterpenoids, phenolic acids, essential oils.

and helps the yellow jaundice; expels poison, provokes women's courses, drives forth the dead child, and after-birth ... The juice or water put into foul ulcers, whether they be cancerous or fistulous, with tents rolled therein, or parts washed and injected therewith, cleanses them thoroughly from the bottom, and heals them up safely. The same juice or water also cleanses the skin wonderfully of all sorts of deformity, as leprosy, morphew, scurf, wheals, pimples, or spots, applied of itself, or used with some powder of Lupines.'

MODERN RESEARCH

As previously mentioned, Yellow toadflax is native in the UK. While the Purple variety (*Linaria purpurea*) has been established in the country since the 17th century and shares some medicinal properties with it, it is the Yellow toadflax that is the focus here. I have found nothing to substantiate Culpeper's use of the herb to provoke menstruation or expel a stillborn child and afterbirth, but other confirmation of its properties can be given:

Anti-dyslipidemic

A 2018 study confirmed the Gerard and Culpeper's observations regarding jaundice and the liver, when it demonstrated that the linarin found in Toadflax exhibits a protective effect against hyperlipidaemia (high cholesterol) and hepatic steatosis (fatty liver) induced by a Western-type diet. The effect of this may be to reverse liver metabolic dysfunction, inflammation and advanced forms of non-alcoholic fatty liver disease.

Diuretic

The fact that Toadflax contains tannins will explain the diuretic use described by Gerard and Culpeper as tannins are implicated in decreasing blood pressure by promoting the excretion of water and electrolytes.

Antihistamine

In another 2018 study, the allergy-preventive effects of the plant were studied, and it was observed that linaric acid and its derivatives showed significant allergy-preventive activities, confirming that this may aid in the development of new agents for the treatment of allergic diseases such as atopic dermatitis, allergic asthma and hay fever.

Antiviral

In 2022, the antiviral activity of an alcohol-based tincture of *Filipendula vulgaris* (Meadowsweet), *Petroselinum crispum* (Parsley), *Apium graveolens* (Celery), *Galium verum* (Cleavers) and *Linaria vulgaris* (Toadflax) with *Calendula officinalis* flowers was evaluated on the following *in vitro* viral infections: human *Herpes* virus-2, hepatitis C and coronavirus of transmissive porcine gastroenteritis (TGEV). The tincture demonstrated high antiviral activity to all tested viruses.

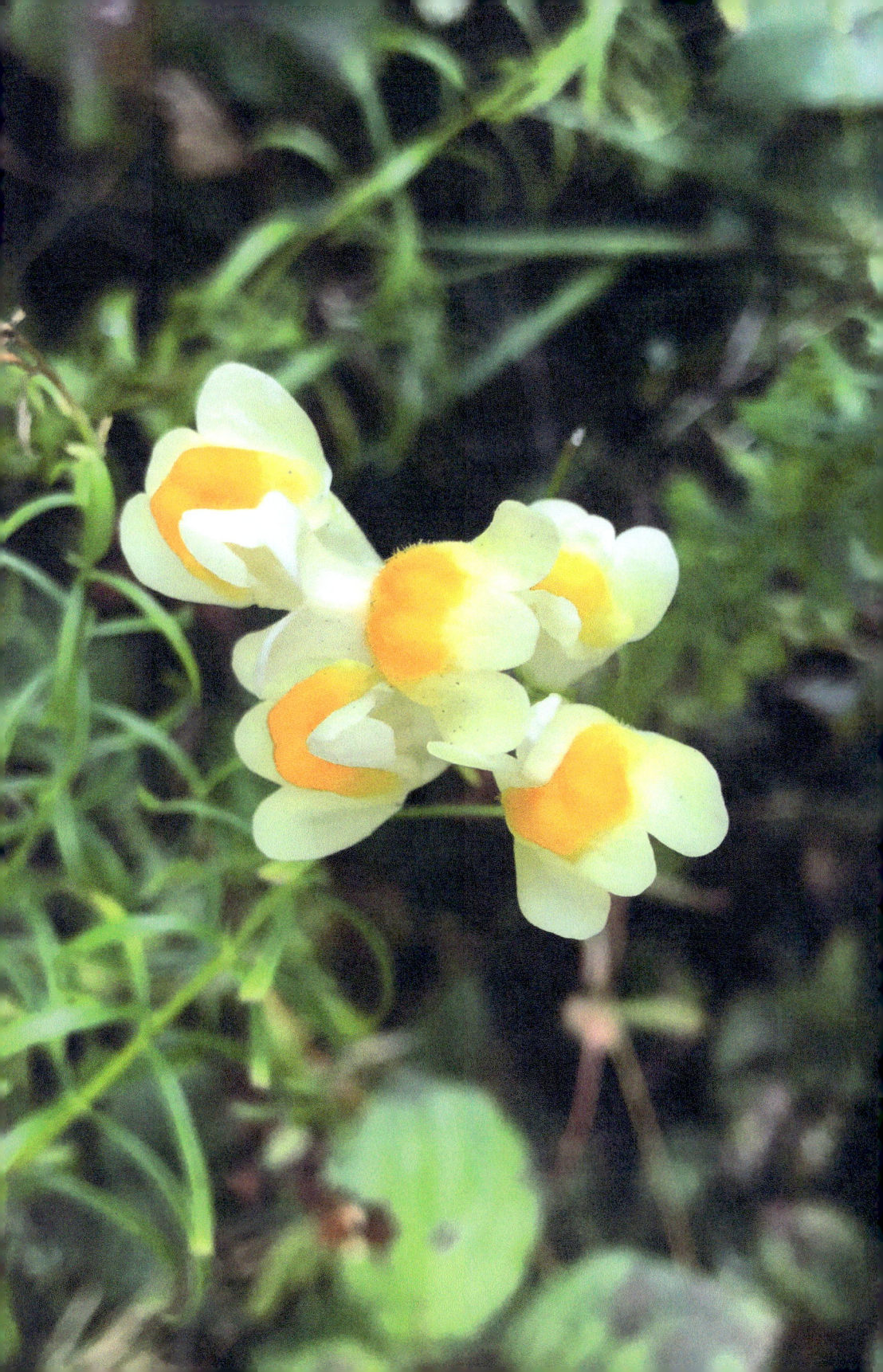

TOPICAL USE

Externally Toadflax is applied to haemorrhoids, skin eruptions, sores and malignant ulcers to take advantage of the astringency provided by the tannin content.

DOSAGE

Tisane – 1tsp/5g, 2–3 times per day.

PRECAUTIONS

The plant should be used with caution. Prolonged use of Toadflax internally should be avoided owing to the presence of compounds that may be toxic in large doses. Not suitable for children or those who are pregnant or lactating.

Toadflax recipes

Medicinal recipes

Toadflax tisane

Pour 250ml boiling water over ½tsp/2.5g of the dried herb and allow to steep for 10–15 minutes. Use to promote digestion and act as a mild diuretic.

Toadflax poultice

- 1tsp fresh Toadflax leaf (if using dried you will need to moisten with water first)
- 2tsp coconut oil
- cheesecloth or cotton bandage

Finely chop the herb into a pulp and add the coconut oil to make a paste. Spread the paste evenly over the desired area and wrap with the cloth or bandage. Use to relieve various skin diseases such as rashes, ulcers, inflammation, wounds and haemorrhoids.

Toadflax infused oil

- 100g leaves and flowers
- 2tbsp alcohol, such as Everclear
- 1l grapeseed oil

Place the herbs in a jar with the alcohol and allow to steep for 10 minutes before adding the oil. Leave for 4 weeks and then strain. Use as a topical treatment to soothe skin irritations, inflammations and minor wounds.

USNEA
Usnea barbata

Usnea is a fascinating lichen, also known as Bearded moss or Old man's beard. It is characterised by its long, stringy and beard-like appearance, and can be found hanging from tree branches in forests and woodlands.

HISTORICAL USES

Nicholas Culpeper's *Herbal* stated that, *'the Tree Mosses are cooling and binding, and partake of a digesting and mollifying quality withal, as Galen saith. But each Moss partakes of the nature of the tree from whence it is taken; therefore, that of the oak is more binding, and is of good effect to stay fluxes in man or woman; as also vomiting or bleeding, the powder thereof being taken in wine. The decoction thereof in wine is very good for women that are troubled with the overflowing of their courses. The same being drank, stays the stomach that is troubled with casting, or hiccough; and, as Avicena saith, it comforts the heart. The powder thereof taken in drink for some time together, is thought available for the dropsy. The oil that has had fresh Moss steeped therein for a time, and afterwards boiled and applied to the temples and forehead, marvellously eases the head-ache coming of a hot cause; as also the distillations of hot rheums or humours in the eyes, or other parts. The ancients much used it in their ointments and other medicines against the*

ETYMOLOGY OF COMMON NAME
Probably derived from the Arabic word *ushnah*, meaning moss or lichen, though it may also mean 'rope-like'.

PLANT LORE
Believed to maintain the 'lungs' of the Earth owing to its sacred relationship with its host tree.

USE
All parts.

EDIBILITY
Technically yes, but it is not particularly pleasant.

HARVEST
When it falls during storms.

MEDICINAL PROPERTIES
Antimicrobial, analgesic, antibacterial, antifungal, anti-inflammatory, antipyretic, anti-tumour.

ACTIVE CONSTITUENTS
Usnic acids, polysaccharides, volatile oils.

lassitude, and to strengthen and comfort the sinews.'

There is much debate about whether Culpeper is referring to Usnea specifically, but we do know that Usnea has been used as far back as 100BC in Chinese medicine and was allegedly used by Hippocrates to treat urinary complaints.

Usnic acid, the main medicinal constituent of Usnea, was first isolated as a prominent secondary lichen metabolite by the German scientist Knop in 1844. It was being developed as a modern pharmaceutical in the 20th century just prior to the advent of the penicillin antibiotics.

MODERN RESEARCH

Owing to its past development as an antibiotic, Usnea has been studied fairly thoroughly and the following properties found:

Antimicrobial

Usnea contains usnic acid, which has potent antimicrobial properties. In fact, against certain bacteria, usnic acid is stronger than the antibiotic penicillin. It is effective against gram-positive bacteria including *Streptococcus, Staphylococcus* and *Pneumococcus,* but unlike many antibiotics, does not harm the gram-negative bacteria that live in the gut and vagina.

In preliminary clinical trials in 1988, a mouthwash containing 1% usnic acid was administered to volunteers. The samples of oral bacterial flora were examined at regular intervals, and it was reported that the growth of *Streptococcus mutans,* involved in the cause of dental decay, was selectively suppressed (Ghione et al.)

Usnic acid has been shown to suppress the growth of gram-positive organisms that are mainly responsible for body odour, and as a result is often an ingredient in deodorants (Ingolfsdottir, 2002).

Other studies have shown that usnic acid is active against methicillin-resistant *Staphylococcus aureus* (MRSA) and therefore has potential for use in the sterilisation of surgical implants and is also active against tuberculosis and chronic bronchitis.

Usnea is also antifungal, working by disrupting the fungal cell membrane and inhibiting cellular processes essential for fungal growth and reproduction. It specifically interferes with the synthesis of ergosterol, a crucial component of fungal cell membranes, leading to cell lysis and death.

It is also beneficial for women with yeast infections, trichomoniasis, bacterial vaginosis and chlamydia. It could be useful for people with chronic fatigue, HIV, *Herpes* and other chronic conditions related to depressed immune systems.

Usnic acid has also been shown to be antiviral against Epstein-Barr virus, herpes simplex type I and polio type 1 viruses in animal tests. In a clinical trial, the effect of a formula containing usnic acid and zinc sulfate was evaluated in

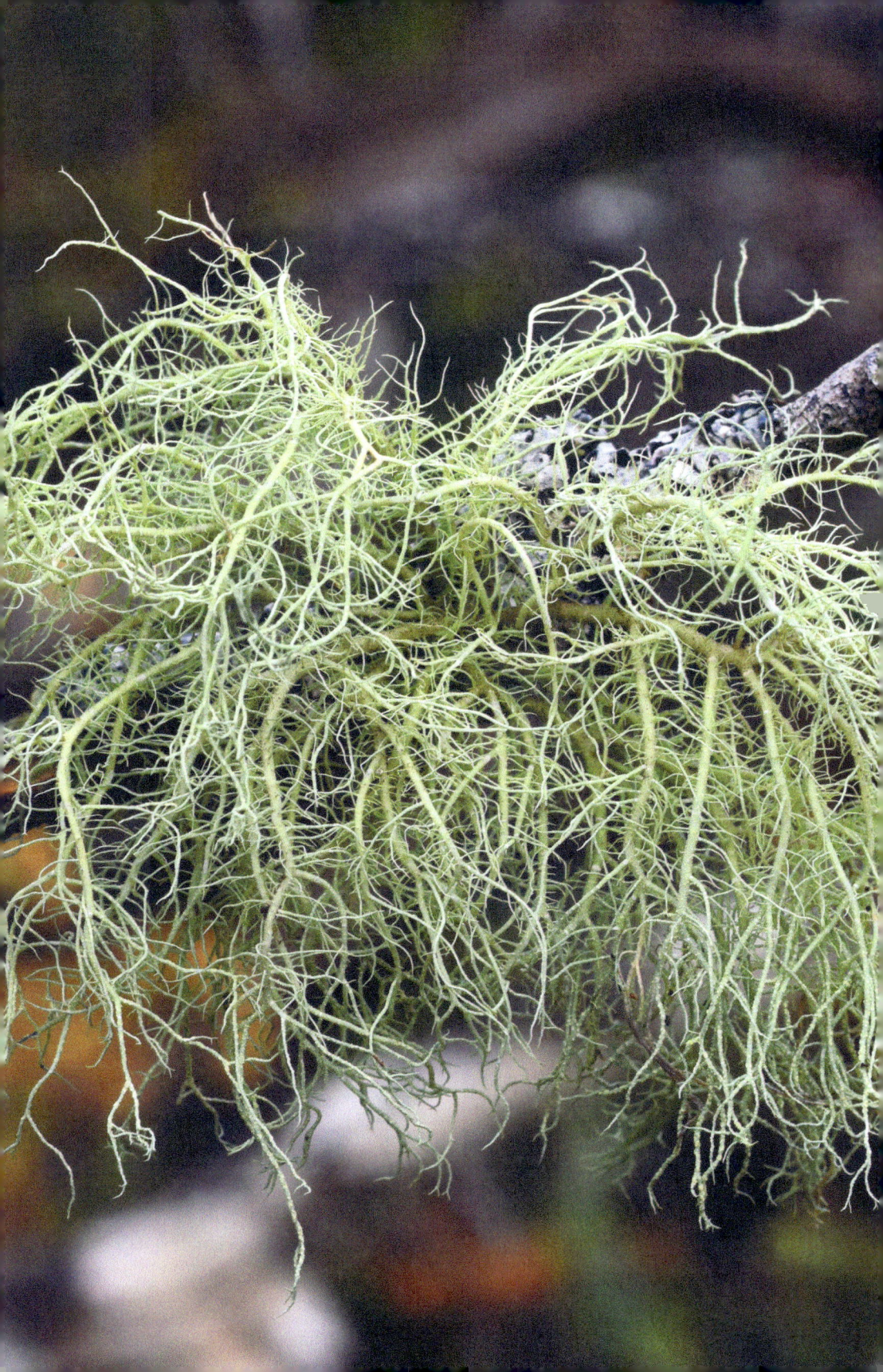

100 women with genital infections of human papilloma virus. The treatment significantly improved the time of healing.

Anticancerogenic
In 2010 and 2013, studies on usnic acid revealed that it may prevent cancer cell growth and kill cancerous cells while selectively avoiding non-cancerous ones. Then, in 2016, cytotoxic activity of the extracts was evaluated in mouse melanoma and rat glioma, and found to decrease the viability of both cells. Research has suggested that usnic acid may have synergistic effects when used in combination with other anti-cancer agents, potentially enhancing the efficacy of conventional cancer treatments (Manojlovic et al 2012)

Anti-obesity
Usnic acid is also used in weight loss products as it is believed to increase the metabolic rate. However, many studies carried out circa 2011 revealed that a potential side effect of these products is liver failure. Durazo et al. 2004 reported on a healthy 28-year-old woman who developed acute liver failure within one month of commencing usnic acid at a dose of 500mg/day for two weeks. Sanchez et al. 2006 also reported severe hepatotoxicity in a husband and wife (both 38 years of age) who were bodybuilders taking a multi-ingredient health supplement containing 150mg usnic acid for three months. Another herbal remedy containing usnic acid is kombucha tea. This is a beverage made by brewing a culture of bacteria and yeast (a SCOBY) in sweet black tea, with some reported liver damage on overconsumption.

TOPICAL USES

Research in rats shows that usnic acid increases markers of wound-healing, such as collagen formation, when applied directly to wounds.

DOSAGE

Tincture – 1:5, 3–4ml daily – 20 drops = 1ml/1tsp = 5ml. However, see below.

PRECAUTIONS

When taken by mouth, Usnea may cause stomach upset and severe liver damage. Children and pregnant or breastfeeding women should completely avoid it, while all others should practise extreme caution. In any event, Usnea should not be used for more than three weeks in a row. Scientific reports on the toxic properties of high doses were published by Pätiälä in 1949. The compound administered at a dose of 3mg daily caused liver pain. With reducing its dosage to 1mg per day, the symptoms were removed.

Usnea recipes

As with most lichens, Usnea is not very water-soluble, so either alcohol or oil must be used to make an extract.

Medicinal recipes
Usnea infused oil
- 100g powdered Usnea
- 2tsp alcohol, such as Everclear
- 100ml grapeseed oil

Place the Usnea in a jar with the alcohol and allow to steep for 10 minutes before adding the oil. Leave for 4 weeks and then strain. Make into a stronger tincture infused salve by using 80ml oil and 20ml tincture, then use a 1:4 ratio of melted beeswax to your tincture/oil mix, ie. 1 part wax to 4 parts liquid as follows:

Weigh or measure out the wax pellets and place them with the herbal infused oil in a double boiler or bain-marie. Heat over a low heat until the wax is fully melted and then stir well. This is the time to slowly add your tincture to the mix, whisking it lightly as you do. Remove from the heat and allow to cool and set completely. Use as a topical antibiotic, antifungal and anti-inflammatory treatment for wounds, burns and athlete's foot. Usnea can also be used in a powder form directly on wounds as an antibiotic.

Usnea poultice
- Fresh Usnea

Clean to remove any dirt or debris then crush or chop the Usnea to release its juices. Apply the crushed Usnea directly to the affected area and cover with a clean cloth or gauze to hold the poultice in place.

Leave it on for 20-30 minutes, then rinse. Repeat as needed for relief from skin inflammation and to promote wound-healing.

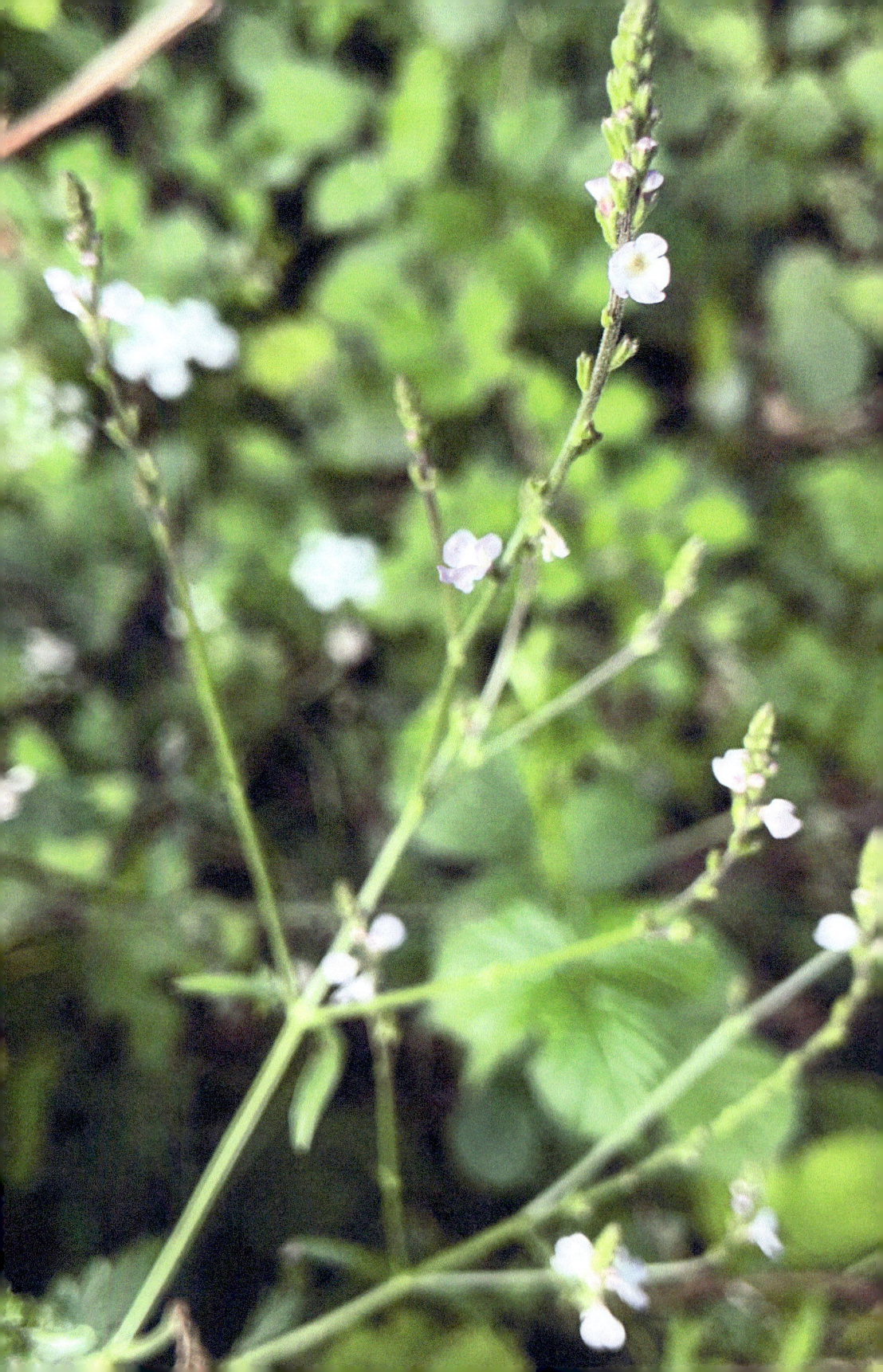

VERVAIN
Verbena officinalis

Vervain is a versatile and historically significant plant with a wide range of traditional uses. It is native to the UK and likely to be found in meadows, grasslands, roadsides and even waste areas.

HISTORICAL USES

The use of vervain for medicinal, ceremonial and superstitious purposes goes back thousands of years. It was a sacred plant to several ancient civilisations, including the Persians, Romans, Greeks and the ancient Egyptians, who believed vervain first sprang from the tears of the goddess Isis as she mourned the death of the god Osiris. The Druids held a sprig of vervain during the act of soothsaying or speaking divine prophecies, having first made offerings to Mother Earth in grand ceremonies surrounding the gathering of the plant (De Cleene and Lejeune, 2002).

Nicholas Culpeper's *Herbal* said, '*Vervain is hot and dry, opening obstructions, cleansing and healing. It helps the yellow jaundice, the dropsy and the gout; it kills and expels worms in the belly, and causes a good colour in the face and body, strengthens as well as corrects the diseases of the stomach, liver, and spleen; helps the cough, wheezings, and shortness of breath,*

ETYMOLOGY OF COMMON NAME
From Celtic *fer* and *faen* meaning 'to drive away the stone'.

PLANT LORE
One of the three most sacred herbs to the Druids. Infused in wine or worn on the head during Midsummer festivals.

USE
All parts.

EDIBILITY
The leaves can be parboiled, seasoned and then eaten.

HARVEST
In summer.

MEDICINAL PROPERTIES
Diaphoretic, antispasmodic, antiparasitic, analgesic and anxiolytic.

ACTIVE CONSTITUENTS
Vervenalini, vervenalini (glycosides), essential oil, alkaloids, tannins, mucus, bitter substance.

LEFT: VERVAIN

and all the defects of the reins and bladder, expelling the gravel and stone. The leaves bruised, or the juice of them mixed with some vinegar, does wonderfully cleanse the skin, and takes away morphew, freckles, fistulas, and other such like inflammations and deformities of the skin in any parts of the body. The distilled water of the herb when it is in full strength, dropped into the eyes, cleanses them from films, clouds, or mists, that darken the sight, and wonderfully strengthens the optic nerves.'

The American herbalist Albert Isaiah Coffin (1790–1866) agreed with Culpeper, writing that *'As an emetic, it ranks next to lobelia; it is also one of the strongest sweating medicines in nature. It is good for colds, coughs and pain in the head, and some years ago was highly esteemed as a remedy for consumption. Vervain will relieve and cure complaints in children which generally accompany teething; it likewise destroys worms. Administered as a tea, it powerfully assists the pains of labour; as a diuretic it increases the urinary discharge.'*

MODERN RESEARCH

As Culpeper mentioned, this plant was used in folk medicine for a great many ailments, and modern research has found or confirmed the following medicinal properties:

Antiparasitic

Both Culpeper and Coffin refer to the antiparasitic properties of Vervain. In a 2022 study, treatment with Vervain showed 74% efficacy in reducing the shed of *Cryptosporidium* spp. oocyst in the stool of infected mice. The antiparasitic properties had been previously shown by a study against *Trichomoniasis vaginalis*, and Teklay et al. (2013) demonstrated that the extract or the juice of roots could be used to treat ascariasis (roundworm infection).

Diuretic

Culpeper and Coffin list the diuretic actions of the plant, which the phytopharmaceutical authors N.G. Bisset and Max Wichtl confirmed in 2001, together with some evidence that vervain can be useful in cases of urinary stones (Mills and Bone, 2000).

Anxiolytic

Vervain is known for its calming properties, and has been used to reduce anxiety and promote relaxation. It is considered a nervine tonic, which means it supports the health and function of the nervous system. A 2016 study on the anticonvulsant, anxiolytic and sedative effects of Vervain found that the extract had an anxiolytic effect comparable to diazepam, which validated its folk use in neurological disorders. While I have found nothing to substantiate Culpeper's findings for cough, wheezings and shortness of breath, it may be that the calming properties of Vervain also ease respiratory issues.

Antibacterial

A 2017 study found that the stems of Vervain proved potent against 24 strains of gram-positive and gram-negative bacteria and that its effect on *Staphylococcus aureus* and *Pseudomonas aeruginosa* was higher than the antibiotic amoxicillin. This was confirmed in a 2020 study using ethanolic extracts of its stems, leaves and roots, which were effective against all the tested gram-positive and gram-negative microorganisms, confirming the use of Vervain as a remedy for microbial infections.

Anti-inflammatory and analgesic

Studies in 1998, 2000 and 2006 confirmed the use described by Coffin of Vervain as an anti-inflammatory and analgesic.

TOPICAL USES

Using Vervain helps relieve discomfort from insect bites and can accelerate the healing process by closing wounds more quickly. You can use fresh Vervain plant, crushed into a pulp, or just soak a clean cloth in a strong version of Vervain tea and apply directly to your skin.

DOSAGE

Infusion – 1tsp/5g, 2–3 times per day.

PRECAUTIONS

Not for use by those with kidney disease or when pregnant/lactating. Excessive doses may cause vomiting.

Vervain recipes

Medicinal recipes

Vervain tisane

Pour 250ml boiling water over 1tsp/5g of the dried herb and allow to steep for 10-15 minutes. Use for the relief of tension and stress and for postviral fatigue. The tisane may also be used as a mouthwash to treat ulcers in the mouth.

Vervain poultice

- 1tsp fresh Vervain leaf (if using dried you will need to moisten with water first)
- 2tsp coconut oil
- cheesecloth or cotton bandage

Finely chop the herb into a pulp and add the coconut oil to make a paste. Spread the paste evenly over the desired area and wrap with the cloth or bandage. Use as a topical anti-inflammatory and analgesic.

Vervain infused oil

- 100g Vervain
- 2tsp alcohol, such as Everclear
- 100ml grapeseed oil

Place the Vervain in a jar with the alcohol and allow to steep for 10 minutes before adding the oil. Leave for 4 weeks and then strain. Use as a remedy for bruises, skin infections, insect bites, eczema and other skin disorders. It has also been used to alleviate sprains and may give relief in nerve pains.

For relaxation

- 1 part Betony
- 1 part Vervain
- 2 parts Lemon balm

Combine and use 1tsp per cup of boiled water. Drink 3 times per day.

VIOLET
Viola odorata

There are several species of *Viola* that are native or naturalised in the UK, but for the purposes of this chapter, I focus on Sweet violet (*Viola odorata*), which is considered the superior medicinal species.

HISTORICAL USES

In her *Physica*, Hildegard of Bingen (1098–1179) explained that Violets are good for the eyes, '*Violet is between hot and cold [and is of an especially sober colour]. Although it is cold, it grows from the* [mild, gentle] *air which after winter is beginning to warm up. It is valuable against fogginess of the eyes. Take good oil, and boil it in a new pot, either in the sun or over a fire. When it boils, put violets in so that it becomes thickened. Put this in a glass vessel and save it. At night put this unguent around the eyelids and eyes. Although it shan't touch the inside of the eyes, it will expel the fogginess.*'

In his *Herball*, John Gerard (1545–1612) said, '*The floures are good for all inflammations, especially of the sides and lungs; they take away the hoarsenesse of the chest, the ruggednesse of the winde-pipe and jawes, and take away thirst.*'

Nicholas Culpeper's *Herbal* stated, '*All the Violets are cold and moist while they are fresh and green, and are used to cool any heat, or distemperature of the*

ETYMOLOGY OF COMMON NAME
From Middle English *violet* and *vyolette*, and the Latin *viola*, meaning 'purple'.

PLANT LORE
In Greek mythology, Persephone was apparently picking violets when Hades kidnapped her to live with him in the underworld.

USE
The leaves and flowers.

EDIBILITY
Both leaves and flowers are used in salads.

HARVEST
When in bloom.

MEDICINAL PROPERTIES
Anti-inflammatory, antihypertensive, expectorant, diuretic, antibacterial and anticancerogenic.

ACTIVE CONSTITUENTS
Flavonoids, saponins, alkaloids, essential oils.

body, either inwardly or outwardly, as inflammations in the eyes, in the matrix or fundament, in imposthumes also, and hot swellings, to drink the decoction of the leaves and flowers made with water in wine, or to apply them poultice-wise to the grieved places: it likewise eases pains in the head, caused through want of sleep; or any other pains arising of heat, being applied in the same manner, or with oil of roses. The green leaves are used with other herbs to make plaisters and poultices to inflammations and swellings, and to ease all pains whatsoever, arising of heat, and for the piles also, being fried with yolks of eggs, and applied thereto.'

Harold Ward's *Herbal Manual* (1936) commented on the '*Remarkable claims* [that] *have been made for violet leaves in the treatment of malignant tumours. The case of Lady Margaret Marsham, of Maidstone, was reported in the* Daily Mail *for November 14th, 1901. This lady, suffering from cancer of the throat, used an infusion, which was left to stand for twelve hours, of a handful of fresh violet leaves to a pint of boiling water. After a fortnight of warm fomentations with this liquid the growth was said to have disappeared. The same newspaper, dated March 18th, 1905, told its readers that violet leaves as a cure for cancer were advocated in the current issue of the* Lancet, *where a remarkable case was reported by Dr William Gordon, M.D. Such accounts as these, although interesting, should be read with considerable reserve.*'

MODERN RESEARCH

With a long history of use, this small plant has been widely studied and been found or confirmed to have the following properties:

Diuretic

In a 2009 study, the aqueous extract of Violet showed significant diuretic activity, and combined butanolic (butyl alcohol) and aqueous extracts showed good laxative effect.

Antihypertensive

The results of a 2012 study showed that the extract of leaves of Sweet violet exhibited blood pressure-lowering effects in rats under anaesthesia. The plant also displayed reduction in body weight and cholesterol levels, which may be related to the absorption of lipids and antioxidant activities. The conclusion of the study was: 'Thus, this study provides a pharmacologic rationale to the medicinal use of Sweet Violet in hypertension and dyslipidaemia and may be a good candidate to be developed as antihypertensive and anti-dyslipidaemic medicine, with therapeutic potential in obesity and metabolic syndrome.'

Expectorant and analgesic

A 2018 review confirmed some of Culpeper's findings of the efficacy of Sweet violet syrup in coughs, insomnia and migraines. It also found that Sweet violet (as a syrup) appears to be a safe treatment for management of

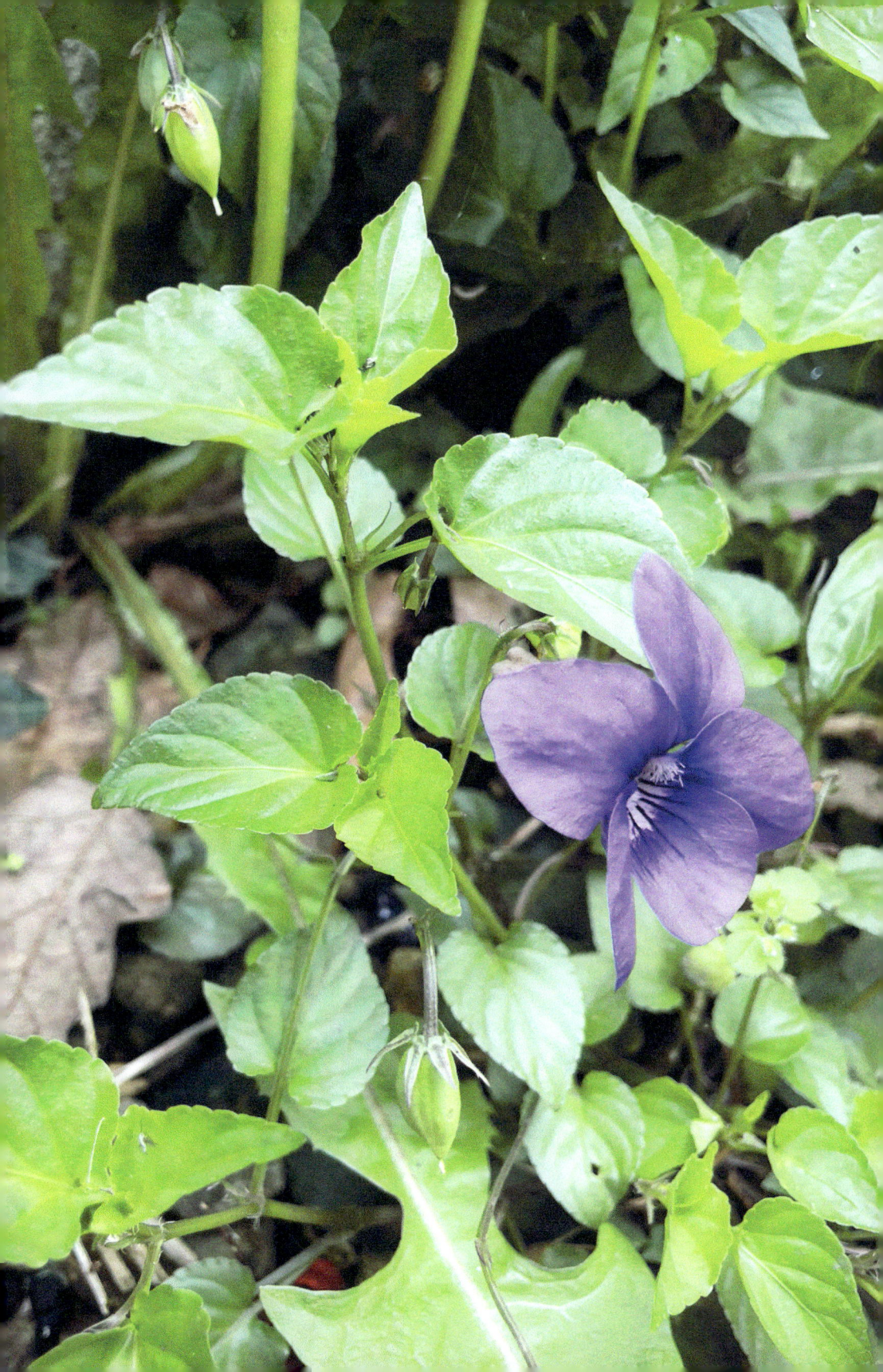

respiratory ailments in children and that efficacy in the treatment of pain, fever, cough, infection and inflammation may make it a suitable treatment.

A 2023 clinical study confirmed the use of Sweet violet syrup in COVID-19 patients when those who received the syrup recovered faster and the mean severity scores of coughs decreased more greatly in comparison to the control group.

Anti-inflammatory

In 2003, an aqueous extract of Sweet violet showed anti-inflammatory properties equal to the effect of hydrocortisone in aiding the resolution of induced lung damage (Koochek et al.).

Sweet violet is also considered effective against various neurodegenerative diseases such as Alzheimer's and Parkinson's disease as well as epilepsy and anxiety, owing to its anti-inflammatory and antioxidant potential (Vishal et al., 2009).

A 2021 study confirmed the above and noted that the methanolic extract of Sweet violet may be therapeutically effective in memory improvement by increasing oxidative stress biomarkers and decreasing pro-inflammatory markers.

Viola odorata has been found to be a rich source of cyclotides, and these cyclotides were studied in 2022 in relation to inflammatory diseases such as multiple sclerosis. They were shown in animal studies to significantly reduce clinical scores, inflammation and demyelination, meaning they could be used as immunomodulatory agents with similar effects to fingolimod, an immunomodulating medication used for the treatment of multiple sclerosis.

Antibacterial

A 2016 study found that Sweet violet has significant bioactive properties against respiratory microorganisms owing to the presence of ionones. When tested, extracts were found to be active against *Haemophilus influenzae*, *Pseudomonas aeruginosa*, *Staphylococcus aureus*, *Staphylococcus pneumoniae* and *Staphylococcus pyogenes* respectively, thereby validating its use as a potential source of natural drug for curing the respiratory diseases caused by selected microorganisms.

Anticancerogenic

As Harold Ward pointed out, the whole aerial part of Sweet violet, including stem, flowers and leaves, is used in cancer treatments and antitumour agents; this owes much to the presence of its cyclotides, which cause cell death by membrane permeabilisation. A 2010 study documented several cyclotides with robust cytotoxicity that may be promising agents against drug-resistant breast cancer (Gerlach et al.).

Cholinergic

There is a study that somewhat backs up Hildegard von Bingen's theory of using Sweet violet for the eyes. In 2019, a randomised, double-blind, placebo-controlled study of 105 patients with dry eye symptoms between the ages of 18 and 60 years were allocated to violet-almond oil, almond oil and placebo groups. The treatment and placebo were administered intranasally, 2 drops three times a day for one month. Results showed that intranasally administered Sweet violet oily extract enhanced tear production and improved tear film stability.

TOPICAL USES

Again, as per Culpeper's findings, Sweet violet is an old remedy for bruises, and is used as a poultice for treatment of headache, cough, colds, bronchitis and fever in different traditional medicines.

DOSAGE

Infusion – 1tsp/5g, 2–3 times per day.

PRECAUTIONS

Higher doses can be laxative. Not suitable for children or those who are pregnant or lactating.

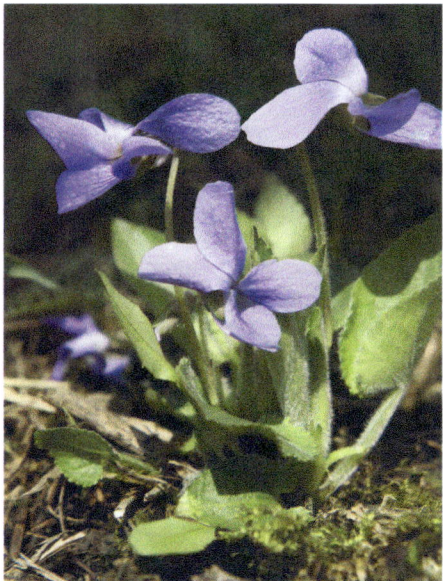

Violet recipes

Medicinal recipes

Sweet violet tisane

Pour 250ml boiling water over 1tsp/5g of the dried herb and allow to steep for 10–15 minutes. Use for the treatment of bronchitis, dry cough, asthma, respiratory and urinary infections.

Sweet violet cough syrup

- 128g fresh Sweet violet crushed flowers and leaves
- 600ml of boiling water
- 500g of sugar

Cover the leaves and flowers with the water and let stand for 12 hours. Strain the leaves, add the sugar and simmer slowly until syrupy before adding to a jar. Use 1tbsp/15g for coughs or slight constipation 2 or 3 times a day.

Sweet violet poultice

- 1tsp fresh flower and leaf (if using dried you will need to moisten with water first)
- 2tsp coconut oil
- cheesecloth or cotton bandage

Finely chop the herb into a pulp and add the coconut oil to make a paste. Spread the paste evenly over the desired area and wrap with the cloth or bandage. Use as a remedy for a headache, cough, colds, bronchitis and fever.

Violet bath tea

- 50g herb
- 1l water

Steep the herb in the water for 15 minutes, then strain and add to the bathwater. The fresh crushed flowers are soothing to the skin and the aroma is very relaxing.

Violet infused oil

- 100g flowers
- 2tbsp alcohol, such as Everclear
- 1l grapeseed oil

Place the herbs in a jar with the alcohol and allow to steep for 10 minutes before adding the oil. Leave for 4 weeks and then strain. Use as a topical treatment for skin irritations, inflammations and minor wounds.

WILLOWHERBS
Epilobium spp.

In the UK alone there are approximately a dozen species of Willowherb, including the three focused on here: Hairy (*Epilobium hirsutum*), Hoary (*Epilobium parviflorum*) and Rosebay (*Epilobium angustifolium*). Willowherbs are typically found in a variety of habitats, including grasslands, woodlands, heathlands and along roadsides. They are often pioneer species, thriving in disturbed or recently cleared areas, and play an important role in ecosystems as they provide nectar for pollinators like bees and butterflies. Additionally, their seeds are a food source for birds.

HISTORICAL USES

Native Americans used the root of some Willowherb species externally, to treat skin infections and rectal bleeding owing to the astringent properties (Raymond, 1945; Shikov et al., 2006).

Nicholas Culpeper's *Herbal* stated, '*All the species of Willow-Herb have the same virtues; they are under Saturn in Aries and are cooling and astringent. The root carefully dried and powdered, is good against bloody fluxes, and other hæmorrhages; and the fresh juice is of the same virtue.*'

In view of the astringent, demulcent and emollient properties, Willowherb infusions were recommended by American herbalists in the 19th and

ETYMOLOGY OF COMMON NAME
Named for the willow-like leaves; it has a downy stem.

PLANT LORE
Willowherb is sometimes called 'fireweed' because it is one of the first plants to colonise areas after wildfires.

USE
All aerial parts.

EDIBILITY
The young shoots and leaves of Rosebay willowherb are edible and can be eaten raw or cooked.

HARVEST
In summer, when in flower.

MEDICINAL PROPERTIES
Astringent, antiprostatic, anti-inflammatory, antioxidant and antimicrobial.

ACTIVE CONSTITUENTS
Phenolic compounds, tannins, phytosterols, polysaccharides, fatty acids.

early 20th centuries as a very effective agent to treat gastrointestinal diseases such as dysentery and diarrhoea, as well as other bowel and intestinal disorders associated with infection, irritation and inflammation.

MODERN RESEARCH

The Willowherbs have been studied for their potential health benefits, including anti-inflammatory, antioxidant and antimicrobial properties. Research has discovered and confirmed the following:

Astringent

As Culpeper said, the leaves have astringent properties and will therefore help to heal wounds. We now know that this is because they contain tannins, which are polyphenolic compounds with astringent properties.

Antimicrobial

Studies have shown that the Willowherbs exert many antimicrobial activities. Hairy willowherb showed strong antibacterial activity against both gram-negative and gram-positive bacteria and on both *Staphylococcus aureus* standard strains and methicillin-resistant *Staphylococcus aureus* (MRSA) strains. Moreover, Hairy willowherb showed synergism with ampicillin or tetracycline antibiotics and increased the antimicrobial effect against *Staphylococcus aureus* standard strains.

Extracts have also shown antiviral activity when a polyphenolic mixture of Hairy willowherb (combined with a water-alcohol extract) was found to have a significant inhibitory effect on the reproduction of influenza viruses (Ivancheva et al., 1992).

The antimicrobial activity of the Hoary willowherb was also confirmed against *Staphylococcus aureus* and *Escherichia coli* by Rauha et al. in 2000, while significant antifungal activity of the root extract against *Candida glabrata*, *Candida lusitaniae* and *Saccharomyces cerevisiae* was detected by Webster et al. in 2008.

In 2012, ethanolic extracts of Rosebay willowherb were found to strongly inhibit the growth of *Escherichia coli*, *Micrococcus luteus*, *Pseudomonas aeruginosa* and *Staphylococcus aureus*, and were more effective than the antibiotics vancomycin and tetracycline. These findings were confirmed by Kosalec et al. in 2013, with the addition of activity against *Bacillus subtilis*, *Proteus mirabilis*, *Candida albicans*, *Candida tropicalis*, *Candida dubliniensis* and *Saccharomyces cerevisiae*.

A 2018 study confirmed that the pharmacological activity and therapeutic effects were thanks to polyphenolic compounds, such as flavonoids and ellagitannins derivates, particularly oenothein B.

Antioxidant

All of the Willowherbs contain antioxidants, including flavonoids and phenolic compounds, which help protect cells from oxidative damage

RIGHT: HAIRY WILLOWHERB

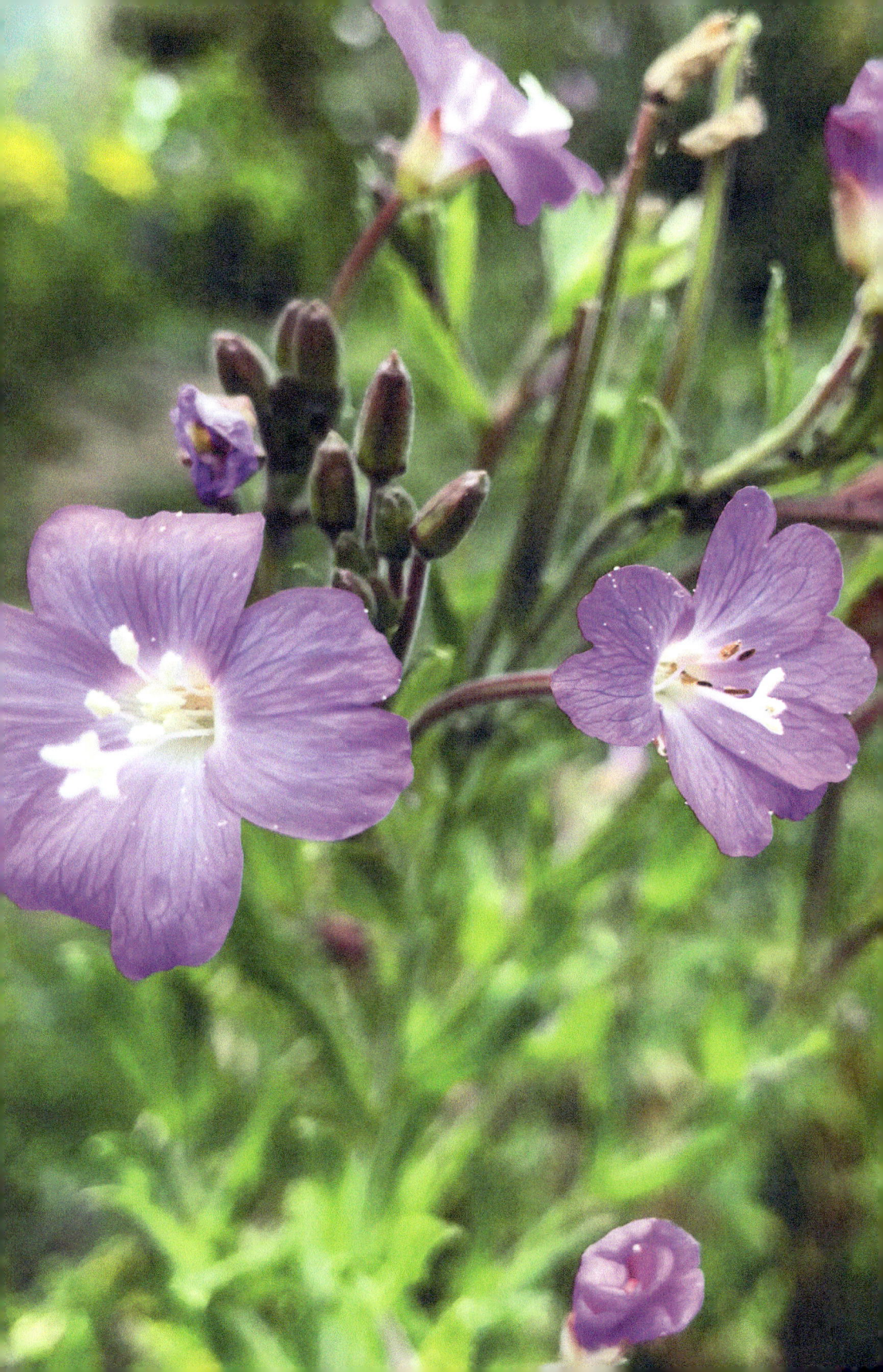

caused by free radicals. The antioxidant levels of Hairy willowherb are very high. In fact, in a 2001 study showed it has the highest antioxidant values of 32 plants tested, owing to the catechins and procyanidins it contains. It was also the only one of the plants selected for testing that contained the bioflavonoid myricetin, which is also found in many berries, walnuts, onions and red grapes as well as other plants, and suggests that it could be used as a natural antioxidant source.

The above was confirmed in 2017 when animals treated with extracts of Hairy willowherb showed significant organ protection and improved serum iron profile when compared to control groups.

Analgesic

Methanolic extracts of Hairy willowherb exhibited antinociceptive activity in mice. Doses of 500mg/kg resulted in higher pain tolerance than doses of diclofenac (50mg/kg) and morphine (5mg/kg). Furthermore, doses of the methanolic extract did not impair locomotors skills of mice (Pourmorad et al., 2007). Similar analgesic activity of Rosebay tincture was then also determined in mice in 2001.

Antiprostatic

In a 2006 study, extracts of five herbal remedies were investigated for treatment of benign prostatic hyperplasia (BPH). The ethanolic extract of Hoary willowherb showed inhibitory effects on both the COX-1 and COX-2 (enzymes that produce inflammatory lipids) catalysed prostaglandin biosynthesis, inhibited growth of *Escherichia coli* and exerted antioxidant activity.

On 2 February 2016 (under EMA/822538/2015) the Committee on Herbal Medicinal Products concluded that, on the basis of its long-standing use, Willowherb can be used by patients with BPH for the relief of lower urinary tract symptoms such as difficulty starting urination or a frequent need to urinate.

Anticancerogenic

A 2021 paper was the first to demonstrate that Hoary willowherb had a strong growth inhibiting property on breast cancer cell lines, and is a potential model to treat human breast cancer cells. The most cytotoxic effect was noted for the methanolic root extract.

Another 2021 study exhibited the antiproliferative activity of Hoary willowherb extracts in colon cancer cell lines. Results confirmed that aqueous and ethanolic extracts can eliminate proliferation of human colorectal carcinoma cells *in vitro* and suggested that Hoary willowherb may have the potential to become a therapeutic agent against colon cancers. Likewise, treatment of androgen-sensitive human prostate adenocarcinoma cells with Willowherb extracts resulted in a significant increase in the number of apoptotic cells. Various Willowherb extracts, including extracts from Rosebay willowherb, caused a similar inhibitory effect on the proliferation of human cancer cell lines and inhibited DNA synthesis in human astrocytoma (brain tumour) cells.

TOPICAL USES

A 2013 study has shown evidence that the antioxidant benefits of Hairy willowherb could be helpful for the treatment of diabetic foot syndrome, a serious complication of diabetes.

Rosebay willowherb is also used as a cleansing, soothing, antiseptic and healing agent to treat minor burns, skin rashes, ulcers and infections, and for treatment of inflammations of the ear, nose and throat. The photoprotective and anti-ageing properties of Rosebay willowherb extract have been revealed in human stress-induced fibroblasts in *in vitro* and *in vivo* models, making it a prospective candidate for additions to skin treatments.

DOSAGE

Tisane – 2tsp/10g. Drink freely.
Decoction – 1tsp root. Drink a half cup, 3 times per day.
Tincture – 1:10 45%, 1–2tsp, 3 times per day.

PRECAUTIONS

Epilobium interferes with the hormone progesterone, so if you are pregnant, taking hormone replacement therapy or on birth control pills, you should avoid using this herb.

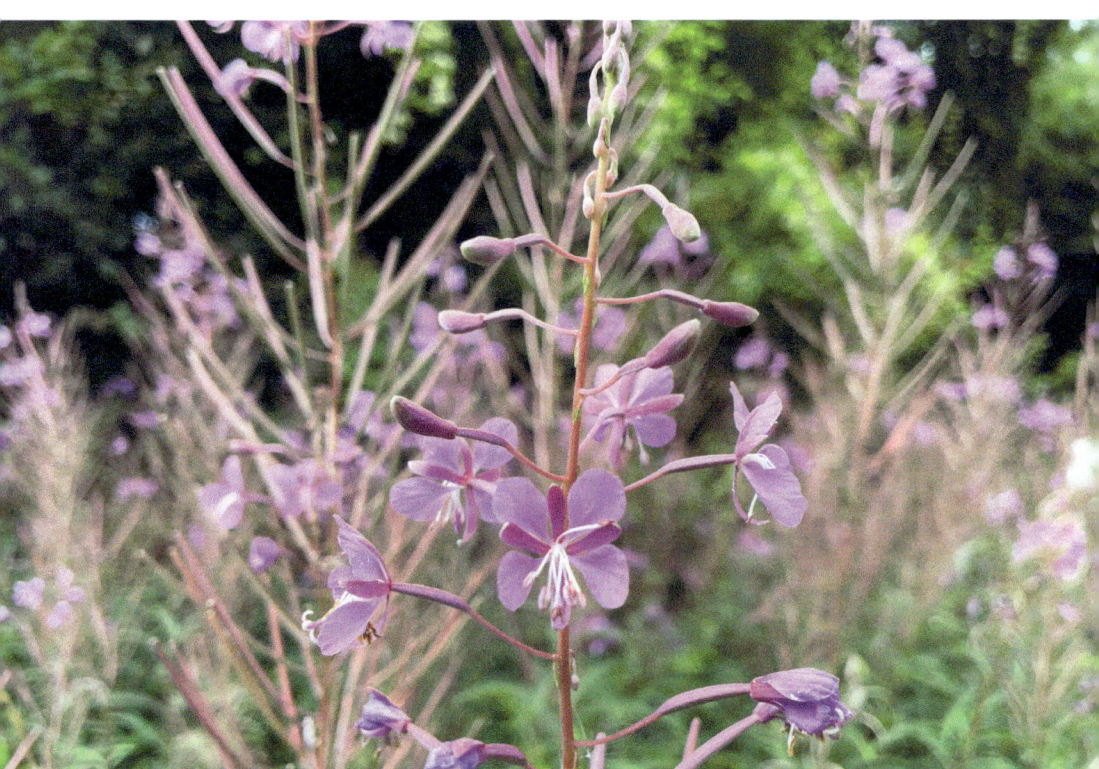

Willowherb recipes

Medicinal recipes

Hoary willowherb tisane

Pour 250ml boiling water over 1tsp/5g of the dried herb and allow to steep for 10-15 minutes. Use for the treatment of leucorrhoea, menorrhagia, uterine haemorrhage and micturition problems associated with prostatic hyperplasia, and for gastrointestinal disorders and mucous membrane lesions of the mouth.

Willowherb infused oil

- 100g dried leaf of any of the Willowherbs
- 2 tbsp alcohol, such as Everclear
- coconut oil

Place the herbs in a jar with the alcohol, muddle and allow to steep for 10 minutes before adding the oil. Infuse in coconut oil in a warm oven (75-100°) for 3-4 hours. Once infused, strain and keep in the fridge between use. Use for acne and seborrheic skin, such as face creams.

Hairy willowherb tincture 1:10 45%

If you are using 40% alcohol, ie. vodka, make a simple tincture by covering 1 part herb to 10 parts fluid.

If you are using Everclear or other 100% proof, use the following method for a specific tincture:

- 100g Hairy willowherb dried root, powdered
- 450ml alcohol
- 550ml water

Divide the root material into two parts of 50g each and cover one part with the alcohol and the other part in a pan with the water. Bring to the boil and simmer for 20-30 minutes. Strain and add to the alcohol mix. Allow to steep for 14 days and then strain and use as an analgesic and antiviral for colds and flu.

Rosebay cordial

- 3-5 handfuls of Rosebay flowers
- 1l water
- 60g caster sugar
- 1 lemon

Squeeze the lemon for the juice and add to a pan, then add the sugar and flowers and pour over 1 litre boiling water. Stir well and leave to cool. Strain into another jug and keep in the refrigerator, ready to use to support digestive health.

WOUNDWORT
Stachys spp.

The Woundworts belong to the larger *Stachys* genus, which includes over 300 species distributed worldwide. Species native to the UK include Hedge woundwort (*Stachys sylvatica*), Marsh woundwort (*Stachys palustris*) and Field woundwort (*Stachys arvensis*). While they share common medicinal uses and habitats, each species has unique characteristics and adaptations. All three also play a role in supporting biodiversity and have a history of traditional medicinal use.

HISTORICAL USES

In her *Physica*, Hildegard of Bingen (1098–1179) advised that '*when a person has outstandingly large ulcers on him, he should cook Woundwort in water and place it, warm, on the ulcers and frequently moisten them in this way. He will become well.*'

In his *Herball*, John Gerard (1545–1612) referred to Clownes Woundwort, meaning Marsh woundwort, but the properties are the same for both Marsh and Hedge woundwort. He said, '*The leaves hereof stamped with Axungia or hogs grease, and applied unto greene wounds in manner of a pultesse, heale them in short time, and in such absolute manner, that it is hard for any that have not had the experience thereof to believe.*'

ETYMOLOGY OF COMMON NAME
Named for the leaves, used in the dressing of wounds.

PLANT LORE
Believed to be Nature's gift to weary travellers, to bind wounds from falls or thorn-ripped flesh.

USE
The stalks and flowers.

EDIBILITY
The tuberous roots of Woundwort can be boiled as a vegetable, as can the tender and young shoots.

HARVEST
In spring and summer.

MEDICINAL PROPERTIES
Astringent, styptic, antibacterial, antioxidant, anti-proliferative.

ACTIVE CONSTITUENTS
Phenolic acids, triterpenes, flavonoids, alkaloids.

Nicholas Culpeper's *Herbal* said simply '*It is inferior to none* in its ability to heal wounds.'

MODERN RESEARCH

The Woundworts are related to Betony, which goes some way to explaining why Culpeper thought so highly of them. This family of plants is a rich source of flavonoids, and the presence of phenolic compounds such as chlorogenic acids has also been shown from the aerial parts of Marsh woundwort, the more studied of the three. So far modern research has found these plants to have the following properties:

Astringent

Woundworts have been traditionally used to arrest bleeding owing to their tannin content. Maude Grieve's *A Modern Herbal* (1931) explained that, '*The bruised leaves, which have an unpleasant odour and an astringent taste, when applied to a wound will stop bleeding and heal the wound, and as is claimed for them by old tradition, the fresh juice is made into a syrup and taken internally to stop haemorrhages, dysentery, etc.*'

Antioxidant

A 2012 study showed that the extract of Hedge woundwort contains essential oils, flavonoids, phenolics and a high extent of antioxidant activity. A study in 2020 confirmed similar compounds in Field woundwort, and the antioxidant properties of Marsh woundwort were also studied in 2022, with results showing that the flowers and leaves had the highest radical-scavenging activities and were more effective at eliminating excess reactive oxygen species that cause oxidative stress in the body.

Anticancerogenic

Following on from the above, the same 2022 study also explored the anti-proliferative activity in the leaves, flowers, stems and roots of Marsh woundwort against lung adenocarcinoma, pancreatic ductal adenocarcinoma, colorectal adenocarcinoma, bladder cancer and acute myeloid leukaemia cells. The most significant results were obtained for leaves and flower extracts and, in particular, the extract from the leaves markedly decreased the metabolic activity of all tested cell lines, meaning the plant has strong potential for further trials of its medicinal effects.

Anti-inflammatory

The 2020 study of Field woundwort above also found it to have an excellent anti-inflammatory activity, close to that of acetylsalicylic acid (aspirin), which was used as a control.

A 2020 study of Hedge woundwort concluded that extracts could improve some symptoms of polycystic ovary syndrome (PCOS) because of the iridoid, flavonoid and sesquiterpene content, together with antioxidant

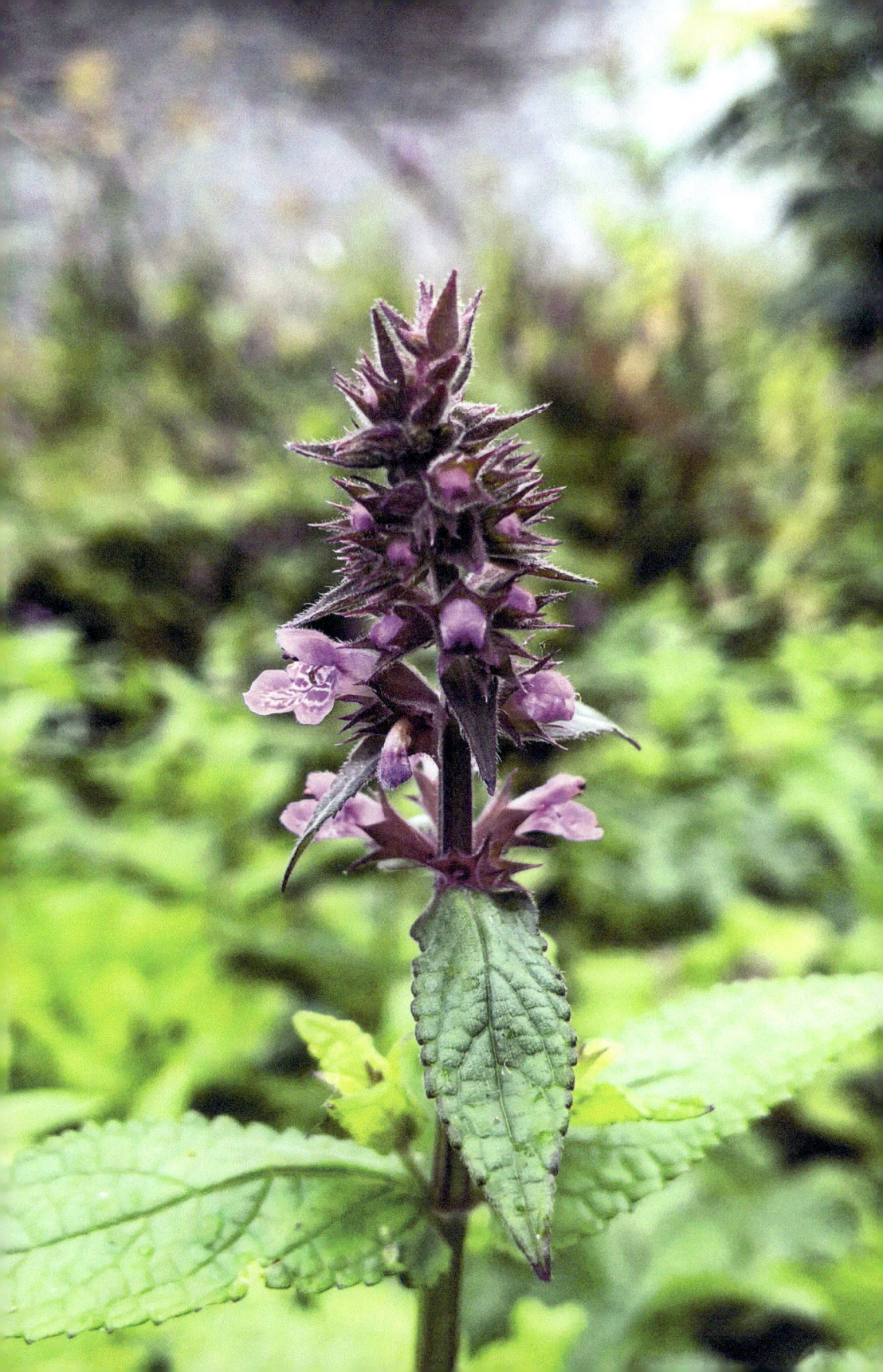

and anti-inflammatory effects. In this experiment, a 500mg/kg dose of extract was considered as the most effective dose. Given that women with PCOS showed high concentrations of inflammation factors, the study assumed that the extract could act as anti-inflammatory and antioxidant agent.

Antibacterial

The *n*-butanol extract of Field woundwort was shown to possess good antibacterial activity against gram-positive and gram-negative strains of bacteria, while the ethanolic extracts of Hedge woundwort indicated potential antibacterial effects against the eye pathogens *Staphylococcus capitis*, *Moraxella nonliquefaciens* and *Cutibacterium acnes* as compared to the standard antibacterial agents such as penicillin, ampicillin and tobramycin.

TOPICAL USES

Woundwort, as the name implies, is very good for dressing cuts and other wounds. The species are also reputed to cure aching joints when made into an ointment, no doubt owing to the anti-inflammatory properties already mentioned.

DOSAGE (as with Betony)

Tisane – 1tsp/5g, 3 times per day with cold water.
Tincture – 2–6ml of 1:5 45% – 20 drops = 1ml/1tsp = 5ml.

PRECAUTIONS

Not suitable for children or those who are pregnant or lactating.

Woundwort recipes

Medicinal recipes

Woundwort tisane

Pour 250ml boiling water over 1tsp/5g of the dried herb and allow to steep for 10–15 minutes. Use externally as a wash for wounds and skin irritations as well as part of the recipe for syrup, below.

Woundwort syrup

- 2tsp/10g Woundwort herb in 500ml of boiling water
- 500g of sugar

Make a tisane as above, using double the amounts stated, ie 2tsp/10g Woundwort herb in 500ml water and let it stand overnight. Warm your tisane over a low heat and bring to a simmer. Then cover partially and reduce the liquid down to half its original volume, ie. 250ml. Add the sugar and stir constantly, but do not let the mix boil. Remove the syrup from the heat cool before using. Syrups keep for up to 2 years unopened. After opening, store in the refrigerator and use within 1 month. Use as an anti-inflammatory and to treat diarrhoea, fevers and internal haemorrhages.

Hedge woundwort infused tincture – 1:5 45%

If you are using 40% alcohol, ie. Vodka, make a simple tincture by covering 1 part herb to 5 parts fluid.

If you are using Everclear or other 100% proof, use the following method for a specific tincture:

- 100g dried Woundwort herb
- 225ml alcohol
- 275ml water

Cover 50g dried herb with 225ml of alcohol. Then steep/infuse another 50g of dried Woundwort in 275ml of water for 15 minutes. Strain thoroughly and top up if the water is less than 275ml. Add the infusion to the dried herb and alcohol mix, and leave for 14 days before straining. Use for PCOS.

Woundwort wound salve

- 100g dried herb
- 2 tbsp alcohol, such as Everclear
- 1l grapeseed oil

Place the herbs in a jar with the alcohol and allow to steep/infuse for 10 minutes before adding the oil. Leave for 4 weeks and then strain. Make into a salve by using a 1:4 ratio of melted beeswax to your oil mix, ie. 1 part wax to 4 parts liquid. Melt the wax pellets in the oil in a double boiler or bain-marie. Remove from the heat and allow to cool and set completely before using to promote healing of wounds and reduce inflammation.

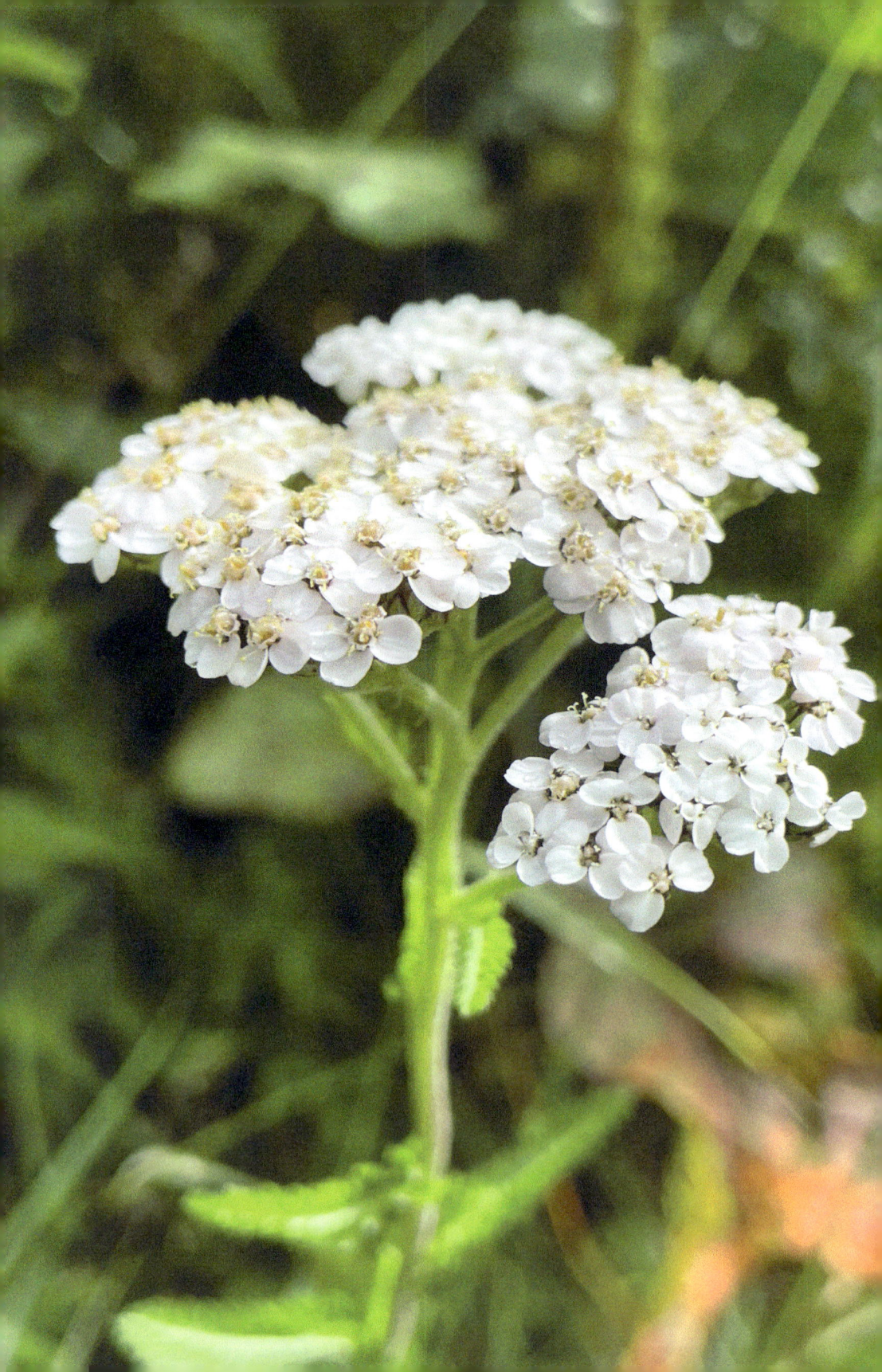

YARROW
Achillea millefolium

Yarrow is a common sight in the UK and can be found in a variety of habitats, including meadows, grasslands, roadsides and disturbed areas. It typically grows to a height of about 1 to 3 feet (30 to 90cm) tall. It blooms from late spring to late summer and is attractive to pollinators like bees, butterflies and hoverflies.

HISTORICAL USES

Yarrow has a long history of use, and DNA analysis has shown it to be among species present in two pressed tablets of plant material recovered from a collection of medical supplies in a Roman ship that sank off the coast of Tuscany, sometime between 140 and 120BCE (Touwaide and Appetiti, pers. comm., 10 February 2011).

Three major surviving Old English medical texts from ca. 950–1000CE all recommended Yarrow, usually as a component in multispecies recipes. These texts were primarily translations of earlier Latin works, though including some influence from pre-Christian Northern European traditions (Pollington, 2000). Uses included the treatment of wounds, inflammation and swellings, diarrhoea, intestinal pain, heartburn, lung disease, toothache, headache, difficult urination, and snake and dog bites.

ETYMOLOGY OF COMMON NAME
A corruption of the Anglo-Saxon name for the plant, *gearwe*, which means 'completeness' or 'effective'.

PLANT LORE
Yarrow has a place of honour in Greek mythology as the plant in whose waters Thetis bathed Achilles in order to make him invincible.

USE
All aerial parts.

EDIBILITY
Fresh flowers and leaves are good in salads, soups and stews.

HARVEST
When in bloom.

MEDICINAL PROPERTIES
Digestive, antimicrobial, astringent and vulnerary.

ACTIVE CONSTITUENTS
Volatile oil, flavonoids, alkaloids, coumarins, tannins, sesquiterpene lactones.

In her *Physica*, Hildegard Von Bingen advised that '*If a person has been wounded by a blow, the wound should be cleaned in wine. Then Yarrow cooked gently in water, and that water squeezed out, should tie gently, while warm over the cloth which covers the wound. It will take away putrid matter and the ulcer from the wound and the wound will be healed. As the wound starts to heal, remove the bandage and place the cooked/warm yarrow directly on the wound and it heals even faster, without complications. For those who have suffered internal injury, drink yarrow powder in warm water. As the person begins to heal, drink the powder in warm wine to accelerate the cure.*'

Nicholas Culpeper's *Herbal* noted of Yarrow that '*As a medicine it is drying and binding. A decoction of it boiled with white wine, is good to stop the running of the reins in men, and whites in women; restrains violent bleedings, and is excellent for the piles. A strong Tisane made of the leaves, and drank plentifully; and equal parts of it, and of toad flax, should be made into a poultice with pomatum, and applied outwardly. This induces sleep, eases the pain, and lessens the bleeding. An ointment of the leaves cures wounds, and is good for inflammations, ulcers, fistulas, and all such runnings as abound with moisture.*'

In his 1936 *Herbal Manual* Harold Ward said of it, '*The herb is extremely useful in colds and acute catarrhs of the respiratory tract generally. As it has the effect of opening the pores, thus permitting free perspiration, Yarrow is taken at the commencement of influenza and in other feverish conditions. An infusion of 1 ounce to 1 pint of boiling water is drunk warm in wineglass doses. As a very popular remedy for influenza, it is usually combined with Elder flowers and Peppermint in equal quantities. It was sometimes prescribed by the old herbalists as a tonic in nervous debility, but there are many better herbal medicines for this condition.*'

MODERN RESEARCH

A vast array of literature shows that Yarrow has an esteemed status in herbs for its diverse activity spectrum, which includes:

Digestive

In 1990 the German Commission E, a scientific advisory board, approved the use of Yarrow as a digestive and for dyspeptic ailments as it stimulates and enhances digestion while its astringent properties protect the gut.

Contraceptive

Takzare et al. (2011) studied the effect of ethanol extract of Yarrow flowers on spermatogenesis in adult male Wistar rats. The extracts were administered for 22 days, on every other day. A dose of 800mg/kg caused thickness in seminiferous tubules, a decrease in cell accumulation, severe disarrangement, degenerative cells and severe decrease in sperm count. These results suggest that Yarrow exhibits temporary antifertility activity in adult male animals.

Antimicrobial

A 2016 study showed that Yarrow essential oils had an inhibitory effect on MRSA, *Staphylococcus aureus*, *Pseudomonas aeruginosa*, *Escherichia coli* and *Bacillus cereus*. The biggest inhibition zone was against MRSA and the smallest against *Pseudomonas aeruginosa*.

Vulnerary

Native Americans and early North American settlers used Yarrow for its astringent qualities in wound-healing and bleeding. Cavalcanti et al. confirmed this use in 2006 by demonstrating that an aqueous extract of Yarrow efficiently healed chronic ulcers in rodents. Mucosal damage was reduced up to 75% after 7 days of treatment.

A 2018 clinical trial was performed on 140 pregnant women. They were randomly divided into four groups, each group containing 35 women: there were two control groups and two case groups including St John's wort ointment and Yarrow ointment. Results showed that there was significant difference between groups in post-episiotomy pain level postpartum, with the pain level, redness, oedema and ecchymosis in the groups who used St John's wort ointment and Yarrow ointments being far less than in the control group and therefore confirming hese plants to be useful for episiotomy treatment.

Anti-neurodegenerative

Yarrow has also been shown to aid certain brain disorders, such as multiple sclerosis, Alzheimer's, Parkinson's and encephalomyelitis owing to its flavonoid content. A review found that while almost all recent reports showed beneficial therapeutic properties on epilepsy, Alzheimer's disease, multiple sclerosis, Parkinson's disease and stroke, clinical trials of Yarrow were still awaited. However, considering the few side effects of Yarrow on main brain functions, as well as its availability for supplemental use, one can suggest using it in neurodegenerative disorders.

Antiviral

In 2023, Yarrow's virucidal activity was studied in relation to COVID-19. The Yarrow-treated SARS-nCoV-2 cell exhibited the disintegration of the virus membrane and provides a scientific basis for further explaining the mechanism underlying Yarrow's antiviral and anti-inflammatory properties.

Anti-inflammatory

Yarrow contains flavonoids, coumarins and sesquiterpene lactones, such as achillin and achillicin, which have anti-inflammatory properties. Recent findings have confirmed the traditional uses mentioned by the historical writers. In the most relevant study, a gel containing 6% Yarrow extract was equal to a diclofenac sodium gel in reducing carrageenan-induced paw oedema (by nearly 50%) in albino rats (Maswadeh et al., 2006).

TOPICAL USES

The above findings were again demonstrated in 2017 studies that showed that Yarrow extracts had an evident anti-inflammatory property and significant anti-inflammatory effect in an *in vivo* double-blind study. The skin parameters assessed in the study were restored after 3 and 7-day treatment with the tested extracts and showed promise in the use of preparations designed for topical application as anti-inflammatories that have a positive impact on the skin pH and its moisture content.

A 2022 review of Yarrow covered several studies that have confirmed that the topical application of Yarrow extracts improves the healing process of various skin injuries. This was related to the antibacterial, anti-inflammatory, antioxidant and moisturising effects of Yarrow extract.

DOSAGE

Tisane – 1–2tsp per cup of boiled water, up to 3 times per day.
Tincture – 1:5 25%, – 2–4ml – 20 drops = 1ml/1tsp = 5ml.

PRECAUTIONS

Pregnant women should not take Yarrow, because its ability to relax the smooth muscle of the uterus could cause miscarriage. Furthermore, people with bleeding disorders, undertaking surgery or who take blood thinners should avoid Yarrow because it may increase the risk of bleeding.

Yarrow recipes

Medicinal recipes

Yarrow tisane

Pour 250ml boiling water over 1tsp/5g of the dried herb and allow to steep for 10–15 minutes. Use to reduce temperatures at the onset of fevers and flu. Also use for high blood pressure, stomach cramps and to prevent blood clots. Also as an antiviral in cases of COVID-19.

Yarrow tincture 1:5 25%

If you are using 40% alcohol, ie. vodka, you will need to dilute this in the ratio of 60ml water to every 100ml of vodka to make a 25% medium and then cover 1 part herb to 5 parts fluid.

If you are using Everclear or other 100% proof, use the following method for a specific tincture:

- 100g dried Yarrow herb
- 125ml alcohol
- 375ml water

Cover 50g dried herb with 125ml of alcohol. Then steep/infuse another 50g of dried Yarrow in 375ml of water for 15 minutes. Strain thoroughly and top up if the water is less than 275ml. Add the infusion to the dried herb and alcohol mix, and leave for 14 days before straining. Use for respiratory ailments, at the onset of fevers and for congestion and digestive complaints.

Yarrow infused oil

- 100g dried Yarrow flower and leaf
- 2 tbsp alcohol, such as Everclear
- 1l grapeseed oil

Place the herbs in a jar with the alcohol and allow to steep/infuse for 10 minutes before adding the oil. Leave for 4 weeks and then strain. Use as an anti-inflammatory and for wounds and skin injuries.

Yarrow infused honey

- fresh Yarrow flowers
- honey

Fill a clean, dry jar with fresh Yarrow flowers. Pour honey over the flowers until they are fully covered. Stir gently to release any air bubbles. Seal the jar and let it sit in a warm, sunny spot for 1–2 weeks to infuse. Strain the Yarrow flowers from the honey and transfer the infused honey to a clean jar. Use the Yarrow-infused honey as a sweetener for tea, drizzle it over yogurt or spread it on toast.

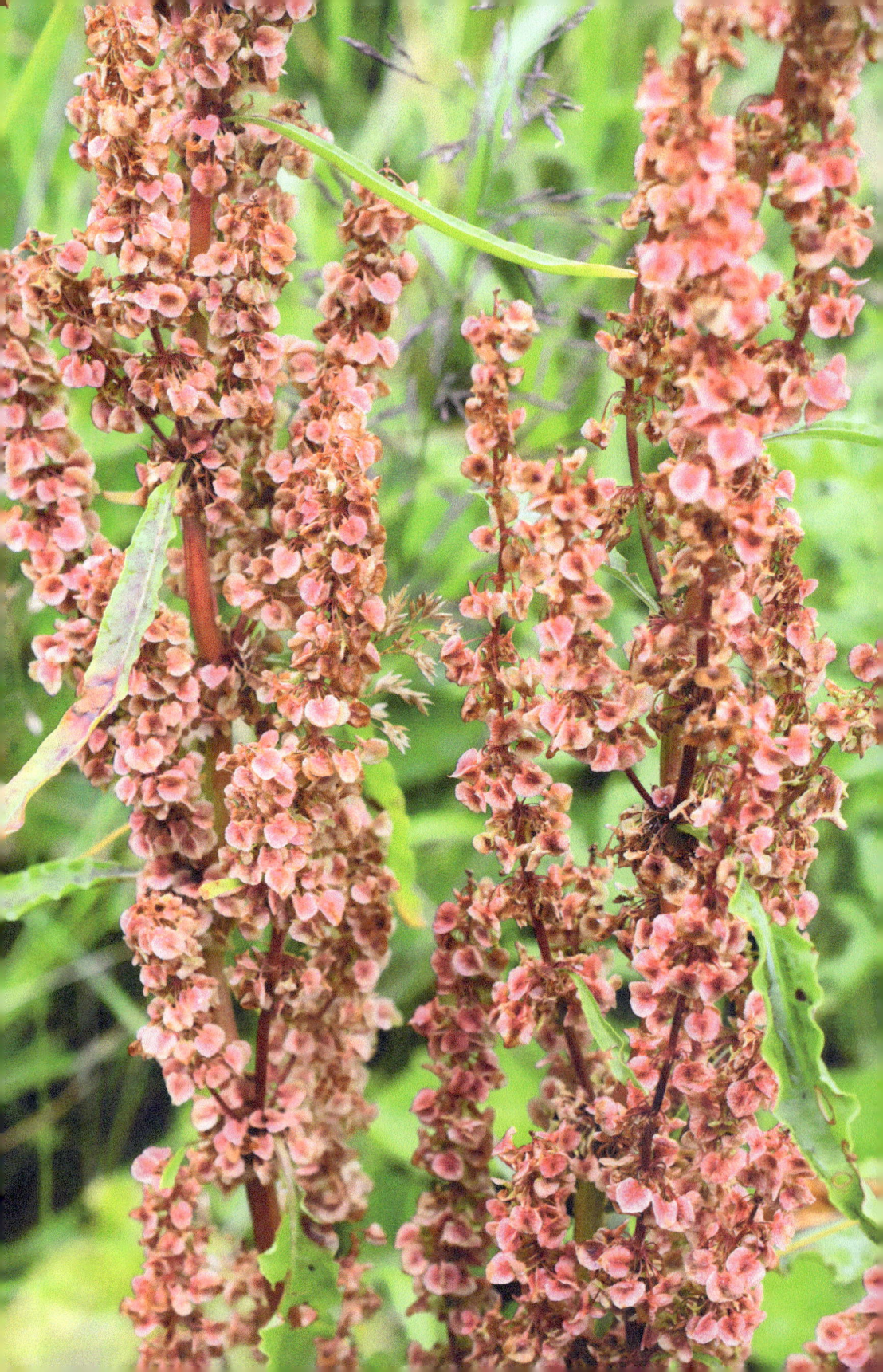

YELLOW DOCK
Rumex crispus

Yellow dock, or Curly dock as it is also known, belongs to the large genus *Rumex* in the family commonly known as Docks or Sorrels. There are over 200 species of *Rumex* worldwide, and several of them are found in the UK. It has a long history of culinary and medicinal use.

HISTORICAL USES

Nicholas Culpeper's *Herbal* states that, '*the yellow dock-root is best to be taken when either the blood or liver is affected by choler. All of them have a kind of cooling (but not all alike) drying quality, the sorrel being most cold, and the bloodworts most drying. Of the burdock, I have spoken already by itself. The seed of most of the other kinds, whether the gardens or fields, do stay lasks and fluxes of all sorts, the loathing of the stomach through choler, and is helpful for those that spit blood. The roots boiled in vinegar helpeth the itch, scabs, and breaking out of the skin, if it be bathed therewith. The distilled water of the herb and roots have the same virtue, and cleanseth the skin from freckles, morphew, and all other spots and discolourings therein.*'

Fray's Golden Recipes for the Use of All Ages (1897) provided a favourite country remedy that was of '*great value in the treatment of skin diseases ... Clean and bruise half-a-pound of common yellow*

ETYMOLOGY OF COMMON NAME
From the Old English *docce*. Yellow refers to the root colour.

PLANT LORE
In some traditions, Yellow dock was associated with fertility and love. It was believed that carrying or wearing Yellow dock leaves or seeds could attract love or enhance fertility.

USE
The root.

EDIBILITY
The leaves can be added to salads, cooked as a potherb or put in soups. Only the very young leaves should be used, preferably before the stems have developed.

HARVEST
In autumn.

MEDICINAL PROPERTIES
Antimicrobial, antiparasitic, laxative, hepatic, anticancerogenic, anti-inflammatory, detoxing and tonic.

ACTIVE CONSTITUENTS
Anthraquinone, tannins, flavonoids, phenolic acids.

LEFT: YELLOW DOCK

dock root, simmer for two hours in three gills of water, strain and evaporate to half a tea-cupful. Add gradually six ounces of prepared lard and an ounce of yellow wax, which have been previously melted together. Stir the whole till cold and apply freely.'

MODERN RESEARCH

Studies of *Rumex* species have already identified 268 compounds, including quinones, flavonoids, tannins, stilbenes, naphthalenes, terpenes, diterpene alkaloids, lignans and other classes of phytochemical compounds.

In addition, and as Culpeper mentions, Yellow dock is nourishing. It contains a form of bio-chelated iron, which the body can readily absorb, and this makes it an important herb for those with low iron and conditions related to anaemia such as fatigue and low energy. Other properties attributed to Yellow dock are as follows:

Antimicrobial and antiparasitic

A 2013 study found that Yellow dock contains nepodin, which is a potential antimalarial compound that prolonged the survival time of mice while inhibiting the parasites.

A 2019 study revealed that extracts of Yellow dock have therapeutic potentials against some microbes (fungal and bacteria) and parasites (*Trypanosoma* and *Plasmodium*). The study showed that the overall antibacterial potency of the extracts of the root was significantly higher than the extracts of the leaf, while the antifungal potency was higher in the leaf extracts. Nevertheless, the verification of the antimicrobial and antiparasitic potential of Yellow dock extracts shows that it could be a potential source for new antibacterial, antifungal, anti-trypanosomal and anti-plasmodial drugs.

A 2022 study measuring antimicrobial activity from the root against methicillin-resistant *Staphylococcus aureus* (MRSA) showed that multiple constituents contribute to the antimicrobial activity of Yellow dock against MRSA, in particular the anthraquinone emodin (Pelzer et al., 2022).

Laxative

A 2020 study declared that Yellow dock possesses antioxidant, antimicrobial and antifungal activities, and showed that Yellow dock dried roots are a gentle and safe laxative, useful for treatment of mild constipation, owing to the anthraquinones that give the roots their yellow-coloured pigment.

Anticancerogenic

Wegiera et al. (2012) provided evidence for cytotoxicity and induction of apoptosis by various *Rumex* species, including Yellow dock, and reported that the mechanism for the anticancer effect needed to be further investigated.

In 2015 and 2016, it was shown that water extracts of Yellow dock root were effective at antiproliferation of colorectal cancer cells. Then, in 2023, extracts from the root and leaves were investigated again and showed that the leaf extract was the most potent fraction, causing a significant amount of cytotoxicity to the cancer cells and making the leaves a promising anti-cancer agent.

Anti-inflammatory

In a 2014 study by Im et al., the anti-inflammatory effects of ethanol extract of Yellow dock were investigated, and the authors showed that the extract significantly decreased nitric oxide production and the levels of other inflammatory factors, suggesting that an ethyl acetate extract might be beneficial in the treatment of chronic inflammatory diseases.

These results were confirmed in 2020 when anti-inflammatory tests revealed that high antioxidant activity correlated with inhibitory effects on nitric oxide production, and that once again the ethyl acetate extract of Yellow dock reduced the secretion of pro-inflammatory cytokines.

TOPICAL USES

Yellow dock leaves are astringent, rich in iron and used as poultice for sores and hives. Application of a compress helps with skin irritations, and rubbing the leaves on the skin can relieve the itchy symptoms of a stinging nettle rash.

Reuter et al. (2010) stated that Yellow dock can be used in acne treatment and is also useful for treating a wide range of skin problems such as fungal disorders, spring eruption and scrofula. This confirms Fray's recommendations.

DOSAGE

Decoction – 1tbsp/15g in 475ml water, taken up to 3 times per day.
Tincture – 1–2ml of the 1:5 45% tincture, taken up to 3 times per day.

PRECAUTIONS

The fresh root may cause vomiting. The plant causes dermatitis in some. Do not exceed recommended dose as this can upset the digestive system. Not suitable for children or those who are pregnant or lactating.

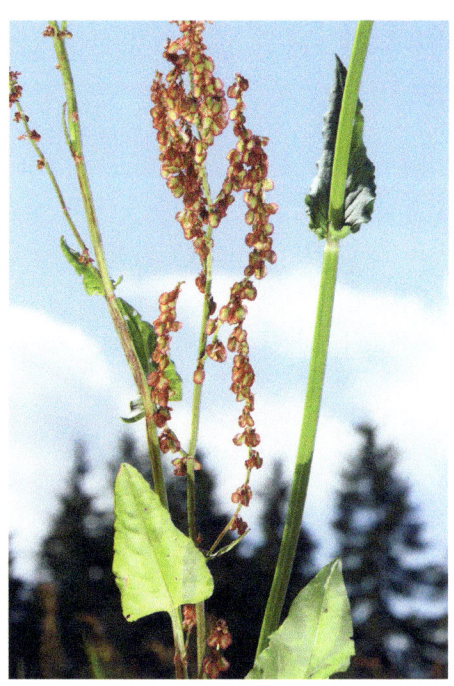

Yellow dock recipes

Medicinal recipes

Yellow dock decoction

Put 15g of Yellow dock root to a pan. Add 475ml of water. Bring the water to a gentle boil, reduce heat and simmer for 20-40 minutes. Remove from heat and allow to cool a bit. Carefully strain off the herbs and drink for anaemia as well as to improve digestion.

Yellow dock compress

Soak cotton pads in the decoction and use as a compress on acne, eczema, psoriasis, hives and other skin irritations.

Yellow dock decocted tincture 1:5 45%

If you are using 40% alcohol, ie. vodka, make a simple tincture by covering 1 part herb to 5 parts fluid.

If you are using Everclear or other 100% proof, use the following method for a specific tincture:

- 100g dried Yellow dock root
- 125ml alcohol
- 375ml water

Divide your powdered root into two equal 50g parts. Cover 50g with 125ml alcohol and place the other 50g in 375ml water. Bring the water to a gentle boil, reduce heat and simmer for 20-40 minutes. Remove from heat and allow to cool a bit, then strain thoroughly and top up if the water is less than 375ml. Add the decoction to the alcohol mix and leave for 14 days before straining. Use for its blood cleansing and detoxifying properties.

Yellow dock vinegar

Slice fresh Yellow dock roots thinly and place in a jar. Cover with apple cider vinegar. Allow to macerate for at least 4 weeks, then strain. Dilute 1-2 tablespoons in a glass of water or juice and use to support digestion, stimulate appetite and promote overall wellness.

BIBLIOGRAPHY

Agrawal, P.K., Agrawal, C. and Blunden, G. Quercetin: Antiviral Significance and Possible COVID-19 Integrative Considerations. *Natural Product Communications* 15 (2020): 12.

Al-Snafi, A. The Pharmacological importance of *Bellis perennis* – A Review. *International Journal of Phytotherapy* 5 (2015): 63–69.

Aliev, R.K. A Wound-Healing Preparation from the Leaves of the Large Plantain (*Plantago major* L.). *American Journal of Pharmacy* 1825 (1950): 24–26.

Allen, D.E. and Hatfield, G. *Medicinal Plants in Folk Tradition: An Ethnobotany of Britain & Ireland*. Portland, OR: Timber Press, 2004.

Alzoreky, N. and Nakahara, K. Antioxidant Activity of Some Edible Yemeni Plants Evaluated by Ferrylmyoglobin/ABTS*+ Assay. *Food Science and Technology Research* 7 (2001): 141–144.

Amabeoku, G.J., Leng, M.J. and Syce, J.A. Antimicrobial and Anticonvulsant Activities of *Viscum capense*. *Journal of Ethnopharmacology* 61 (1998): 237–241.

Ansari. Traditional Use of Kahu (*Lactuca scariola* L.): A Review. 1881.

Atmaca, H., Bozkurt, E., Cittan, M. and Tepe, H.D. Effects of *Galium aparine* Extract on the Cell Viability, Cell Cycle, and Cell Death in Breast Cancer Cell Lines. *Journal of Ethnopharmacology* 186 (2016): 305–310.

Bald. *Leechbook*. Translation in *Leechdoms, Wortcunning, and Starcraft of Early England*, ed. O. Cockayne. Rolls Series. 3 vols. London: Longmans, 1864–66. Vol. 2.

Barnes, J., Anderson, L.A. and Phillipson, J.D. St John's Wort (*Hypericum perforatum* L.): A Review of Its Chemistry, Pharmacology, and Clinical Properties. *The Journal of Pharmacy and Pharmacology* 53, no. 5 (2001): 583–600.

Bartram, T. *Bartram's Encyclopedia of Herbal Medicine*. London: Robinson, 1998.

Beara, I.N., Marko, B.L, Nenad, M., Ksenija, M., Lučic, D., Knezevic-Vukcevic, S. and Slavica. S. Comparative Analysis of Phenolic Profile, Antioxidant, Anti-inflammatory and Cytotoxic Activity of Two Closely-Related Plantain Species: *Plantago altissima* L. and *Plantago lanceolata* L. *LWT – Food Science and Technology* 47 (2012): 64–70.

Becker, A., Zaiter, A., Petit, J., Karam, M.C., Sudol, M., Baudelaire, E., Scher, J. and Dicko, A. How Do Grinding and Sieving Impact Physicochemical Properties, Polyphenol Content, and Antioxidant Activity of *Hieracium pilosella* L. Powders? *Journal of Functional Foods* 35 (2017): 666–672.

Beckert, S. and Hensel, A. Proteinase-Inhibiting Activity of an Extract of *Rumex acetosa* L. Against Virulence Factors of *Porphyromonas gingivalis*. *Planta Medica* 79 (2013).

Bello, O.M. and Naidoo, R. Wild Vegetable *Rumex acetosa* Linn.: Its Ethnobotany, Pharmacology, and Phytochemistry – A Review. *South African Journal of Botany* 125 (2019): 149–160.

Bespalov, V.G., Kudryashova, E.Y., Brusentsev, E.B. and Vinokurova, G.A. Chemoprevention of Radiation-Induced Carcinogenesis Using Decoction of Meadowsweet (*Filipendula ulmaria*) Flowers. *Pharmaceutical Chemistry Journal* 52 (2019): 860–862.

Best, M.R. and Brightman, F.H., trans. Book of Secrets of Albertus *Magnus: Of the Virtues of Herbs, Stones, and Certain Beasts, also a Book of the Marvels of the World*. York Beach, ME: Weiser Books, 2008.

Bingen, Hildegard Von. *Physica: The Complete English Translation of Her Classic Work on Health and Healing*. First published 1158. Reproduction, Rochester, VT: Healing Arts Press, 1998.

Bisset, N.G. and Wichtl, M. *Herbal Drugs and Phytopharmaceuticals*. Stuttgart: Medpharm Scientific Publishers, 2001: 638–640.

Blagojević, P., Radulović, G., Palic, M. and Stojanović, Z. Chemical Composition of the Essential Oils of Serbian Wild-Growing *Artemisia absinthium* and *Artemisia vulgaris*. *Journal of Agricultural and Food Chemistry* 54, no. 13 (2006): 4780–4789.

Boerhaave, H. *Materia Medica: Or, a Series of Prescriptions, Adapted to the Sections of His Practical Aphorisms Concerning the Knowledge and Cure of Diseases*. Originally published 1741. Classic Reprint, 2020.

Boone, C.W., Steele, V.E. and Kelloff, G.J. Screening for Chemopreventive (Anticarcinogenic) Compounds in Rodents. *Mutation Research* 267, no. 2 (1992): 251–255.

Boskabady, M.H., Aslani, P., Kiani, M.J. and Azizi, M.H. Antitussive Effect of *Plantago lanceolata* in Guinea Pigs. *Iranian Journal of Medical Sciences* 31 (2006): 143–146.

British Herbal Pharmacopoeia. Published by the British Herbal Medicine Association and produced by the Association's Scientific Committee, 1976.

British Herbal Pharmacopoeia. Compiled by M.J. Willoughby and S. Mills, ed. British Herbal Medicine Association Scientific Committee. British Herbal Medicine Association, 1996.

Brookes, Dr R. *The General Dispensatory, Containing a Translation of the Pharmacopoeias of the Royal Colleges of Physicians.* Originally published 1753. Reproduction, 2018.

Cakılcıoglu, U., Sengun, M.T. and Turkoglu, I. An Ethnobotanical Survey of Medicinal Plants of Yazıkonak and Yurtbasi Districts of Elazığ Province, Turkey. *Journal of Medicinal Plant Research* 4 (2010): 567–572.

Cameron, M.L. *Anglo-Saxon Medicine.* Cambridge: Cambridge University Press, 2006.

Carroll, M.E., Zangerl, R.L. and Berenbaum, M.R. Brief Communication. Heritability Estimates for Octyl Acetate and Octyl Butyrate in the Mature Fruit of the Wild Parsnip. *Journal of Heredity* 91 (2000): 68–71.

Castleman, M. *The New Healing Herbs: The Classic Guide to Nature's Best Medicines Featuring the Top 100 Time-Tested Herbs.* Emmaus, PA: Rodale Press, 2001.

Chen, X.C. Utilization of *Lonicera japonica. Forest By-Product and Specialty in China* 92 (2008): 37–39. (In Chinese)

Chen, Z., Zhao, Y., Zhang, M., Yang, X. and Wei, X. Structural Characterization and Antioxidant Activity of a New Polysaccharide from *Bletilla striata* Fibrous Roots. *Carbohydrate Polymers* 227 (2019): 115362.

Cheng, X., Liu, Y., Xu, L. and Xu, J. Experimental Study of the Inhibitory Effects of *Chelidonium majus* L. Extractive on *Streptococcus mutans* In Vitro. *Shanghai Kou Qiang Yi Xue* 15, no. 3 (2006): 318–320.

Chevallier, A. *Encyclopedia of Medicinal Plants*. London: Dorling Kindersley, 1996.

Chilo, R. and Raju, N. Evaluation of Diuretic Activity of Fractional Extracts of *Ajuga remota* Benth (Lamiaceae) in Albino Mice. *Department of Pharmacy, College of Health Science, Mettu University, Oromia, Ethiopia* 33, no. 54B (2021).

Chipeva, V.A, Petrova, L., Sinapova, V. and Lazarova, D. Antimicrobial Activity of Extracts from In Vivo and In Vitro Propagated *Lamium album* L. Plants. *African Journal of Traditional, Complementary, and Alternative Medicines* 10, no. 6 (2013): 559–562.

Choi, J., Park Y.G., Yun, M.S. and Seol, J.W. Effect of Herbal Mixture Composed of *Alchemilla vulgaris* and *Mimosa* on Wound Healing Process. *Biomedicine and Pharmacotherapy* 106 (2018): 326–332.

Christensen, R. and Bliddal. H. Is Phytalgic® a Goldmine for Osteoarthritis Patients or Is There Something Fishy about This Nutraceutical? A Summary of Findings and Risk-of-Bias Assessment. *Arthritis Research & Therapy* 12, no. 105 (2010).

Clare, B A., Conroy, T.L. and Spelman, F.E. The Diuretic Effect in Human Subjects of an Extract of *Taraxacum officinale* Folium Over a Single Day. Journal of Alternative and Complementary Medicine 15, no. 8 (2009): 929–934.

Clement, K., Covertson, C., Johnson, M.J. and Dearing, K. St. John's Wort and the Treatment of Mild to Moderate Depresson: A Systematic Review. *Holistic Nursing Practice* 20, no. 4 (2006): 197–203.

Coffin, A.I. Botanic Guide to Health, and the Natural Pathology of Disease. London: British Medico-Botanic Establishment, 29th ed. (1855).

Coles, W. *Adam in Eden, or Nature's Paradise. The History of Plants, Fruits, Herbs, and Flowers*. 1657. Wellcome Collection.

Colgate, E C., Miranda, C.L., Stevens, J.F., Bray, T.M. and Ho, E. Xanthohumol, a Prenylflavonoid Derived from Hops Induces Apoptosis and Inhibits NF-kappaB Activation in Prostate Epithelial Cells. *Cancer Letters* 246, nos. 1–2 (2007): 201–209.

Cuéllar, M.J., Giner, R.M., Recio, M.C., Just, M.J., Mañez, S., Cerdá, S. and Ríos, J.L. Screening of Antiinflammatory Medicinal Plants Used in Traditional Medicine Against Skin Diseases. *Phytotherapy Research* 12 (1998): 18–23.

Culpeper, N. *Herbal.* London: Milner & Co. Originally published 1653. Reproduction, circa 1850.

De Cleene, M. and Lejeune, M.C. *Verbena officinalis*, Vervain. *Medical Herbs*, 327–336. December 2011.

De Vico, G., Di Miceli, G., Faggio, G. and Caruso, E. *Urtica dioica* (Stinging Nettle): A Neglected Plant with Emerging Growth Promoter/Immunostimulant Properties for Farmed Fish. *Frontiers in Physiology* 9 (2018): 285.

DeGrandi-Hoffman, G., Ahumada, F., Probasco, G. and Schantz, L. The Effects of Beta Acids from Hops (*Humulus lupulus*) on Mortality of Varroa destructor (Acari: Varroidae). *Experimental and Applied Acarology* 58 (2012): 109–120.

DeGrandi-Hoffman, G., Ahumada, F., Curry, R., Probasco, G. and Schantz, L. Population Growth of Varroa destructor (Acari: Varroidae) in Commercial Honey Bee Colonies Treated with Beta Plant Acids. *Experimental and Applied Acarology* 64 (2014): 171–186.

Del Rio, J.A., Fuster, M.D., Sabater, F., Porras, L., Garcia-Lidon, A. and Ortuno, A. Selection of Citrus Varieties Highly Productive for the Neohesperidin Dihydrochalcone Precursor. *Food Chemistry* 59, no. 3 (1997): 433–437.

Delaveau, P. Fumeterre. *Les Actualites Pharmaceutiques* 172 (1980): 33–34.

Dhouibi, R., Affes, H., Ben Salem, M., Hammami, S., Sahnoun, Z., Zeghal, K.M. and Ksouda, K. Screening of Pharmacological Uses of *Urtica dioica* and Others Benefits. *Progress in Biophysics and Molecular Biology* 150 (2020): 67–77.

Ding, Y. and Wen, H. Dandelion Root Extract Protects NCM460 Colonic Cells and Relieves Experimental Mouse Colitis. *Journal of Natural Medicines* 72, no. 1 (2018): 123–130.

Dioscorides. *De Materia Medica Libri Quinque*. Originally published AD 50. Reproduction, 2014.

Divine Farmer's Materia Medica. A Translation of the "Shen Nong Ben Cao Jing" (Great Masters Series). Originally published circa AD 2. Reproduction, 1998.

Dombrádi, V. and Földeák, G. Anti-Leukemic Activity of a Four-Plant Mixture in a Leukemic Rat Model. *Clinical Phytoscience* 4 (1965).

Duke, J.A. and Ayensu, E.S. *Medicinal Plants of China.* Algonac, MI: Reference Publications, 1985.

Eddouks, M., El Bousta, M. and Mrabet, A. Ethnopharmacological Survey of Medicinal Plants Used for the Treatment of Diabetes Mellitus, Hypertension, and Cardiac Diseases in the Southeast Region of Morocco (Tafilalet). *Journal of Ethnopharmacology* 82, no. 2–3 (2002): 97–103.

Ellis, D. *Medicinal Herbs and Poisonous Plants.* Originally published 1918. Reproduction, 2010.

Ergene, B., Bakar, F., Saltan, G., Nebioğlu, S.N. and Acikara Bahadir, Ö. Antibacterial and Antifungal Activity of *Heracleum sphondylium* subsp. Artvinense. *African Journal of Biotechnology* 5, no. 11 (2006): 1087–1089.

Ergene, B., Acikara Bahadir, Ö., Bakar, F., Saltan G. and Nebioğlu, S. Antioxidant Activity and Phytochemical Analysis of *Alchemilla persica* Rothm. *Journal of Faculty of Pharmacy of Ankara* 39, no. 2 (2010): 145–154.

Ericksen, B.R. *Nutrition and Human Metabolism.* Wadsworth Learners, 2000. Arizona, 67–80.

Erzsébet, I., Tóth, F. and Tóth-Fáber, E. *Primula veris* L. Kivonatok Fitokémiai és Antimikróbás Hatásának Vizsgálata. *Bulletin of Medical Sciences* 2021.

ESCOP Monographs, 2nd ed. Supplement. *Agrimoniae Herba*— Agrimony Herb. European Directorate for the Quality of Medicines, 2005. Accessed 12 January 2023. https://www.escop.com/downloads/agrimoniae-herba-agrimony/

European Directorate for the Quality of Medicines. *European Pharmacopoeia.* Strasbourg: Maisonneuve, 2000. Accessed 4 November 2024. https://www.ema.europa.eu/en/news/public-statement-risk-drug-interactions-hypericum-perforatum-st-johns-wort-antiretroviral-medicinal-products.

European Medicines Agency. Assessment Report on *Chelidonium majus* L., Herba. Based on Article 10a of Directive 2001/83/EC as Amended (Well-Established Use). 2011. Accessed 4 November 2024. https://www.ema.europa.eu/en/documents/herbal-report/final-assessment-report-chelidonium-majus-l-herba_en.pdf.

Farokhi, S. Histopathologic Changes of Lung in Asthmatic Male Rats Treated with Hydro-Alcoholic Extract of *Plantago major* and Theophylline. *Avicenna Journal of Phytomedicine* 3, no. 2 (2013): 143–151.

Fayyaz, A., Khan, R.A. and Rasheed, S. Study of Analgesic and Anti-Inflammatory Activity from Plant Extracts of *Lactuca scariola* and *Artemisia absinthium*. Journal of Islamic Academy of Sciences 5, no, 2 (1992): 111–114.

Felter, H.W. *The Eclectic Materia Medica, Pharmacology and Therapeutics*. Cincinnati: J.K. Scudder, 1922.

Felter, H.W. and Lloyd, J.U. *King's American Dispensatory*. 18th ed. Cincinnati: Ohio Valley Co., 1898.

Fernie, W. *Herbal Simples: Approved for Modern Uses of Cure*. Originally published 1895, 2nd ed. 1897, Wellcome Library.

Fluckinger, F.A. *Pharmazeutische Chemie*. Berlin: R. Gaertner's Verlag, 1888.

Foster, S. St. John;s Wort. 2000. Accessed 4 November 2024 http://www.stevenfoster.com/education/monograph/hypericum.html.

Fostok, S.F., Ezzeddine, R.A., Homaidan, F.R., Al-Saghir, J.A., Salloum, R.G., Saliba, N.A. and Talhouk, R.S. Interleukin-6 and Cyclooxygenase-2 Downregulation by Fatty-Acid Fractions of *Ranunculus constantinopolitanus. BMC Complementary and Alternative Medicine* 9 (2009): 44.

Fray, E. *Fray's Golden Recipes for the Use of All Ages*. Liverpool: William M'Call; London: E. Seale, 1897.

Gálvez, M., Cordero, M., Cortes, F. and Ayus, M.Y. Cytotoxic Effect of *Plantago* spp. on Cancer Cell Lines. *Journal of Ethnopharmacology* 88 (2003): 125–130.

Gastaldo, P. *Compendio della Flora Officinale Italiana*. Padova: Piccin, 1987.

Geetha, K.M., Bhaskara Gopal, P.V.V.S. and Murugan, V. Antiepileptic Activity of Aerial Parts of *Viscum articulatum* (Viscaceae) in Rats. *Journal of Pharmacy Research* 3 (2010): 2886–2887.

Geetha, K M., Murugan, V., Pavan Kumar, P. and Wilson, B. Antiepileptic Activity of *Viscum articulatum* Burm and Its Isolated Bioactive Compound in Experimentally Induced Convulsions in Rats and Mice. *European Journal of Biomedical and Pharmaceutical Sciences* 5 (2018): 311–318.

Gerard, J. *Gerard's Herball: The History of Plants with Descriptions, Origins, Location and Characteristics of Almost 200 Herbs*. Originally published 1597. Reproduction, 1985.

Gerenčer, M., Spirić, V., Savić, L. and Krstulović, M.S. In Vitro and In Vivo Anti-Retroviral Activity of the Substance Purified from the Aqueous Extract of *Chelidonium majus* L. *Antiviral Research* 72, no. 2 (2006): 153–156.

Gerhauser, C. Broad Spectrum Anti-Infective Potential of Xanthohumol from Hop (*Humulus lupulus* L.) in Comparison with Activities of Other Hop Constituents and Xanthohumol Metabolites. *Molecular Nutrition & Food Research* 49, no. 11 (2005): 1012–1019.

Gerlach, S.L., Rathinakumar, R., Chakravarty, G., Göransson, U., Wimley, W.C., Darwin, S.P. and Mondal, D. Anticancer and Chemosensitizing Abilities of Cycloviolacin O2 from *Viola odorata* and Psyche Cyclotides from *Psychotria leptothyrsa*. *Biopolymers* 94, no. 5 (2010): 617–625.

German Commission E. Monographs. Accessed 4 November 2024. https://www.heilpflanzen-welt.de/german-commission-e-monographs-list/.

Gescher, K., Hensel, A., Hafezi, W., Derksen, A. and Kühn, J. Oligomeric Proanthocyanidins from *Rumex acetosa* L. Inhibit the Attachment of Herpes Simplex Virus Type-1. *Antiviral Research* 89 (2011): 9–18.

Ghale-Salimi, M., Eidi, M., Ghaemi, N. and Khavari-Nejad, R.A. Inhibitory Effects of Taraxasterol and Aqueous Extract of *Taraxacum officinale* on Calcium Oxalate Crystallization: In Vitro Study. *Renal Failure* 40, no. 1 (2018): 298–305.

Ghione, M., Parrello, D. and Grasso, L. Usnic Acid Revisited: Its Activity on Oral Flora.

Chemioterapia 7 *(1988): 302–305.*

Giachetti, D., Taddei, I., Cenni, A. and Taddei, E. Diuresis from Distilled Water Compared with that from Vegetable Drugs. *Planta Medica* 55 (1989): 2–10.

Giannetti, B.M., Staiger, C., Bulitta, M. and Predel, H.G. Efficacy and Safety of Comfrey Root Extract Ointment in the Treatment of Acute Upper or Lower Back Pain: Results of a Double-Blind, Randomised, Placebo-Controlled, Multicentre Trial. *British Journal of Sports Medicine* 44, no. 9 (2010): 637–641.

Gokadze, S. I. et al. *Georgian Medical News* 218 (2013): 72–77.

Gorman, M.W. Economic Botany of Northwestern Alaska. *Pittonia* 3 (1896): 464–465.

Graça, V.C., Barros, L., Calhelha, R.C., Dias, M.I., Carvalho, A.M., Santos-Buelga, C., Santos, P.F. and Ferreira, I.C. Chemical Characterization and Bioactive Properties of Aqueous and Organic Extracts of *Geranium robertianum* L. *Food & Function* 7, no. 9 (2016): 3807–3814.

Grieve, M. *A Modern Herbal*. Originally published 1931, Reproduced Vintage Publishing, 1974.

Grigorescu, E., Stanescu, U., Basceanu, V. and Aur, M.M. Phytochemical and Microbiologic Control of Some Plant Species Used in Folk Medicine II: *Plantago lanceolata*, *Plantago media*, and *Plantago major*. *Revista de Medicina Chirurgicala* 77 (1973): 835–841.

Grube, B., Grünwald, J., Krug, L. and Staiger, C. Efficacy of a Comfrey Root (*Symphyti offic.* radix) Extract Ointment in the Treatment of Patients with Painful Osteoarthritis of the Knee: Results of a Double-Blind, Randomised, Bicenter, Placebo-Controlled Trial. *Phytomedicine* 14, no. 1 (2007): 2–10.

Gu, J.W., Hasuo, H., Takeya, M. and Akasu, T. Effects of Emodin on Synaptic Transmission in Rat Hippocampal CA1 Pyramidal Neurons In Vitro. *Neuropharmacology* 49 (2005): 103–111.

Guillén, M.E.N., Emim, J.A., Souccar, C. and Lapa, A.J. Analgesic and Anti-inflammatory Activities of the Aqueous Extract of *Plantago major* L. *Pharmaceutical Biology* 35. (2008): 99–104.

Gupta, G., Kazmi, I., Afzal, M., Rahman, M., Saleem, S., Ashraf, S., Khusroo, M.J., Nazeer, K., Ahmed, S., Mujeeb, M., Ahmed, Z. and Anwar, F. Sedative, Antiepileptic and Antipsychotic Effects of *Viscum album* L. (Loranthaceae) in Mice and Rats. *Journal of Ethnopharmacology* 141 (2012): 810–816.

Hailu, W. and Engidawork, E. Evaluation of the Diuretic Activity of the Aqueous and 80% Methanol Extracts of *Ajuga remota* Benth (Lamiaceae) Leaves in Mice. *BMC Complementary and Alternative Medicine* 14 (2014): 135.

Hajhashemi, V., Sajjadi, S.E. and Heshmati, M. Antiinflammatory and Analgesic Properties of *Heracleum persicum* Essential Oil and Hydroalcoholic Extract in Animal Models. *Journal of Ethnopharmacology* 124, no. 3 (2009): 475–480.

Halkes, A.B.A., Beukelman, C.J., Kroes, B.H., Van den Berg, A.J.J., Labadie, R.P. and Van Dijk, H. In Vitro Immunomodulatory Activity of *Filipendula ulmaria*. *Phytotherapy Research* 11, no. 7 (1998): 518–523.

Han, K.H., Park, J.M., Jeong, M., Han, Y.M., Go, E.J., Park, J., Kim, H., Han, J.G., Kwon, O. and Hahm, K.B. Heme Oxygenase-1 Induction and Anti-Inflammatory Actions of *Atractylodes macrocephala* and *Taraxacum herba* Extracts Prevented Colitis and Were More Effective than Sulfasalazine in Preventing Relapse. *Gut and Liver* 11, no. 5 (2017): 655–666.

Harborne, J.B. and Baxter, H. *Phytochemical Dictionary and Handbook of Bioactive Compounds from Plants*. London: Taylor and Francis, 1993.

Hartwell, J.L. Plants Used Against Cancer: A Survey. *Lloydia* 34 (1971): 204–255.

Heyerick, A., Vervarcke, S., Depypere, H., Bracke, M. and De Keukeleire, D. A First Prospective, Randomized, Double-Blind, Placebo-Controlled Study on the Use of a Standardized Hop Extract to Alleviate Menopausal Discomforts. *Maturitas* 54, no. 2 (2006): 164–175.

Hill, J. *The British Herbal – An History of Plants and Trees, Natives of Britain, Cultivated for Use, or Raised for Beauty*. London: Osborne & Shipton, 1756.

Hoffmann, D. *Medical Herbalism. The Science and Practice of Herbal Medicine*. Rochester, VT: Inner Traditions/Bear, 2003.

Hool, R.L. *Common Plants and Their Uses in Medicine*. Bolton: Lancashire Branch of the National Association of Medical Herbalists, 1922.

Huber, R., Ditfurth, A.V., Amann, F., Güthlin, C., Rostock, M. and Trittler, R. Clinical Efficacy of an Extract of *Echinacea*. *Phytomedicine* 14, no. 8 (2007): 507–515.

Hussain, M., Raza, S.M. and Janbaz, K.H. A Pharmacologically Mechanistic Basis for the Traditional Uses of *Rumex acetosa* in Gut Motility Disorders and Emesis. *Bangladesh Journal of Pharmacology* 10 (2015): 548.

Im, N.K., Jung, Y.S., Choi, J.H., Yu, M.H. and Jeong, G.S. Inhibitory Effect of Leaves of *Rumex crispus* L. on LPS-Induced Nitric Oxide Production and the Expression of iNOS and COX-2 in Macrophages. *Natural Products Sciences* 20 (2014): 51–57.

Ingólfsdóttir, K. Usnic Acid. *Phytochemistry* 61, no. 7 (2002): 729–736.

Ivancheva, S., Manolova, N., Serkedjieva, J., Dimov, V. and Ivanovska, N. Polyphenols from Bulgarian Medicinal Plants with Anti-Infectious Activity. In *Plant Polyphenols*, ed. R.W. Hemingway and P.E. Laks. Boston, MA: Springer, 1992: 59–70.

Ivanov, S.A., Garbuz, S., Malfanov, I.L. and Ptitsyn, L.R. Screening of Russian Medicinal and Edible Plant Extracts for Angiotensin I-Converting Enzyme (ACE I) Inhibitory Activity. *Russian Journal of Bioorganic Chemistry* 39 (2013): 743–749.

Jahodář, J. Medicinal Plants in Modern Medicine or What Mathioli Did Not Know Yet. Havlíček Brain Team, 2010 (in Czech).

Jang, S.A., Park, D.W., Kwon, J.E., Song, H.S., Park, B., Jeon, H., Sohn, E.H., Koo, H.J. and Kang, S.C. Quinic Acid Inhibits Vascular Inflammation in TNF-α-stimulated Vascular Smooth Muscle Cells. *Biomedicine & Pharmacotherapy = Biomedecine & pharmacotherapie* 96, (2017): 563–571.

arić, S., Kostić, O., Mataruga, Z., Pavlović, D., Pavlović, M., Mitrović, M. and Pavlović, P. Traditional Wound-Healing Plants Used in the Balkan Region (Southeast Europe). *Journal of Ethnopharmacology* 211 (2018): 311–328.

Jin, J., Kang, W., Zhong, C., Qin, Y., Zhou, R., Liu, H., Xie, J., Chen, L., Qin, Y. and Zhang, S. The Pharmacological Properties of *Ophiocordyceps xuefengensis* Revealed by Transcriptome Analysis. *Journal of Ethnopharmacology* 219 (2018): 195–201.

Jones, W.H.S. Pliny *Natural History*, with an English Translation in Ten Volumes. Vol. VII, Libri XXIV–XXVII. London: Harvard University Press, 1966.

Jung, S.M., Schumacher, H.R., Kim, H., Kim, M., Lee, S.H. and Pessler, F. Reduction of Urate Crystal-Induced Inflammation by Root Extracts from Traditional Oriental Medicinal Plants: Elevation of Prostaglandin D2 Levels. *Arthritis Research and Therapy* 9, no. 4 (2007): R64.

Kabiruddin, H. *Kitabul Advia, Mukhzanul Mufredat*. Daftar al-Masih, Hyderabad, (1951): 289–290.

Karakaş, F., Yidirim, A.B., Bayram, R., Yavuz, M.Z., Gepdiremen, A. and Turker, A. Antiproliferative Activity of Some Medicinal Plants on Human Breast and Hepatocellular Carcinoma Cell Lines and their Phenolic Contents. *Tropical Journal of Pharmaceutical Research* 14 (2015): 1787.

Karakas, F.P., Turker, A.U., Karakaş, A., Mshvildadze, V., Pichette, A. and Legault, J. In Vitro Cytotoxic, Antibacterial, Anti-inflammatory and Antioxidant Activities and Phenolic Content in Wild-grown Flowers of Common Daisy—A Medicinal Plant. *Journal of Herbal Medicine* 8 (2017): 31–39.

Kéry, A., Horváth, J., Nász, I., Verzár-Petri, G., Kulcsár, G. and Dán, P. Antiviral Alkaloid in *Chelidonium majus* L. *Acta Pharmaceutica Hungarica* 57 (1987): 19–25.

Khorasani A. *Makhzan-al' advieh*. Islamic Culture Press Center. Tehran, Iran: 1371: 159–160.

Kiasalari, Z., Khalili, M., Roghani, M. and Sadeghian, A. Antiepileptic and Antioxidant Effect of *Brassica nigra* on Pentylenetetrazol-Induced Kindling in Mice. *Iranian Journal of Pharmaceutical Research* 11, no. 4 (2012): 1209–1217.

Koch, W. and Koch, G. Östrogene Hormone in Hopfen und Bier. *Medizinische Wochenschrift* 95 (1953): 845.

Koll, R., Buhr, M., Dieter, R., Pabst, H., Predel, H.G., Petrowicz, O., Giannetti, B. and Klingenburg, S. Efficacy and Tolerance of a Comfrey Root Extract (*Extr. Rad. Symphyti*) in the Treatment of Ankle Distortions: Results of a Multicenter, Randomized, Placebo-Controlled, Double-Blind Study. *Phytomedicine* 11, no. 6 (2004): 470–477.

Kosalec, I., Kopjar, N. and Kremer, D. Antimicrobial Activity of Willowherb (*Epilobium angustifolium* L.) Leaves and Flowers. *Current Drug Targets* 14, no. 9 (2013): 986–991.

Kozuharova, E., Kutzanova, R., Vasileva, K. and Goranova, P. New Records of the Remedial Properties of Vascular Plants, Some Traditionally Accepted as Medicinal Plants and Some Less Familiar to Ethnobotanists. *Phytologia Balcanica: International Journal of Balkan Flora and Vegetation* 18 (2012): 123–129.

Krasnov, E.A., Kaminskij, I.P., Kadyrova, T.V., Pekhen'ko, V.G. and Adekenov, S.M. Antimicrobial Activity of Extracts from the Aerial Part of *Centaurea scabiosa* (Asteraceae). *Rastitelnye Resursy* 48 (2012): 262–266.

Kühn, K.G. *Claudi Galeni Opera Omnia.* Published in twenty volumes between 1821 and 1833. Reproduced by Cambridge Library Collection – Classics.

Kujawska, M., Klepacki, P. and Łuczaj, Ł. Fischer's Plants in Folk Beliefs and Customs: A Previously Unknown Contribution to the Ethnobotany of the Polish-Lithuanian-Belarusian Borderland. *Journal of Ethnobiology and Ethnomedicine* 13 (2017): 20.

Kumarasamy, Y., Middleton, M., Reid, R.G., Nahar, L. and Sarker, S.D. Biological Activity of Serotonin Conjugates from the Seeds of *Centaurea nigra*. *Fitoterapia* 74, no. 6 (2003).

Lee, J.J., Ahn, K.S., Rhee, J.S. and Ryu, H.Y. Effects of Betaine, Coumarin, and Flavonoids on Mucin Release from Cultured Hamster Tracheal Surface Epithelial Cells. *Phytotherapy Research* 18, no. 4 (2004): 301–305.

Lee, S.J., Son, K.H., Chang, H.W., Kang, S.S. and Kim, H.P. Anti-Inflammatory Activity of *Lonicera japonica*. *Phytotherapy Research* 12 (1998): 445–447.

Lee, S.J., Chung, H.Y., Maier, C.G.A., Wood. A.R., Dixon, R.A. and Mabry, T.J. Estrogenic Flavonoids from *Artemisia vulgaris* L. *Journal of Agricultural and Food Chemistry* 46 (1998): 3325–3329.

Li, S. *Compendium of Materia Medica: Bencao Gangmu.* 2 vols. Originally published 1578. Reproduction, 2023.

Li, Z.J., Zhang, Y.H., Zheng, W.H., Yang, J.H., Yao, S.B. and Li, W.C. Bellisosides A–F, Six Novel Acylated Triterpenoid Saponins from *Bellis perennis* (Compositae). *Tetrahedron* 61, no. 9 (2005): 2175–2180.

Lin, M.Y., Liu, M.F., Hsu, L.F. and Tsai, P.S. Effects of Self-Management on Chronic Kidney Disease: A Meta-Analysis. *International Journal of Nursing Studies* 74 (2017): 128–137.

Linchenko, N.A. Gosudarstvennaia farmakopeia SSSR X izdaniia kak standart na lekarstvennoe rastitel'noe syr'e [The 10th edition of the USSR Government Pharmacopoeia as a standard for medicinal plant raw material]. Farmatsiia, 18 no. 6 (1969): 5–8.

Liu, H., Zhang, Z., Yang, Y., Wang, X. and Li, W. Nuclear Import of Proinflammatory Transcription Factors Is Required for Massive Liver Apoptosis Induced by Bacterial Lipopolysaccharide. *Journal of Biological Chemistry* 279, no. 46 (2004): 48434–48442.

Liu, J., Burdette, J.E., Xu, H., Gu, C., Van Breemen, R.B., Bhat, K.P., Booth, N., Constantinou, A.I., Pezzuto, J.M., Fong, H.H. and Farnsworth, N.R. Evaluation of Estrogenic Activity of Plant Extracts for the Potential Treatment of Menopausal Symptoms. *Journal of Agricultural and Food Chemistry* 49, no. 5 (2001): 2472–2479.

Liu, J., Burdette, J.E., Xu, H., Gu, C., Van Breemen, R.B., Bhat, K.P., Booth, N., Constantinou, A.I., Pezzuto, J.M., Fong, H.H. and Farnsworth, N.R. Protective Effect of Polysaccharides-Enriched Fraction from *Angelica sinensis* on Hepatic Injury. *Life Sciences* 66, no. 19 (2000): 1777–1786.

Lotan, A.M., Gronovich, Y., Lysy, I., Binenboym, R., Eizenman, N., Stuchiner, B., Goldstein, O., Babai, P. and Oberbaum, M. *Arnica montana* and *Bellis perennis* for Seroma Reduction Following Mastectomy and Immediate Breast Reconstruction: Randomized, Double-Blind, Placebo-Controlled Trial. *European Journal of Plastic Surgery* 43 (2020): 285–294.

Ma, J., Leung, J.C., Chan, K.W., Wong, R.S.H., Chan, M.S.K. and Li, J.J.S. Antiviral Chinese Medicinal Herbs Against Respiratory Syncytial Virus. *Phytotherapy Research* 16, no. 2 (2002): 127–134.

Manojlovic, N., Rankovic, B., Kosanic, M., Vasiljevic, P. and Stanojkovic, T. Chemical Composition of Three Parmelia Lichens and Antioxidant, Antimicrobial and Cytotoxic Activities of Some of Their Major Metabolites. *Phytomedicine* 19 (2012): 1166–1172.

Marques, T.H.C., De Melo, C.H.S. and De Freitas, R.M. In Vitro Evaluation of Antioxidant, Anxiolytic and Antidepressant-Like Effects of the *Bellis perennis* Extract. *Brazilian Journal of Pharmacognosy* 22 (2012): 1044–1052.

Maswadeh, H., Shaaban, K.A.J., Al-Azzam, K.D. and Abdurahman, R.D. Anti-Inflammatory Activity of *Achillea* and *Ruscus* Topical Gel on Carrageenan-Induced Paw Edema in Rats. *Pharmaceutical Biology* 44, no. 5 (2006): 362–368.

Matsumoto, K., Hosono-Nishiyama, H. and Yamada, H. Evaluation of the Antiviral Activity of *Artemisia* and Its Active Components. *Planta Medica* 72, no. 3 (2006): 276–278.

Matteson, A. *Occult Family Physician and Botanic Guide to Health*, published by the author in 1894. Reproduction, 1996.

Mazzio, E.A. and Soliman, K.F. In Vitro Screening for the Tumoricidal Properties of International Medicinal Herbs. *Phytotherapy Research* 23, no. 3 (2009): 385–398.

Menzies-Trull, C. *Herbal Medicine: Keys to Physiomedicalism Including Pharmacopoeia.* Faculty of Physiomedical Herbal Medicine, 2003.

Meyrick, W. *The New Family Herbal; or, Domestic Physician*. Originally published in 1790. Reproduction, 2018.

Mills, E., Ernst, E., Singh, R., Ross, C. and Wilson K. Health Food Store Recommendations: Implications for Breast Cancer Patients. *Breast Cancer Research* 5 (2003): R170–R174.

Mills, S. and Bone K. *Principles and Practice of Phytotherapy: Modern Herbal Medicine*. 2nd ed, Edinburgh: Churchill Livingstone, 2000.

Mimica-Dukić, N. Native Plants in Serbia as a Source of New Anti-Inflammatory Agents – The Case of Polygonaceae Family. XV Optima Meeting, 6–11 June 2016.

Mincheva, I, Zaharieva, M.M., Batovska, D., Najdenski, H., Ionkova, I. and Kozuharova, E. Antibacterial activity of extracts from *Potentilla reptans* L. *Pharmacia* 66, no. 1 (2019): 7–11.

Miyamoto, K., Kishi, N., Murayama, T., Furukawa, T. and Koshiura, R. Induction of Cytotoxicity of Peritoneal Exudate Cells by Agrimoniin, a Novel Immunomodulatory Tannin of *Agrimonia pilosa* Ledeb. *Cancer Immunology, Immunotherapy* 27 (1988): 59–62.

Moerman, D.E. *Native American Ethnobotany*. Portland, OR: Timber Press, 1998.

Morali, G., Morali, N. and Salvatore, L.V.G.L. Open, Non-Controlled Clinical Studies to Assess the Efficacy and Safety of a Medical Device in Form of Gel Topically and Intravaginally Used in Postmenopausal Women with Genital Atrophy. *Gynaecological Therapeutics* 21 (2006): 120–128.

Morikawa, T., Kawaguchi, Y., Nakagawa, T. and Yokoyama, S.S.T. Oleanane-Type Triterpene Saponins with Collagen Synthesis-Promoting Activity from the Flowers of *Bellis perennis*. *Phytochemistry* 114 (2015): 76–82.

Neagu, A., Niculescu, A.E.R., Toma, E.A., Dragan, I.C.M. and Ciornea, R.C. Phytochemical Study of Some *Symphytum officinalis* Extracts Concentrated by Membranous Procedures. *U.P.B. Scientific Bulletin*, Series B 73, no. 3 (2011): 47–54.

NIMH. National Institute of Medical Herbalists. Accessed 28 October 2024. https://nimh.org.uk/.

Ofokansi, K.C., Esimone, C.O. and Anele, C.R. Evaluation of the In Vitro Combined Antibacterial Effect of the Leaf Extracts of *Bryophyllum pinnatum* (Fam: Crassulaceae) and *Ocimum gratissimum* (Fam: Labiatae). *Plant Production Research Journal* 9 (2005): 23–27.

Okwu, D.E. and Okwu, M.E. Chemical Composition of *Spondias mombin* Linn Plant Parts. *Journal of Sustainable Agriculture and the Environment* 6, no. 2 (2004): 140–147.

Osbaldeston, T.A. and Wood, R.P.A. *Dioscorides de Materia Medica: Being a Herbal with Many Other Materials Written in Greek in the Firſt Century of the Common Era.* An Indexed Version in Modern English. Book 2. Johannesburg: Ibidis Press, 2000.

Ottenweller, J., Putt, K., Blumenthal, E.J., Dhawale, S. and Dhawale, S.W. Inhibition of Prostate Cancer-Cell Proliferation by Essiac. *Journal of Alternative & Complementary Medicine* 10, no. 4 (2004): 687–691.

Overk, C. R., Yao, P., Chadwick, L.R., Nikolic, D., Sun, Y., Cuendet, M.A., Deng, Y., Hedayat, A.S., Pauli, G.F., Farnsworth, N.R., Van Breemen, R.B. and Bolton, J.L. Comparison of the In Vitro Estrogenic Activities of Compounds from Hops (*Humulus lupulus*) and Red Clover (*Trifolium pratense*). *Journal of Agricultural and Food Chemiſtry* 53, no. 16 (2005): 6246–6253.

Pallag, A., Filip, G.A., Olteanu, D., Clichici, S., Baldea, I., Jurca, T., Micle, O., Vicaș, L., Marian, E., Soriţău, O., Cenariu, M. and Mureșan, M. *Equisetum arvense* L. Extract Induces Antibacterial Activity and Modulates Oxidative Stress, Inflammation, and Apoptosis in Endothelial Vascular Cells Exposed to Hyperosmotic Stress. *Oxidative Medicine and Cellular Longevity* (2018): 3060525.

Panahi, Y., Dadjo, Y., Pishgoo, B., Akbari, A. and Sahebkar, A. Clinical Evaluation of the Anti-Inflammatory Effects of *Heracleum persicum* Fruits. *Comparative Clinical Pathology* 24 (2015): 971–974.

Papageorgiou, S., Varvaresou, A., Tsirivas, E. and Demetzos, C. New Alternatives to Cosmetics Preservation. *Journal of Cosmetic Science* 61, no. 2 (2010): 107–123.

Pareek, A., Suthar, M., Rathore, G.S. and Bansal, V. Feverfew (*Tanacetum parthenium* L.): A Systematic Review. *Pharmacognosy Review*s 5, no. 9 (2011): 103–110.

Parfitt, K., ed. *Martindale: The Complete Drug Reference.* 32nd ed. London: Pharmaceutical Press, 1999.

Park, H.W., Choi, S.U., Baek, N.I., Kim, S.H., Eun, J.S., Yang, J.H. and Kim, D.K. Guaiane Sesquiterpenoids from *Torilis japonica* and Their Cytotoxic Effects on Human Cancer Cell Lines. *Archives of Pharmacal Research* 29 (2006): 131–134.

Park, W.S., Son, E.D., Nam, G.W., Kim, S.H., Noh, M.S., Lee, B.G., Jang, I.S., Kim, S.E., Lee, J.J. and Lee, C.H. Torilin from *Torilis japonica*, as a New Inhibitor of Testosterone 5 Alpha-reductase. *Planta Medica* 69, no. 5 (2003): 459–461.

Patiala, R. Application of Usnic Acid to a Case of *Lupus Vulgaris*. *Annales Medicinae Experimentalis Biologiae Fennicae* 27 (1949): 151.

Paul, A., Das, J., Das, S., Samadder, A. and Khuda-Bukhsh, A.R. Poly (Lactide-Co-Glycolide) Nano-Encapsulation of Chelidonine, an Active Bioingredient of Greater Celandine (*Chelidonium majus*), Enhances Its Ameliorative Potential Against Cadmium Induced Oxidative Stress and Hepatic Injury in Mice. *Environmental Toxicology and Pharmacology* 36, no. 3 (2013): 937–947.

Paun, G., Neagu, E., Moroeanu, V., Ungureanu, O., Cretu, R., Ionescu, E., Tebrencu, C.E., Ionescu, R., Stoica, I. and Radu, G.L. Phytochemical Analysis and In Vitro Biological Activity of *Betonica officinalis* and *Salvia officinalis* Extracts. *Romanian Biotechnological Letters* 22, no. 4 (2017): 12751–12761.

Pelzer, C.V., Houriet, J., Crandall, W.J., Todd, D.A., Cech, N.B. and Jones, D.D., Jr. More Than Just a Weed: An Exploration of the Antimicrobial Activity of *Rumex crispus* Using a Multivariate Data Analysis Approach. *Planta Medica* 88, no. 9–10 (2022): 753–761.

Peter-Horvath, M. *Chemical Abstracts* 62 (1965): 3105.

Pilipović, S., Bosnić, T., Redžić, S. and Mijanović, M. Topical Anti-Inflammatory Effect of Acetone Rhizome/Root Extract of *Potentilla malyana* Borbas. *Planta Medica* 73 (2007): 829–830.

Pilipović, S., Grujić-Vasić, J., Ibrulj, A., Redžić, S. and Bosnić, T. Anti-Inflammatory Effect of Rhizome and Root of *Potentilla erecta* (L.) Raeuschel and *Potentilla alba* L. (Rosaceae). Society of Medicinal Plant Research meeting, Florence (2005): Abstract P164.

Piwowarski, J.P., Granica, S., Zwierzyńska, M., Stefańska, J., Schopohl, P., Melzig, M. F. and Kiss, A.K. Role of Human Gut Microbiota Metabolism in the Anti-Inflammatory Effect of Traditionally Used Ellagitannin-Rich Plant Materials. *Journal of Ethnopharmacology* 155, no. 1 (2014): 801–809.

Pliny. *Naturalis Historia*. Originally published in AD 77–79. Reproduced by Penguin Classics, 1991.

Pollington, S. *Leechcraft: Early English Charms, Plant-Lore and Healing*. Norfolk: Anglo-Saxon Books, 2000.

Pourmorad, F., Ebrahimzadeh, M.A., Mahmoudi, M. and Yasini, S. Antinociceptive Activity of Methanolic Extract of *Epilobium hirsutum*. *Pakistan Journal of Biological Science*s 10, no. 16 (2007): 2764–2767.

Predel, H.G., Giannetti, B., Koll, R., Bulitta, M. and Staiger, C. Efficacy of a Comfrey Root Extract Ointment in Comparison to a Diclofenac Gel in the Treatment of Ankle Distortions: Results of an Observer-Blind, Randomized, Multicenter Study. *Phytomedicine* 12, no. 10 (2005): 707–714.

Prior, R. Fruits and Vegetables in the Prevention of Cellular Oxidative Damage. *American Journal of Clinical Nutrition* 78 (2003): 572S–578S.

Quer, P.F. *Plantas Medicinales*. Barcelona, España: Editora Labor S.A., 1985.

Quinlan, F.J.B. *Galium aparine* as a Remedy for Chronic Ulcers. *British Medical Journal* 1 (1883): 1173.

Râcz–Kotilla, E., Râcz, G. and Solomon, A. The Action of *Taraxacum officinale* Extracts on the Body Weight and Diuresis of Laboratory Animals. *Planta Medica* 26 (1974): 212–217.

Rahman, A. and Kang, S.C. In Vitro Control of Food-Borne and Food Spoilage Bacteria by Essential Oil and Ethanol Extracts of *Lonicera japonica* Thunb. *Food Chemistry* 116 (2009): 670–675.

Rainsford, K.D. *Aspirin and the Salicylates*. London: Butterworths, 1984.

Raiola, A., Errico, A., Petruk, G., Monti, D.M., Barone, A. and Rigano, M.M. Bioactive Compounds in Brassicaceae Vegetables with a Role in the Prevention of Chronic Diseases. *Molecules* 23, no. 1 (2018): 15.

Rauha, J.P., Remes, S., Heinonen, M., Hopia, A., Kähkönen, M., Kujala, T., Pihlaja, K., Vuorela, H. and Vuorela, P. Antimicrobial Effects of Finnish Plant Extracts Containing Flavonoids and Other Phenolic Compounds. *International Journal of Food Microbiology* 56, no. 1 (2000): 3–12.

Ravn, H. and Brimer, L. Structure and Antibacterial Activity of Plantamajoside, a Caffeic Acid Sugar Ester from *Plantago major* subsp. major. *Phytochemistry* 27 (1988): 3433–3437.

Raymond, M. Notes Ethnobotaniques sur les Tete-de-Boule de Manouan. *Contributions de l'Institute Botanique de l'Universitt de Montréal* 55 (1945): 113–134.

Redvers, A., Laugharne, R., Kanagaratnam, G. and Srinivasan, G. How Many Patients Self-Medicate with St John's Wort? *Psychiatric Bulletin* 25 (2001): 254–256.

Reisch, J., Spitzner, W. and Schulte, K.E. Zur Frage der mikrobiologischen Wirksamkeit einfacher Acetylen-Verbindungen [On the Problem of the Microbiological Activity of Simple Acetylene Compounds]. *Arzneimittelforschung* 17, no. 7 (1967): 816–825.

Reuter, S., Gupta, S.C., Chaturvedi, M.M. and Aggarwal, B.B. Oxidative Stress, Inflammation, and Cancer: How Are They Linked? *Free Radical Biology and Medicine* 49, no. 11 (2010): 1603–1616.

Riehemann, K., Behnke, B. and Schulze-Osthoff, K. Plant Extracts from Stinging Nettle (*Urtica dioica*), an Antirheumatic Remedy, Inhibit the Proinflammatory Transcription Factor NF-kappaB. *FEBS Letters* 442, no. 1 (1999): 89–94.

Rohde, E.S. *A Garden of Herbs*. London, Boston: P.L. Warner, Publisher to the Medici Society. Originally published 1921; Reproduction, 1969.

Rugman, F., Meecham, J. and Edmondson, J. *Mercurialis perennis* (Dog's Mercury) Poisoning: A Case of Mistaken Identity. *British Medical Journal* 287, no. 6409 (1983): 1924.

Salah, N., Miller, N.J. and Paganga, G. Polyphenolic Flavanols as Scavengers of Aqueous Phase Radicals and as Chain-Breaking Antioxidants. *Archives of Biochemistry and Biophysics* 322 (1995): 339–346.

Samuelsen, A.B. The Traditional Uses, Chemical Constituents and Biological Activities of *Plantago major* L.: A Review. *Journal of Ethnopharmacology* 71, no. 1–2 (2000): 1–21.

Sarker, S.D. and Nahar, L. Natural Medicine: The Genus Angelica. *Current Medicinal Chemistry* 11, no. 11 (2004): 1479–1500.

Sarno, F., Pepe, G., Termolino, P., Carafa, V., Massaro, C., Merciai, F., Campiglia, P., Nebbioso, A. and Altucci, L. *Trifolium repens* Blocks Proliferation in Chronic Myelogenous Leukemia via the BCR-ABL/ STAT5 Pathway. *Cells* 9, no. 2 (2020): 379.

Savona, G., Piozzi, F., Hanson, J.R. and Siverns, M. Structures of Three New Diterpenoids from *Ballota* Species. *Journal of the Chemical Society, Perkin Transactions* 1, no. 3 (1977): 322–324.

Scambia, G., Mancuso, S., Capelli, A. and Ranelletti, F. Type II Oestrogen Binding Sites in Acute Lymphoid and Myeloid Leukemias: Growth Inhibitory Effect of Oestrogen and Flavonoids. *British Journal of Haematology* 75 (1990): 489–495.

Schulz, V., Hänsel, R. and Tyler, V.E. *Rational Phytotherapy: A Physicians' Guide to Herbal Medicine*. 3rd ed. Berlin: Springer-Verlag, 1998.

Senejoux, F., Demougeot, C., Cuciureanu, M., Miron, A., Cuciureanu, R., Berthelot, A. and Girard-Thernier, C. Vasorelaxant Effects and Mechanisms of Action of *Heracleum sphondylium* L. (Apiaceae) in Rat Thoracic Aorta. *Journal of Ethnopharmacology* 147, no. 2 (2013): 536–539.

Sharifi-Rad, J., Tayeboon, G., Niknam, F. and Sharifi-Rad, M. *Veronica persica* Poir. Extract: Antibacterial, Antifungal and Scolicidal Activities, and Inhibitory Potential on Acetylcholinesterase, Tyrosinase, Lipoxygenase and Xanthine Oxidase. *Cellular and Molecular Biology* (Noisy-le-Grand) 64, no. 8 (2018): 50–56.

Shikov, A.N., Poltanov, E.A., Dorman, HJ., Makarov, V.G., Tikhonov, V.P. and Hiltunen, R. Chemical Composition and In Vitro Antioxidant Evaluation of Commercial Water-Soluble Willow Herb (*Epilobium angustifolium* L.) Extracts. *Journal of Agricultural and Food Chemistry* 54, no. 10 (2006): 3617–3624.

Shishehgar, M., Rezaie, A. and Nazeri, M. Study of Sedation, Pre-Anesthetic and Anti-Anxiety Effects of Hop (*Humulus lupulus* L.) Extract Compared with Diazepam in Rats. *Journal of Animal and Veterinary Advances* 11, no. 14 (2012): 2570–2575.

Short, T. *Medicina Britannica: Or, A Treatise on Such Physical Plants as Are Generally to Be Found in the Fields or Gardens in Great-Britain: Containing a Particular Account of Their Nature, Virtues, and Uses*. Originally published London, Printed for R. Manby and H. Shute Cox, 1746. Reproduction, 2023.

Siatka, T. and Kašparová, M. Seasonal Variation in Total Phenolic and Flavonoid Contents and DPPH Scavenging Activity of *Bellis perennis* L. Flowers. *Molecules* 15, no. 12 (2010): 9450–9461.

Smelcerovic, A. and Spiteller, M. Phytochemical Analysis of Nine *Hypericum* L. Species from Serbia and the F.Y.R. Macedonia. *Pharmazie* 61 (2006): 251–252.

Song, J., Meng, L., Li, S., Qu, L. and Li, X. A Combination of Chinese Herbs, *Astragalus membranaceus* var. *mongholicus* and *Angelica sinensis*, Improved Renal Microvascular Insufficiency in 5/6 Nephrectomized Rrats. *Vascular Pharmacology* 50, no. 5–6 (2009): 185–193.

Stefkov, G., Miova, B., Dinevska-Kjovkarovska, S., Stanoeva, J.P., Stefova, M., Petrusevska, G. and Kulevanova, S. Chemical Characterization of *Centaurium erythrea* L. and Its Effects on Carbohydrate and Lipid Metabolism in Experimental Diabetes. *Journal of Ethnopharmacology* 152, no. 1 (2014): 71–77.

Stevens, J.F. and Page, J.E. Xanthohumol and Related Prenylflavonoids from Hops and Beer: To Your Good Health! *Phytochemistry* 65, no. 4 (2004): 447–449.

Subbotina, M.D., Timchenko, V.N., Vorobyov, M.M., Konunova, Y.S., Aleksandrovih, Y.S. and Shushunov, S. Effect of Oral Administration of Tormentil Root Extract (*Potentilla tormentilla*) on Rotavirus Diarrhea in Children: A Randomized, Double Blind, Controlled Trial. *Pediatric Infectious Disease Journal* 22, no. 8 (2003): 706–711.

Tahvilian, R., Shahriari, S., Faramarzi, A. and Komasi, A. Ethno-Pharmaceutical Formulations in Kurdish Ethno-Medicine. *Iranian Journal of Pharmaceutical Research* 13, no. 3 (2014): 1029–1039.

Tai, J., Cheung, S., Wong, S. and Lowe, C. In Vitro Comparison of Essiac and Floressence on Human Tumor Cell Lines. *Oncology Reports* 11 (2004): 471–476.

Takzare, N., Hosseini, M.-J., Mortazavi, S.H., Safaie, S. and Moradi, R. The Effect of *Achillea millefolium* Extract on Spermatogenesis of Male Wistar Rats. *Human & Experimental Toxicology* 30, no. 4 (2011): 328–334.

Talhouk, R.S., Karam, C., Fostok, S., El-Jouni, W. and Barbour, E.K. (2007). Anti-inflammatory Bioactivities in Plant Extracts. *Journal of Medicinal Food* 10, no. 1 (2007): 1–10.

Tammaro, F. *Flora Officinale d'Abruzzo*. Chieti: Giunta Regionale d'Abruzzo, Centro Servizi Culturali, 1984.

Tan, G.T., Pezzuto, J.M., Kinghorn, A.D. and Hughes, H. Evaluation of Natural Products as Inhibitors of Human Immunodeficiency Virus Type 1 (HIV-1) Reverse Transcriptase. *Journal of Natural Products* 54, no. 1 (1991): 143–154.

Tasić-Kostov, M., Arsić, I., Pavlović, D., Stojanović, S., Najman, S., Naumović, S. and Tadić, V. Towards a Modern Approach to Traditional Use: In Vitro and In Vivo Evaluation of *Alchemilla vulgaris* L. Gel Wound Healing Potential. *Journal of Ethnopharmacology* 238 (2019): 111789.

Thornton, R. *A Family Herbal or Familiar Account of the Medicinal Properties of British and Foreign Plants*. 2nd ed, printed for R. and E. Crosby and Co, London, 1814.

Tilford, G.L. *Edible and Medicinal Plants of the West*. Missoula, MN: Mountain Press Publishing, 1997.

Tkachev, E., Korolyuk, E.A. and Letchamo, W. Volatile Oil-Bearing Flora of Siberia VIII: Essential Oil Composition and Antimicrobial Activity of Wild *Solidago virgaurea* L. from the Russian Alta. *Journal of Essential Oil Research* 18, no. 1 (2006): 46–50.

Todorov, D., Hinkov, A., Shishkova, K. and Shishkov, S. Antiviral Potential of Bulgarian Medicinal Plants. *Phytochemistry Reviews* 13 (2014): 525–538.

Tosun, F., Akyüz Kızılay, Ç., Şener, B. and Vural, M. The Evaluation of Plants from Turkey for In Vitro Antimycobacterial Activity. *Pharmaceutical Biology* 43, no. 1 (2005): 58–63.

Touwaide, A. and Appetiti, E. 2000-Year-Old Medicine Revealed. Institute for Medical Traditions, 2011. Accessed June 2024. https://medicaltraditions.org/institute/news/168-research-breakthrough-2000-year-old-medicine-revealed.

Tsyvunin, V., Shtrygol, S., Prokopenko, Y., Georgiyants, V. and Blyznyuk, N. Influence of Dry Herbal Extracts on Pentylenetetrazole-Induced Seizures in Mice: Screening Results and Relationship 'Chemical Composition-Pharmacological Effect'. *Scientific Pharmacology* 1 (2016): 18–28.

Tunón, H., Olavsdotter, C. and Bohlin, L. Evaluation of Anti-Inflammatory Activity of Some Swedish Medicinal Plants: Inhibition of Prostaglandin Biosynthesis and PAF-Induced Exocytosis. *Journal of Ethnopharmacology* 48, no. 2 (1995): 61–76.

Turner, R. *Botanologia: The British Physician, or, The Nature and Vertues of English Plants, Exactly Describing Such Plants as Grow Naturally in Our Land.* Originally published 1664. Reproduced, 2010.

Ullah, N., Ahmad, I. and Ayaz, S. In Vitro Antimicrobial and Antiprotozoal Activities, Phytochemical Screening and Heavy Metals Toxicity of Different Parts of *Ballota nigra*. *BioMed Research International* 2014 (2014): 321803.

Umek, A., Kreft, S., Kartnig, T. and Heydel, B. Quantitative Phytochemical Analyses of Six *Hypericum* Species Growing in Slovenia. *Planta Medica* 65, no. 5 (1999): 388–390.

Uzun, Y., Koyuncu, F.T., Akman, O.T. and Öztürk, G. Traditional Medicine in Sakarya Province (Turkey) and Antimicrobial Activities of Selected Species. *Journal of Ethnopharmacology* 95, no. 2 (2014): 287–296.

Vahlensieck, M. The Effect of *Chelidonium majus* Herb Extract on Choleresis in the Isolated Perfused Rat Liver. *Zeitschrift für Gastroenterologie* 33, no. 9 (1995): 637–641.

Vasas, A., Orbán-Gyapai, O. and Hohmann, J. The Genus Rumex: Review of Traditional Uses, Phytochemistry, and Pharmacology. *Journal of Ethnopharmacology* 175 (2015): 25–41.

Vishal, R., Srivastava, A. and Kumar, S. Diuretic, Laxative and Toxicity Studies of *Viola odorata* Aerial Parts. *Pharmacologyonline* 1 (2009): 739–748.

Vlase, L., Mocan, A., Hanganu, D., Benedec, D., Gheldiu, A. and Crișan, G. Comparative Study of Polyphenolic Content, Antioxidant and Antimicrobial Activity of Four *Galium* Species (Rubiaceae). *Digest Journal of Nanomaterials and Biostructures* 9, no. 3 (2014): 1085–1094.

Voigts, L.E. Anglo-Saxon Plant Remedies and the Anglo-Saxons. *Isis* 70, no. 2 (1979): 250–268.

Warburg, O. On the Primary Causes and on the Secondary Causes of Cancer. German presentation, 1966. Accessed May 2023. https://mediatheque.lindau-nobel.org/laureates/warburg.

Ward, H. *Herbal Manual: The Medicinal, Toilet, Culinary and Other Uses of 130 of the Most Commonly Used Herbs*. London: L N. Fowler & Co., 1936.

Watkins, F., Pendry, B., Sanchez-Medina, A. and Corcoran, O. Antimicrobial Assays of Three Native British Plants Used in Anglo-Saxon Medicine for Wound Healing Formulations in 10th Century England. *Journal of Ethnopharmacology* 144, no. 2 (2012): 408–415.

Wdowiak L. Srodki roślinne i inne remedia stosowane w chorobach oczu na ziemiach polskich w czasach zaborów. In *Lek Roślinny – Historia i Współczesność*, vol. 4, eds B. Płonka-Syroka B. and A. Syroka. Wrocław: Wydawnictwo Quaestio, 2015): 117–130.

Webster, D., Taschereau, P., Belland, R.J., Sand, C. and Rennie, R.P. Antifungal Activity of Medicinal Plant Extracts; Preliminary Screening Studies. *Journal of Ethnopharmacology* 118, no. 1 (2008): 138–143.

Wegiera, M., Smolarz, H.D. and Bogucka-Kocka, A. *Rumex* L. Species Induce Apoptosis in 1301, EOL-1 and H-9 Cell Lines. *Acta Poloniae Pharmaceutica* 69, no. 3 (2012): 487–499.

Weiss, R.F. and Volker, F. Herbal Medicine. 2nd ed. Stuttgart, Germany: Thieme, 1988.

Wojnicz, D., Kucharska, A.Z., Sokół-Łętowska, A., Kicia, M. and Tichaczek-Goska, D. Medicinal Plants Extracts Affect Virulence Factors Expression and Biofilm Formation by the Uropathogenic *Escherichia coli*. *Urological Research* 40, no. 6 (2012): 683–697.

Yarnell, E., Abascal, K. and Rountree, R. *Clinical Botanical Medicine*. New Rochelle, NY: Mary Ann Liebert, 2003.

Yip, E.C.H., Chan, A.S.L., Pang, H., Tam, Y.K. and Wong, Y.H. Protocatechuic Acid Induces Cell Death in HepG2 Hepatocellular Carcinoma Cells Through a c-Jun N-terminal Kinase-dependent Mechanism. *Cell Biology and Toxicology* 22 (2006): 293–302.

Youngken, H.W., Jr., Neva A.C., Dauben, H.J., Jr., Chang, Y.W. and Wenkert, E. The Muscle Relaxant Effects Produced by *Potentilla anserina* Extracts; Fractionation Studies. *Journal of the American Pharmaceutical Association* 38, no. 8 (1949): 448–451.

Yu-Wen S, Chiou, W.F., Chao, S.H., Lee, M.H., Chen, C.C. and Tsai, Y.C. Ligustilide Prevents LPS-induced iNOS Expression in RAW 264.7 Macrophages by Preventing ROS Production and Down-regulating the MAPK, NF-κB and AP-1 Signaling Pathways. *International Immunopharmacology* 11, no. 9 (2011): 1166–1172.

Zhang, H., Rothwangl, K., Mesecar, A.D., Sabahi, A., Rong, L. and Fong, H.H. Lamiridosins, Hepatitis C Virus Entry Inhibitors from *Lamium album*. *Journal of Natural Products* 72, no. 12 (2009): 2158–2162.

Zhao, R., Chen, Z., Jia, G., Li, J., Cai, Y. and Shao, X. Protective Effects of Diosmetin Extracted from *Galium verum* L. on the Thymus of U14-bearing Mice. *Canadian Journal of Physiology and Pharmacology* 89, no. 9 (2011): 665–673.

Zielińska-Pisklak, M. and Szeleszczuk, Ł. Pierwiosnek nie tylko zwiastun wiosny! (Primrose Is Not Only a Harbinger of Spring!) *Lek w Polsce* 23 (2013): 1–4.

Zuo, G.Y., Meng, F.Y., Hao, X.Y., Zhang, Y.L., Wang, G.C. and Xu, G.L. Antibacterial Alkaloids from *Chelidonium majus* Linn (Papaveraceae) Against Clinical Isolates of Methicillin-Resistant *Staphylococcus aureus*. *Journal of Pharmaceutical Sciences* 11: (2008): 90–94.

INDEX

abortifacient 150, 160, 371
abscesses, 82, 104, 113, 122, 139, 195, 196
Achillea millefolium, 405
Acinetobacter johnsoni., 254
acne, 4, 5, 16, 20, 21, 55, 56, 85, 97, 121, 138, 142, 147, 173, 240, 246, 342, 344, 398, 413, 414
ADHD, 241
Aegopodium podagraria, 189
ageing, 101, 185, 186, 235, 258, 268, 348, 397
Agrimonia eupatoria, 1
Agrimony, 1
Agrobacterium tumefaciens, 254
Ajuga reptans, 47
Alchemilla vulgaris, 253
allergies, 154, 157, 184, 187, 302, 331, 346
Alliaria petiolata, 179
alopecia, 212, 334
Alzheimer's, 390, 407
amenorrhoeal, 30
anaemia, 298, 358, 412, 414
Anagallis arvensis, 319
analgesic, 13, 30, 74, 78, 114, 120, 124, 160, 194, 208, 216, 224, 226, 228, 268, 272, 300, 306, 310, 313, 315, 316, 350, 361, 385, 386, 388, 396, 398
Anemone, 7
Anemonoides nemorosa, 7
Angelica (wild), 11
Angelica sylvestris, 11
antacid, 272

Anthriscus sylvestris, 119
anti- inflammatory, 13, 30, 58, 90, 115, 143, 146, 171, 187, 189, 194, 228, 230, 251, 258, 262, 265, 278, 289, 310, 313, 367, 370, 390, 413
antiandrogenic, 301
antibacterial, 3, 18, 34, 130, 136, 195, 209, 212, 262, 278, 295, 301, 316, 385, 390, 402, 420, 426, 430, 431, 434, 435, 440
anticancerogenic, 4, 9, 14, 24, 34, 44, 48, 54, 58, 64, 69, 79, 94, 101, 120, 130, 136, 147, 180, 198, 209, 212, 216, 224, 232, 239, 254, 272, 279, 284, 288, 312, 322, 324, 331, 350, 361, 380, 390, 396, 400, 412
anticoagulant, 160
anticonvulsant, 110, 208, 282, 415
antidepressant, 360, 429
antidiabetic, 3, 34, 44, 69, 78, 84, 140, 184, 234, 262, 301, 334, 350
anti-dyslipidaemic, 44, 288, 374
antiestrogenic, 301
antifungal, 14, 70, 84, 96, 190, 200, 254, 346, 370, 378, 381, 394, 412
antihaemorrhagic, 330
anti-hepatic, 3
antihistamine, 298, 374
antihyperglycaemic, 150, 316, 342
antihypertensive, 130, 228, 244, 282, 342, 388
anti-hyperuricaemia, 185
antihypoxic, 366
anti-inflammatory, 3, 9, 25, 30, 38, 44,

48, 52, 58, 64, 69, 74, 82, 89, 100, 120, 124, 130, 134, 140, 150, 154, 164, 170, 190, 194, 208, 211, 220, 224, 228, 232, 258, 268, 272, 278, 295, 300, 324, 330, 336, 340, 346, 350, 354, 385, 390, 400, 407, 413, 416, 424, 426, 436
anti-ischaemic, 25
antimicrobial, 8, 14, 25, 38, 44, 54, 62, 69, 74, 82, 89, 94, 110, 124, 170, 181, 185, 190, 202, 216, 220, 226, 228, 232, 238, 248, 254, 288, 306, 336, 340, 346, 350, 354, 366, 370, 378, 394, 407, 412, 415, 418, 427, 429, 432, 433, 437, 438, 439
anti-neurodegenerative, 407
anti-obesity, 82, 184, 301, 312, 380
antiparasitic, 212, 238, 306, 320, 326, 384, 412
anti-plasmodial, 412
antiprostatic, 396
antipruritic, 82
antiseptic, 9, 79, 84, 129, 138, 181, 185, 234, 279, 320, 397
antispasmodic, 8, 164, 294
anti-trypanosomal, 412
antitussive, 90, 104, 143, 268, 294, 310, 417
antiulcerogenic, 89, 268
antiviral, 58, 147, 282, 295, 320, 324, 358, 374, 407, 415, 422, 426, 429, 437
anxiety, 14, 16, 30, 31, 42, 46, 82, 124, 136, 170, 241, 254, 308, 316, 318, 360, 363, 384, 390
anxiolytic, 14, 42, 82, 136, 170, 316, 384, 429
aphrodisiac, 230
Aquilegia vulgaris, 109
Arctium lappa, 51

Arctium minus, 51
Artemisia vulgaris, 287
arthritis, 13, 16, 69, 115, 143, 160, 162, 167, 185, 196, 232, 241, 258, 260, 285, 300, 302, 303, 306
Ascaridia galli, 294
Aspergillus flavus, 307
Aspergillus niger, 48, 110, 185, 202, 232, 288, 346, 350, 370
asthma, 8, 14, 16, 82, 120, 180, 196, 210, 258, 281, 296, 303, 313, 374, 392
astringent, 2, 18, 38, 48, 58, 88, 110, 130, 184, 224, 254, 262, 394, 400
athlete's foot, 14, 69, 200, 381
Avens, 17
Avicena, 377

Bacillus cereus, 82, 89, 170, 220, 232, 407
Bacillus subtilis, 8, 14, 20, 25, 44, 94, 146, 202, 232, 320, 346, 350, 370, 394
Ballota nigra, 41
Bedstraws, 23
Bellis perennis, 133
benign prostatic hyperplasia, 301, 396
Betonica officinalis, 27
Betony, 27
bile stimulant, 174
Bindweed, 33
Bistort, 37
Bistorta officinalis, 37
Black horehound, 41
bleeding, 5, 8, 21, 24, 30, 31, 33, 38, 58, 82, 88, 93, 110, 116, 146, 148, 243, 246, 248, 254, 256, 261, 262, 264, 265, 297, 298, 300, 310, 324, 330, 331, 332, 333, 377, 393, 400, 406, 407, 408
blepharitis, 157
blisters, 9, 342, 344

bloating, 13, 16, 78, 80, 122, 138, 230, 288
blood pressure, 28, 30, 56, 120, 130, 176, 230, 244, 302, 374, 388, 409
bronchitis, 5, 14, 16, 82, 124, 180, 208, 228, 230, 303, 310, 313, 378, 391, 392
bruises, 2, 18, 30, 68, 82, 113, 117, 120, 126, 129, 133, 134, 137, 138, 146, 147, 163, 195, 196, 226, 247, 253, 265, 318, 333, 334, 336, 348, 358, 363, 386, 391
Bugle, 47
Burdock, 51
Burnet, 57
burns, 9, 10, 26, 35, 38, 51, 52, 58, 60, 82, 90, 117, 131, 147, 167, 202, 208, 234, 280, 289, 330, 331, 361, 367, 381, 397
Buttercup, 61

Calystegia sepium, 33
Calystegia sylvatica, 33
Candida albicans, 8, 44, 48, 89, 94, 185, 190, 220, 232, 288, 307, 320, 346, 350, 394
Capsella bursa-pastoris, 329
Cardamine pratensis, 257
cardiogenic, 20
cardioprotective, 90, 126, 209
carminative, 13, 120
Celandine (greater), 67
Celandine (lesser), 73
cellulitis, 120, 122
Centaurea nigra, 247
Centaurea scabiosa, 247
Centaurium erythraea, 77
Centaury, 77
cervical dysplasia, 274
Chamomile, 305

Chelidonium majus, 67
chicken pox, 342, 344
Chickweed, 81
chilblains, 246
chlamydia, 378
cholecystitis, 174
cholelithiasis, 174
cholestasis, 194
cholesterol, 3, 44, 174, 288, 291, 302, 312, 374, 388
cholinergic, 390
Cinquefoils, 87
Cleavers, 93
Clover, 99
Coffin, Albert, 114, 384, 385, 418
cognitive support, 334
colic, 18, 60, 64, 78, 169, 177, 179, 181, 198, 201, 278, 282, 294, 315, 352
colitis, 2, 9, 21, 38, 40, 58, 60, 89, 92, 116, 140, 142, 256, 280
Coltsfoot, 103
Columbine, 109
Comfrey, 113
common cold, 10, 11, 13, 14, 18, 52, 65, 97, 116, 134, 154, 160, 162, 184, 189, 190, 230, 231, 235, 246, 257, 268, 270, 285, 326, 327, 337, 339, 370, 387, 402, 411, 412
Conium maculatum, 215
conjunctivitis, 4, 5, 154, 157
constipation, 4, 51, 56, 78, 80, 143, 174, 412
contraceptive, 279, 406
cough, 2, 8, 13, 14, 16, 41, 90, 92, 103, 104, 107, 119, 120, 124, 127, 159, 179, 181, 194, 196, 201, 202, 208, 210, 223, 227, 228, 230, 231, 244, 268, 270, 293, 294, 296, 310, 345, 346, 358, 383, 384, 388, 390, 391, 392

COVID-19, 106, 143, 268, 324, 360, 390, 407, 409, 415
Cow parsley, 119
Cowslip, 123
cradle cap, 176
Cranesbill, 129
crohn's, 18, 21, 132
Cryptococcus neoformans, 307
Culpeper, Nicholas, 2, 3, 4, 7, 8, 13, 14, 17, 23, 24, 25, 28, 30, 33, 34, 37, 41, 42, 47, 48, 52, 54, 58, 61, 64, 68, 74, 77, 81, 88, 89, 93, 94, 99, 100, 104, 109, 110, 114, 120, 123, 124, 126, 129, 130, 133, 139, 145, 146, 149, 150, 154, 159, 160, 163, 164, 169, 173, 179, 180, 181, 183, 184, 185, 189, 193, 194, 197, 198, 201, 202, 207, 208, 211, 215, 219, 223, 224, 227, 228, 231, 232, 237, 238, 243, 244, 247, 248, 253, 254, 257, 258, 261, 262, 267, 268, 271, 272, 278, 281, 282, 287, 289, 293, 294, 297, 298, 300, 301, 305, 310, 315, 316, 319, 323, 324, 329, 330, 333, 339, 340, 345, 346, 349, 350, 353, 358, 361, 365, 369, 370, 373, 374, 377, 378, 383, 384, 387, 388, 391, 393, 394, 400, 406, 411, 412, 419
Cutibacterium acnes, 402
cystitis, 5, 14, 38, 40, 94, 97, 184, 272, 313
Cytomegalovirus, 358
cytotoxic, 9, 24, 54, 69, 96, 101, 130, 136, 147, 170, 190, 209, 220, 254, 312, 340, 350, 380, 396

Daisy, 133
Dandelion, 139
dandruff, 79, 80, 97, 278
Deadnettles, 145
decongestant, 184
dental surgery, 256, 300
depression, 42, 46, 218, 228, 240, 319, 357, 360
dermatitis, 10, 35, 142, 161, 164, 176, 177, 214, 226, 240, 374, 413
detoxification, 56, 94, 97, 167, 174, 191, 340
detoxifier, 54, 102
diabetes, 3, 15, 34, 37, 44, 78, 84, 140, 150, 184, 190, 220, 232, 262, 281, 302, 334, 342, 352, 397
diaphoretic, 180
diarrhoea, 5, 18, 21, 31, 37, 48, 50, 57, 60, 84, 88, 89, 92, 130, 132, 142, 170, 172, 177, 205, 214, 224, 250, 254, 256, 262, 313, 336, 352, 394, 403, 405
digestive, 4, 8, 13, 14, 17, 18, 31, 46, 78, 80, 82, 85, 120, 139, 143, 170, 172, 177, 180, 193, 202, 219, 226, 228, 230, 250, 253, 258, 275, 278, 280, 288, 296, 308, 350, 365, 369, 398, 406, 409, 413
Dioscorides, 1, 3, 7, 33, 35, 41, 52, 67, 68, 73, 77, 87, 93, 94, 197, 243, 277, 287, 319, 357, 419, 431
diuretic, 2, 14, 24, 26, 51, 82, 93, 119, 120, 130, 140, 143, 148, 150, 164, 177, 183, 184, 187, 189, 198, 202, 205, 208, 224, 227, 238, 244, 257, 258, 260, 300, 330, 340, 374, 376, 384, 388
diverticulitis, 21
Dog's mercury, 149
dyskinesia, 174
dyslipidaemia, 352, 388
dysmenorrhea, 132, 254
dyspepsia, 18, 143, 241, 363

earache, 295, 296
Echinococcus granulosus, 346
Ectromelia, 254
eczema, 4, 15, 16, 30, 35, 36, 54, 60, 68, 82, 84, 85, 87, 90, 100, 106, 121, 122, 142, 164, 167, 173, 176, 177, 180, 210, 214, 226, 246, 254, 264, 270, 302, 348, 354, 356, 386, 414
emmenagogue, 14, 160, 254, 289
encephalomyelitis, 407
Enterobacter aerogenes, 146
Enterobacter cloacae, 136
Enterococcus faecalis, 44, 124, 146, 216, 336
Epidermophyton floccosum, 55
epilepsy, 28, 88, 110, 124, 176, 281, 282, 285, 331, 390, 407
Epilobium angustifolium, 393
Epilobium hirsutum, 393
Epilobium parviflorum, 393
episiotomy, 244, 407
Epstein-Barr virus, 360, 378
Equisetum arvense, 243
Escherichia coli, 8, 18, 44, 54, 82, 146, 170, 181, 185, 190, 202, 209, 216, 220, 228, 232, 248, 278, 288, 306, 320, 350, 366, 370, 394, 396, 407, 439
Eupatorium cannabinum, 219
Euphorbia helioscopia, 349
Euphorbia peplus, 349
Euphrasia officinalis, 153
expectorant, 13, 90, 124, 127, 134, 138, 181, 195, 205, 208, 227, 336, 337, 346
Eyebright, 153
eyewash, 4, 5, 265

fatigue, 60, 100, 102, 288, 291, 298, 378, 386, 412
febrifuge, 220
Fernie, William, 8, 42, 62, 64, 68, 94, 134, 136, 146, 149, 154, 164, 194, 195, 198, 216, 219, 220, 238, 268, 294, 295, 353, 365, 421
Feverfew, 159
fevers, 17, 18, 47, 77, 78, 87, 88, 146, 160, 180, 219, 220, 222, 271, 345, 369, 403, 409
fibroids, 254, 256, 330
Figwort, 163
Filipendula ulmaria, 271
Fleabane, 169
flu, 14, 16, 107, 124, 184, 196, 220, 235, 327, 398, 409
fractures, 116, 117, 246
Fray's Golden Recipes for the Use of All Ages, 2, 52, 78, 100, 129, 411, 421
frostbite, 90
Fumaria officinalis, 173
Fumitory, 173
fungal infections, 55, 71, 90, 200, 322
Fusarium oxysporium, 254

Galen, 73, 77, 243, 257, 287, 357, 377
Galium aparine, 93
Galium mollugo, 23
Galium odoratum, 365
Galium verum, 23
gallbladder, 80, 174, 177
gallstones, 143, 174, 194, 313
Garlic mustard, 179
gas, 13, 16, 18, 78, 80, 122, 230, 288
gastroduodenitis, 3
gastroenteritis, 71, 322, 374
gastrointestinal, 1, 5, 64, 78, 116, 132, 152, 169, 170, 202, 239, 265, 272,

275, 277, 278, 288, 289, 306, 308,
   317, 394, 398
Geranium molle, 129
Geranium pratense, 129
Geranium robertianum, 223
Geranium sylvaticum, 129
Gerard, John, 1, 3, 7, 8, 11, 14, 28, 30, 37,
   38, 41, 47, 48, 52, 54, 57, 58, 61, 68, 73,
   77, 87, 99, 103, 109, 110, 113, 123, 133,
   134, 137, 145, 153, 159, 173, 183, 189,
   193, 194, 197, 207, 208, 219, 231, 243,
   244, 271, 272, 278, 293, 310, 315, 319,
   323, 333, 334, 339, 349, 353, 357, 361,
   373, 374, 387, 399, 422
Geum urbanum, 17
gingivitis, 38
Glechoma hederacea, 193
gout, 9, 10, 15, 28, 42, 46, 56, 89, 92,
   99, 107, 133, 146, 150, 185, 187, 189,
   190, 191, 194, 215, 218, 272, 285,
   288, 293, 303, 309, 370, 383
Ground elder, 189
Ground ivy, 193
Groundsel, 197

haematuria, 38, 330
Haemophilus influenzae, 390
haemorrhage, 58, 320, 330, 398
haemorrhoids, 38, 40, 60, 74, 75, 121,
   131, 164, 191, 211, 313, 327, 376
haemostatic, 300
hayfever, 154, 298
headache, 8, 11, 28, 30, 31, 62, 119, 124,
   134, 138, 160, 162, 196, 232, 238, 279,
   280, 285, 308, 318, 367, 391, 392, 405
heartburn, 16, 78, 80, 280, 336, 337, 405
Heartsease, 207
heat rash, 354
Hedge bedstraw, 23

Hedge parsley, 211
Helicobacter pylori, 181, 278, 307
Hemlock, 215
Hemp agrimony, 219
hepatitis, 3, 147, 295, 374
hepatobiliary, 28
hepatopathy, 174
hepatoprotective, 100, 110, 140, 174,
   194, 234, 262, 320, 366
hepatotoxicity, 222, 336, 380
Heracleum sphondylium, 227
Herb robert, 223
herpes, 14, 89, 147, 295, 324, 326, 327,
   340, 346, 358, 360, 366, 374, 378
hiatus hernia, 116
Hildegard of Bingen, 27, 30, 67, 77, 81,
   87, 119, 120, 145, 147, 153, 159,
   189, 193, 194, 215, 223, 224, 237,
   309, 387, 390, 399, 406, 416
Hippocrates, 87, 149, 357, 378
HIV-1, 58, 69, 358, 437
Hogweed, 227
Honeysuckle, 231
Hops, 237
Horsetail, 243
hot flushes, 101, 102, 239, 254, 256, 281
Humulus lupulus, 237
hyperacidity, 142, 275
hyperglycaemia, 239, 316, 334, 352
Hypericum hirsutum, 357
Hypericum perforatum, 357
hyperpigmentation, 204, 212
hypertension, 30, 120, 162, 174, 228,
   244, 282, 285, 318, 342, 388
hyperuricaemia, 185

IBS, 18, 21, 38, 60, 92, 142, 177
indigestion, 13, 41, 78, 138, 162, 174,
   260, 275, 278, 280, 336

infections, 11, 18, 20, 21, 38, 62, 65, 69, 70, 71, 75, 88, 110, 136, 147, 164, 187, 190, 212, 220, 226, 232, 235, 250, 251, 262, 278, 303, 307, 312, 354, 374, 378, 380, 385, 386, 392, 393, 397
insect bites, 111, 117, 122, 169, 172, 214, 226, 264, 280, 302, 309, 318, 327, 348, 385, 386
insect deterrent, 161, 307
insect repellent, 159, 223, 226, 305, 372
insecticide, 42
insomnia, 16, 33, 34, 239, 285, 308, 318, 331, 360, 366, 367, 388
ischaemia, 90
itching, 84, 85, 164, 181, 271, 298, 313

jaundice, 2, 28, 30, 38, 47, 67, 68, 78, 93, 94, 100, 109, 139, 193, 194, 197, 227, 228, 238, 329, 340, 373, 374, 383
joint pain, 64, 65, 89, 122, 127, 230, 275, 318, 372

keratitis, 354
kidney stones, 130, 187, 198, 303, 313, 332
Klebsiella pneumoniae, 8, 44, 82, 146, 202, 216, 288, 350
Knapweed, 247

Lactuca serriola, 315
Lady's mantle, 253
Lady's smock, 257
Lamium album, 145
Lamium galeobdolon, 145
Lamium purpureum, 145
laxative, 33, 34, 36, 78, 129, 166, 177, 200, 312, 388, 391, 412
lentigo, 45

lice, 110, 111, 371
Linaria purpurea, 374
Linaria vulgaris, 373
listeria, 14, 89, 228, 232, 346, 366
liver disease, 3, 220, 234, 262, 374
Lonicera japonica, 231
Lonicera peryclymenum, 231
Loosestrife, 261
lupus, 121
lymphatic, 24, 94, 97, 100, 164, 167
Lysimachia vulgaris, 261

Mallow, 267
Malva sylvestris, 267
mastitis, 89, 92, 218, 320
Matricaria discoidea, 305
Meadowsweet, 271
melasma, 45
menopause, 100, 102, 239, 241, 256
menorrhagia, 14, 254, 330, 398
menstrual cramps, 291
menstruation, 14, 15, 33, 110, 132, 159, 253, 256, 281, 291, 374
Mentha aquatica, 277
Mentha arvensis, 277
Mentha piperita, 277
Mentha spicata, 277
Mercurialis perennis, 149
metabolic, 239
Microsporum gypseum, 55, 69
Mint, 277
Mistletoe, 281
Moraxella nonliquefaciens, 402
Mouse-ear, hawkweed, 201
moxibustion, 289
MRSA, 44, 131, 212, 378, 394, 407, 412
Mugwort, 287
Mullein, 293
multiple sclerosis, 390, 407

muscle relaxant, 174
Mycobacterium smegmatis, 248
Mycobacterium tuberculosis, 3, 8, 124
myocardial dysfunction, 25
myocardial infarction, 366

natriuretic, 300
nausea, 21, 41, 46, 152, 277, 280, 290, 336
nephrolithiasis, 332
Nettle, 297
neuralgia, 90, 162, 281, 363, 367
neuritis, 162
neuroprotective, 20, 34
nootropic, 371

obesity, 69, 82, 238, 301, 388
oestrogenic, 100, 239
onychomycosis, 354
osteoarthritis, 114, 289, 295, 300, 324
osteoperosis, 324

Paracelsus, 282, 357
parasites, 214, 294, 412
Parkinson's disease, 20, 45, 331, 390, 407
Penicillium italicum, 254
perimenopausal, 256
periodontitis, 316, 340
Pineappleweed, 305
Plantago lanceolata, 309
Plantago major, 309
Plantain, 309
Pliny, 1, 7, 67, 113, 173, 174, 277, 282, 287, 297, 319, 357, 426, 433
PMS, 89, 330
pneumonia, 25, 354
polycystic ovary syndrome, 30, 301, 400
Polygonatum multiflorum, 333
Polygonatum odoratum, 333
Porphyromonas gingivalis, 316, 340, 416

postpartum, 254, 330, 407
Potentilla anserina, 87
Potentilla erecta, 87
Potentilla reptans, 87
Prickly lettuce, 315
Primula veris, 123
Propionibacterium acnes, 240
prostate, 44, 190, 198, 212, 216, 246, 254, 301, 303, 317, 342, 396
prostatitis, 148
Proteus hauseri, 146
Proteus mirabilis, 44, 394
Prunella vulgaris, 323
pruritus, 256, 322
Pseudomonas aeruginosa, 18, 38, 54, 70, 89, 94, 124, 146, 170, 185, 190, 202, 209, 216, 228, 232, 288, 346, 350, 354, 385, 390, 394, 407
psoriasis, 4, 26, 36, 82, 84, 85, 90, 96, 100, 101, 121, 142, 164, 167, 176, 177, 209, 210, 244, 354, 356
Pulicaria dysenterica, 169
purgative, 68
pyrrolizidine alkaloids, 104, 107, 114, 198, 200, 220

Raillietina spiralis, 294
Ranunculus acris, 61
Ranunculus bulbosus, 61
Ranunculus ficaria, 73
Ranunculus repens, 61
rashes, 4, 84, 92, 110, 142, 164, 176, 214, 234, 235, 251, 254, 256, 264, 265, 302, 342, 344, 356, 376, 397
rheumatism, 9, 10, 13, 16, 62, 64, 65, 71, 120, 127, 134, 150, 162, 218, 258, 260, 285, 298, 372
Rhizoctonia solani, 254
ringworm, 69, 198, 312, 322

Rohde, Eleanour, 294, 365, 366, 434
rosacea, 90, 142
Rotavirus, 88, 436
roundworms, 294
Rumex acetosa, 343
Rumex crispus, 411

Saccharomyces cerevisiae, 394
Salmonella enteritidis, 232, 278, 288
Salmonella typhi, 44, 82, 350
Sanguisorba minor, 57
Sanguisorba officinalis, 57
SARS-CoV-2, 142, 268, 324
Scarlet pimpernel, 319
sciatica, 15, 52, 62, 64, 77, 88, 127, 146, 169, 190, 191, 194, 281, 285, 288, 303, 361
scolicidal, 346
Scrophularia auriculata, 163
Scrophularia nodosa, 163
seasonal affective disorder, 360
sedative, 34, 36, 42, 77, 124, 127, 134, 136, 138, 160, 170, 172, 193, 228, 237, 238, 239, 282, 285, 306, 310, 315, 316, 318, 320, 360, 366, 384
Self-heal, 323
Senecio vulgaris, 197
septicaemia, 25, 354
Serratia marcescens, 254
Shepherd's purse, 329
shingles, 89, 224, 227, 313, 342, 344, 363
sinusitis, 157, 184, 196, 230, 313
Solidago canadensis, 183
Solidago virgaurea, 183
Solomon's seal, 333
soporific, 306
sore throats, 4, 5, 21, 40, 50, 88, 92, 230, 231, 235, 256, 270

Sorrels, 339
Speedwell, 345
spermicidal, 320
sprains, 113, 115, 117, 167, 246, 337, 372, 386
Spurges, 349
St John's wort, 357
Stachys arvensis, 399
Stachys palustris, 399
Stachys sylvatica, 399
Staphylococcus aureus, 3, 8, 14, 20, 44, 55, 62, 70, 82, 94, 110, 124, 136, 146, 170, 181, 185, 190, 202, 212, 216, 228, 232, 248, 262, 278, 279, 288, 306, 336, 346, 350, 361, 366, 370, 378, 385, 390, 394, 407, 412, 440
Staphylococcus capitis, 402
Staphylococcus epidermidis, 14, 110, 136, 146, 262, 301, 336
Staphylococcus pyogenes, 390
Stellaria holostea, 353
Stellaria media, 81
stimulant, 8, 58
Stitchwort, 353
stomatitis, 38
Streptococcus mutans, 378
Streptococcus pneumoniae, 150
stroke, 44, 133, 281, 342, 366, 407
styes, 157
styptic, 330
Symphytum officinale, 113

Tanacetum parthenium, 159
Tanacetum vulgare, 369
Tansy, 369
tapeworm, 294, 346
Taraxacum officinale, 139
temporal arteritis, 285
Thornton, Robert, 18, 88, 281, 298, 370

tinnitus, 194, 196, 371
Toadflax, 373
tonic, 18, 26, 33, 34, 56, 78, 80, 93, 94, 97, 114, 119, 120, 143, 196, 214, 226, 230, 248, 254, 260, 296, 303, 334, 366, 384, 406
tonsillitis, 69, 71, 94, 97
toothache, 67, 68, 92, 278, 405
Torilis japonica, 211
trichomoniasis, 3, 378
trichophyton, 55, 69, 198, 322
Trifolium pratense, 99
Trifolium repens, 99
Tussilago farfara, 103

ulcers, 2, 7, 8, 15, 20, 21, 24, 38, 40, 41, 47, 48, 50, 52, 54, 67, 78, 79, 88, 92, 93, 94, 96, 106, 116, 132, 139, 146, 147, 164, 169, 180, 181, 183, 184, 194, 202, 207, 215, 224, 243, 246, 254, 256, 265, 268, 272, 278, 310, 323, 336, 340, 344, 348, 358, 369, 374, 376, 386, 397, 399, 406, 407
urethritis, 97
urinary tract infections, 3, 34, 55, 184, 187, 320
uroprotective, 320
Urtica dioica, 297
Usnea, 377
Usnea barbata, 377
uterine stimulant, 160
UTI, 5, 34, 36, 354

Vaccinia, 254
vaginal discharge, 148
vaginosis, 378
varicose veins, 74, 75, 121
Verbascum thapsus, 293
Verbena officinalis, 383

Veronica officinalis, 346
Veronica persica, 346
Vervain, 383
Viola odorata, 387
Viola tricolor, 207
Violet, 387
Viscum album, 281
vitiligo, 152
vomiting, 37, 46, 84, 152, 200, 219, 250, 253, 290, 377, 385, 413
vulnerary, 3, 48, 52, 57, 58, 114, 129, 130, 134, 146, 147, 164, 195, 244, 248, 310, 320, 334, 345, 407

Ward, Harold, 5, 18, 55, 56, 68, 88, 208, 248, 253, 268, 324, 329, 330, 358, 365, 370, 388, 390, 406, 439
warts, 1, 9, 65, 68, 70, 74, 152, 294, 317, 322, 352
Willowherbs, 393
Woodruff, 365
wounds, 1, 2, 4, 5, 10, 17, 24, 25, 26, 28, 30, 33, 35, 36, 38, 47, 48, 50, 60, 71, 77, 78, 82, 84, 88, 93, 94, 111, 113, 115, 116, 117, 119, 122, 126, 129, 131, 132, 134, 138, 146, 148, 152, 163, 164, 167, 169, 181, 183, 184, 185, 186, 193, 194, 195, 196, 197, 204, 205, 214, 218, 222, 224, 228, 230, 235, 243, 246, 247, 248, 250, 251, 253, 254, 255, 256, 261, 262, 264, 265, 279, 301, 310, 312, 313, 323, 324, 326, 327, 329, 332, 333, 334, 348, 356, 358, 361, 363, 369, 376, 380, 381, 385, 392, 394, 399, 400, 402, 403, 405, 406, 409
Woundwort, 399

Yarrow, 405
Yellow dock, 411